# Pocket Guide & Toolkit to DeJong's Neurologic Examination

**William W. Campbell, MD, MSHA**

Professor and Chairman
Department of Neurology
Uniformed Services University of Health Sciences
Bethesda, Maryland

Chief, Clinical Neurophysiology
Walter Reed Army Medical Center
Washington, DC

 Wolters Kluwer | Lippincott Williams & Wilkins
Health

Philadelphia · Baltimore · New York · London
Buenos Aires · Hong Kong · Sydney · Tokyo

*Acquisitions Editor:* Frances DeStefano
*Managing Editor:* Leanne McMillan
*Project Manager:* Nicole Walz
*Senior Manufacturing Manager:* Ben Rivera
*Marketing Manager:* Kimberly Schonberger
*Art Director:* Risa Clow
*Cover Designer:* Larry Didona
*Production Services:* International Typesetting and Composition

© **2008 by Lippincott Williams & Wilkins, a Wolters Kluwer business**
**530 Walnut Street**
**Philadelphia, PA 19106**
**LWW.com**

Printed in the USA

**Library of Congress Cataloging-in-Publication Data**

Campbell, William W. (William Wesley)
  Pocket guide and toolkit to Dejong's neurologic examination / William W. Campbell.
    p. ; cm.
  Includes bibliographical references and index.
  ISBN 13: 978-0-7817-7359-1
  ISBN 10: 0-7817-7359-8
  1. Neurologic examination—Handbooks, manuals, etc.   I. Campbell, William W. (William Wesley). DeJong's the neurologic examination.   II. Title.
  [DNLM: 1. Neurologic Examination—Handbooks. WL 39 C192p 2008]
  RC348.C353 2008
  616.8'0475—dc22

                                                                      2007038508

Care has been taken to confirm the accuracy of the information presented and to describe generally accepted practices. However, the authors, editors, and publisher are not responsible for errors or omissions or for any consequences from application of the information in this book and make no warranty, expressed or implied, with respect to the currency, completeness, or accuracy of the contents of the publication. Application of this information in a particular situation remains the professional responsibility of the practitioner.

The authors, editors, and publisher have exerted every effort to ensure that drug selection and dosage set forth in this text are in accordance with current recommendations and practice at the time of publication. However, in view of ongoing research, changes in government regulations, and the constant flow of information relating to drug therapy and drug reactions, the reader is urged to check the package insert for each drug for any change in indications and dosage and for added warnings and precautions. This is particularly important when the recommended agent is a new or infrequently employed drug.

Some drugs and medical devices presented in this publication have Food and Drug Administration (FDA) clearance for limited use in restricted research settings. It is the responsibility of health care providers to ascertain the FDA status of each drug or device planned for use in their clinical practice.

The publishers have made every effort to trace copyright holders for borrowed material. If they have inadvertently overlooked any, they will be pleased to make the necessary arrangements at the first opportunity.

To purchase additional copies of this book, call our customer service department at **(800) 638-3030** or fax orders to **(301) 223-2320**. International customers should call **(301) 223-2300**. Visit Lippincott Williams & Wilkins on the Internet: at LWW.com. Lippincott Williams & Wilkins customer service representatives are available from 8:30 am to 6 pm, EST.

                                                                      10 9 8 7 6 5 4 3 2 1

*To Wes, Matt and Shannon; to Russell N. DeJong, neurologist extraordinaire; and to Anne Sydor.*

# Contents

SECTION E
# The Motor Examination

SECTION F
# The Sensory Examination

SECTION G
# The Reflexes

SECTION H
# Coordination and Gait

SECTION I
# The Autonomic Nervous System

SECTION J
# Special Methods of Examination

# Introduction

# CHAPTER 1

## Introduction

**T**his book is written as a companion and supplement to *DeJong's The Neurologic Examination, 6th edition*. The book has been streamlined, all reference to basic science removed, and the essentials of the clinical examination presented. In addition, novel to medical books as far as I am aware, there are appendices (a "Toolkit") that contain some commonly used and handy instruments and forms that are often useful in the examination of the neurologic patient, especially in regard to neuro-ophthalmology. These include: a simple red lens for diplopia testing, a multi-pinhole for assessing visual acuity, pocket vision screeners for examining near visual acuity at near and at a distance of about 6 feet, a primitive but usable version of an OKN tape, 4 red squares with dots to assess color vision in all 4 quadrants, selected color vision plates, an Amsler grid for evaluating central scotomas, a copy of the Blessed memory-orientation questionnaire, and copies of the Glasgow coma scale, the Hunt and Hess scale for evaluating subarachnoid hemorrhage patients, and a diagram of the brachial plexus. Commercial interests would not allow the inclusion of the Folstein mini-mental examination.

The hope is that the Toolkit will elevate the *Pocket Guide* from a mere abbreviated textbook on the neurologic examination to a useful clinical tool for examining patients. With the *Pocket Guide* and its accompanying Tools, along with the usual instruments found in the neurologist's black bag, the examiner should find at hand all the reasonable tools with which to do a complete neurologic examination, to include detailed neuro-ophthalmologic assessment.

The larger textbook, *DeJong's The Neurologic Examination,* remains the definitive source for all aspects, common and abstruse, for a discussion of the examination. The *Pocket Guide* is intended as a brief version, pocket or bag portable, that contains the essentials of the examination as well as many of the tools that are often hard to find when needed most.

## NEUROLOGIC DIFFERENTIAL DIAGNOSIS

Pathologic processes behave in certain ways depending on their location in the nervous system, and in certain other ways related to their inherent natures. Neurologists deal in two basic clinical exercises: where is the lesion in the nervous system and what is the lesion in the nervous system: differential diagnosis by location and differential diagnosis by pathophysiology or etiology. The anatomic diagnosis and the etiologic diagnosis aid and support each other. In general, the neurologic examination aids primarily in establishing the anatomic or localization diagnosis and the history aids in the etiologic diagnosis, but there is overlap. The examination also serves to indicate the severity of the abnormality. A dependence on neuro-imaging and other tests as the primary approach to diagnosis causes many errors. Defining the patient's illness first in terms of anatomy and likely etiology helps insure the appropriate use of neurodiagnostic studies.

The first consideration should be whether the patient has an organic disease or whether the symptoms are likely psychogenic. If the disorder is organic, consider whether the condition is a primary neurologic disease, a neurologic complication of a systemic disorder, a neurologic complication of drug or medication use, or the effects of a toxin.

## ANATOMICAL DIAGNOSIS

The patterns of abnormality found on examination help to localize a disease process to a particular part of the nervous system. Clinical features that are particularly helpful in neurologic differential diagnosis include the distribution of any weakness, the presence or absence of sensory symptoms, the presence or absence of pain, the presence or absence of cranial nerve abnormalities and whether they are ipsilateral or contralateral to the other abnormalities on examination, the status of the reflexes, the presence of pathological reflexes, involvement of bowel and bladder function, and the presence or absence of symptoms that clearly indicate cortical involvement. Weakness may be unilateral or bilateral, symmetric or asymmetric, primarily proximal or primarily distal; each of these patterns has differential diagnostic significance. The pattern of sensory abnormalities also provides significant information.

In trying to make an anatomical localization, it may be helpful to organize the nervous system by considering sequentially more peripheral or central structures, beginning either at the cerebral cortex or the muscle. Consider each level where disease tends to have a characteristic and reproducible clinical profile. For example, disease involving the muscle, neuromuscular junction, peripheral nervous system, nerve roots, spinal cord, brainstem, and hemispheres each tend to produce a characteristic clinical picture. Some diseases cause multifocal or diffuse abnormalities, and these are often particularly challenging.

At each major level, disease processes tend to have characteristic clinical features, although with some degree of overlap. By trying to localize the disease process to one or two likely levels, such as muscle or neuromuscular junction, one can then think more systematically about the etiologic possibilities.

## MUSCLE DISEASE

Common muscle diseases include muscular dystrophies and inflammatory, metabolic, toxic, and congenital myopathies. Patients with muscle disease usually have symmetric, proximal weakness. Deep tendon reflexes (DTRs) are usually intact but may be depressed when weakness is severe. There are no pathological reflexes. Patients may or may not have muscle pain, tenderness or soreness; usually they do not. There is no sensory loss; bowel and bladder dysfunction generally do not occur, there are no defects in coordination, mentation, or higher cortical function.

## NEUROMUSCULAR JUNCTION (NMJ) DISORDERS

NMJ diseases include myasthenia gravis (MG), Lambert-Eaton syndrome, botulism, hypermagnesemia, and others. The most common condition by far is MG. Patients with NMJ disorders usually have symmetric, proximal muscle weakness, which can simulate a myopathy, but in addition often have bulbar involvement. Most commonly patients have weakness of eye movement causing double vision, or ptosis of one or both eyelids. They may have trouble talking and swallowing, with a tendency to nasal regurgitation of fluids. Such symptoms and signs of bulbar weakness are one of the main differences between an NMJ disease and a myopathy. There is no pain or sensory loss. DTRs are normal in MG but may be depressed in Lambert-Eaton syndrome and other presynaptic disorders. There are no pathological reflexes.

## PERIPHERAL NEUROPATHY

Common causes of peripheral neuropathy include diabetes mellitus, alcoholism, and GBS. Most patients with polyneuropathy have symmetric, predominantly distal weakness, sensory loss, depressed or absent DTRs, no pathologic reflexes, and no bowel or bladder dysfunction. Pain is a common accompaniment and often a major clinical feature. Proximal weakness can occur with some neuropathies.

## PLEXUS DISEASE

Diseases involving the brachial plexus are much more common than those involving the lumbosacral plexus. Most brachial plexopathies are due to trauma. Neuralgic amyotrophy (brachial plexitis, Parsonage-Turner syndrome) is a common inflammatory disorder of the brachial plexus that is notoriously painful. Patients with plexus disorders have a clinical deficit which mirrors the involved structures, so a knowledge of plexus anatomy is vital to deciphering the deficit. There is typically both weakness and sensory loss, accompanied by depressed or absent DTRs in the involved area, no pathologic reflexes, and no bowel or bladder dysfunction.

## NERVE ROOT DISEASE

Most radiculopathies are due to disc herniations or spondylosis. When severe, there are both motor and sensory deficits and a depressed DTR in the distribution of the involved root(s). Pain is common and often severe, usually accompanied limitation of motion of either the neck or lower back, along with signs of root irritability, such as a positive straight leg raising test. There are no pathological reflexes, and no bowel or bladder dysfunction. The presence of these findings suggests there is concomitant spinal cord compression.

## SPINAL CORD DISEASE

Common causes of myelopathy include compression, trauma, and acute transverse myelitis. With transverse myelopathy, there is symmetric involvement causing bilateral weakness below a particular level, producing either paraparesis or quadriparesis. In addition to weakness below the level of the lesion, patients with spinal cord lesions may also have paresthesias, numbness, tingling, and sensory loss with a discrete sensory level, usually on the trunk. Except during the acute phase, patients with spinal cord disease tend to have increased reflexes, along with pathologic reflexes such as the Babinski sign. Patients with spinal cord disease also tend to have difficulty with sphincter control, and bladder dysfunction is often an early and prominent symptom. Pain is not a common feature except for local discomfort due to a vertebral lesion. Peripheral neuropathy may also cause symmetric motor and sensory loss, but DTRs are decreased, sphincter dysfunction is very rare, and there is often pain.

## BRAINSTEM DISEASE

The classic distinguishing feature of brainstem pathology is that deficits are "crossed," with cranial nerve dysfunction on one side and a motor or sensory deficit on the opposite side. There are often symptoms reflecting dysfunction of other posterior fossa structures, such as vertigo, ataxia, dysphagia, nausea and vomiting, and abnormal eye movements. Unless the process has impaired the reticular activating system, patients are normal mentally, awake, alert, able to converse (though perhaps dysarthric), not confused, and not aphasic. DTRs are usually hyperactive with accompanying pathologic reflexes in the involved extremities; pain is rare and sphincter dysfunction occurs only if there is bilateral involvement.

## CRANIAL NERVE DISEASE

Disease may selectively involve one, or occasionally more than one, cranial nerve. The long tract abnormalities, vertigo, ataxia, and similar symptoms and findings that are otherwise characteristic of intrinsic brainstem disease are lacking. Common cranial neuropathies include optic neuropathy due to multiple sclerosis, third nerve palsy due to aneurysm, and Bell palsy. Involvement of more than one nerve occurs in conditions such as Lyme disease, sarcoidosis, and lesions involving the cavernous sinus.

## CEREBELLAR DISEASE

Patients with cerebellar dysfunction suffer from various combinations of tremor, incoordination, difficulty walking, dysarthria and nystagmus, depending on the parts of the cerebellum involved. There is no weakness, sensory loss, pain, hyperreflexia, pathologic reflexes, sphincter dyscontrol, or abnormalities of higher cortical function. When cerebellar abnormalities result from dysfunction of the cerebellar connections in the brainstem there are usually other brainstem signs.

## BASAL GANGLIA DISORDERS

Diseases of the basal ganglia cause movement disorders such as Parkinson disease or Huntington chorea. Movement disorders may be hypokinetic or hyperkinetic, referring to whether movement is in general decreased or increased. Parkinson disease causes bradykinesia and rigidity. Huntington disease in contrast causes increased movements that are involuntary and beyond the patient's control (chorea). Tremor is a frequent accompaniment of basal ganglia disease.

## CEREBRAL HEMISPHERE DISORDERS, CORTICAL V. SUBCORTICAL

Characteristic of unilateral hemispheric pathology is a "hemi" deficit: hemisensory loss, hemi-paresis, hemi-anopsia, or perhaps hemiseizures. Other common manifestations include hyper-reflexia and pathologic reflexes. Pain is not a feature unless the thalamus is involved, and there is no difficulty with sphincter control unless both hemispheres are involved. Within this framework, disease affecting the cerebral cortex behaves differently from disease of subcortical structures. Patients with cortical involvement may have aphasia, apraxia, astereognosis, impaired two point discrimination, memory loss, cognitive defects, focal seizures, or other abnormalities that reflect the essential integrative role of the cortex. Processes affecting the dominant hemisphere often cause language dysfunction in the form of aphasia, alexia, or agraphia. With disease of the non-dominant hemisphere, the patient may have higher cortical function disturbances involving functions other than language, such as apraxia. If the disease affects subcortical structures, the clinical picture includes the hemidistribution of dysfunction but lacks those elements that are typically cortical, e.g., language disturbance, apraxia, seizures, dementia.

## MULTIFOCAL/DIFFUSE DISORDERS

Some disease processes are diffuse or multifocal, producing dysfunction at more than one location, or involve a "system." For example, Devic disease characteristically affects both the spinal cord and the optic nerves, i.e., it is multifocal. ALS is a system disorder causing diffuse dysfunction of the entire motor system from the spinal cord to the cerebral cortex, sparing sensation and higher cortical function.

## DIFFERENTIAL DIAGNOSIS BY ETIOLOGY

From a differential diagnostic standpoint, it is usually most helpful to think first about the localization of the disease process in the nervous system, and secondarily about the etiology. Localization limits the etiologic differential diagnosis, since certain disease processes typically involve or spare particular structures. Knowing the likely location of the pathology generally places the condition into a broad etiologic differential diagnostic category. Occasionally, the etiology is very obvious, such as stroke or CNS trauma and the diagnostic exercise focuses mostly on the localization. Some of the etiologies of primary neurologic disease include neoplasms, vascular disease, infection, inflammation, autoimmune disorders, trauma, toxins, substance abuse, metabolic disorders, demyelinating disease, congenital abnormalities, migraine, epilepsy, genetic and degenerative conditions. Neurologic complications of systemic disease are very common.

Psychiatric disease as an etiologic category requires a caveat. The psychiatric disorders most often of neurologic concern are depression, hysteria, malingering, and hypochondriasis. These are also frequently referred to as functional or nonorganic disorders. Depression tends to exaggerate any symptomatology, neurologic or otherwise. The diagnosis of nonorganic disease can be treacherous. So-called "hysterical signs" on physical examination are often extremely misleading.

# History, Physical Examination, and Overview of the Neurologic Examination

CHAPTER 2

## The Neurologic History

Introductory textbooks of physical diagnosis cover the basic aspects of medical interviewing. This chapter addresses some aspects of history taking of particular relevance to neurologic patients. Important historical points to be explored in some common neurologic conditions are summarized in the tables.

The history is the cornerstone of medical diagnosis, and neurologic diagnosis is no exception. In many instances the physician can learn more from what the patient says and how he says it than from any other avenue of inquiry. A skillfully taken history will frequently indicate the probable diagnosis, even before physical, neurologic, and neurodiagnostic examinations are carried out. Conversely, many errors in diagnosis are due to incomplete or inaccurate histories. In many common neurologic disorders the diagnosis rests almost entirely on the history. The most important aspect of history taking is attentive listening. Ask open ended questions and avoid suggesting possible responses. Although patients are frequently accused of being "poor historians," there are in fact as many poor history takers as there are poor history givers. While the principal objective of the history is to acquire pertinent clinical data that will lead to correct diagnosis, the information obtained in the history is also valuable in understanding the patient as an individual, his relationship to others, and his reactions to his disease.

Taking a good history is not simple. It may require more skill and experience than performing a good neurologic examination. Time, diplomacy, kindness, patience, reserve, and a manner that conveys interest, understanding, and sympathy are all essential. The physician should present a friendly and courteous attitude, center all his attention on the patient, appear anxious to help, word questions tactfully, and ask them in a conversational tone. At the beginning of the interview it is worthwhile to attempt to put the patient at ease. Avoid any appearance of haste. Engage in some small talk. Inquiring as to where the patient is from and what they do for a living not only helps make the encounter less rigid and formal, but often reveals very interesting things about the patient as a person. History taking is an opportunity to establish a favorable patient–physician relationship; the physician may acquire empathy for the patient, establish rapport, and instill confidence. The manner of presenting his history reflects the intelligence, powers of observation, attention, and memory of the patient. The examiner should avoid forming a judgment about the patient's illness too quickly; some individuals easily sense and resent a physician's preconceived ideas about their symptoms. Repeating key points of the history back to the patient helps insure accuracy and assure the patient the physician has heard and assimilated the story. At the end of the history, the patient should always feel as if he has been listened to. History taking is an art; it can be learned partly through reading and study, but is honed only through experience and practice.

The mode of questioning may vary with the age and educational and cultural background of the patient. The physician should meet the patient on a common ground of language and vocabulary, resorting to the vernacular if necessary, but without talking down to the patient. This is sometimes a fine line. The history is best taken in private, with the patient comfortable and at ease.

The history should be recorded clearly and concisely, in a logical, well-organized manner. It is important to focus on the more important aspects and keep irrelevancies to a minimum; the essential factual material must be separated from the extraneous. Diagnosis involves the careful sifting of evidence, and the art of selecting and emphasizing the pertinent data may make it possible to arrive at a correct conclusion in a seemingly complicated case. Recording negative as well as positive statements assures later examiners that the historian inquired into and did not overlook certain aspects of the disease.

Several different types of information may be obtained during the initial encounter. There is direct information from the patient describing the symptoms, information from the patient regarding what previous physicians may have thought, and information from medical records or previous care givers. All these are potentially important. Usually, the most essential is the patient's direct description of the symptoms. Always work from information obtained firsthand from the patient when possible, as forming one's own opinion from primary data is critical. Steer the patient away from a description of what previous doctors have thought, at least initially. Many patients tend to jump quickly to describing encounters with caregivers, glossing over the details of the present illness. Patients often misunderstand much or most of what they have been told in the past, so information from the patient about past evaluations and treatment must be analyzed cautiously. Patient recollections may be flawed because of faulty memory, misunderstanding, or other factors. Encourage the patient to focus on symptoms instead, giving a detailed account of the illness in his own words.

In general, the interviewer should intervene as little as possible, but it is often necessary to lead the conversation away from obviously irrelevant material, obtain amplification on vague or incomplete statements, or lead the story in directions likely to yield useful information. Allow the patient to use his own words as much as possible, but it is important to determine the precise meaning of words the patient uses, clarifying any ambiguity that could lead to misinterpretation. Have the patient clarify what he means by lay terms like "kidney trouble" or "dizziness."

Deciding whether the physician or the patient should control the pace and content of the interview is a frequent problem. Patients do not practice history giving. Some are naturally much better at relating the pertinent information than others. Many patients digress frequently into extraneous detail. The physician adopting an overly passive role under such circumstances often prolongs the interview unnecessarily. When possible, let the patient give the initial part of the history without interruption. In a primary care setting, the average patient tells his story in about five minutes. The average doctor interrupts the average patient after only about 18 seconds. In 44% of interviews done by medical interns, the patient was not allowed to complete their opening statement of concerns. Female physicians allowed fewer patients to finish their opening statement. Avoid interrogation, but keeping the patient on track with focused questions is entirely appropriate. If the patient pauses to remember some irrelevancy, gently encourage them not to dwell on it. A reasonable method is to let the patient run as long as they are giving a decent account, then take more control to clarify necessary details. Some patients may need to relinquish more control than others. Experienced clinicians generally make a diagnosis through a process of hypothesis testing. At some point in the interview, the physician must assume greater control and query the patient regarding specific details of their symptomatology in order to test hypotheses and help to rule in or rule out diagnostic possibilities.

History taking in certain types of patients may require special techniques. The timid, inarticulate, or worried patient may require prompting with sympathetic questions or reassuring comments. The garrulous person may need to be stopped before getting lost in a mass of irrelevant detail. The evasive or undependable patient may have to be queried more searchingly, and the fearful, antagonistic, or paranoid patient questioned guardedly to avoid arousing fears or suspicions. In the patient with multiple or vague complaints, insist on specifics. The euphoric patient may minimize or neglect his symptoms; the depressed or anxious patient may exaggerate, and the excitable or hypochondriacal patient may be overconcerned and recount his complaints at length. The range of individual variations is wide, and this must be taken into account in appraising symptoms. What is pain to the anxious or depressed patient may be but a minor discomfort to another. A blasé attitude or seeming indifference may indicate pathologic euphoria in one individual, but be a defense reaction in another. One person may take offense at questions which another would consider commonplace. Even in a single individual such factors as fatigue, pain, emotional conflicts, or diurnal fluctuations in mood or temperament may cause a wide range of variation in response to questions. Patients may occasionally conceal important information. In some cases, they may not realize the information is important; in other cases, they may be too embarrassed to reveal certain details.

The interview provides an opportunity to study the patient's manner, attitude, behavior, and emotional reactions. The tone of voice, bearing, expression of the eyes, swift play of facial muscles, appearance of weeping or smiling, or the presence of pallor, blushing, sweating, patches of erythema on the neck, furrowing of the brows, drawing of the lips, clenching of the teeth, pupillary dilation, or muscle rigidity may give important information. Gesticulations, restlessness, delay, hesitancy, and the relation of demeanor and emotional responses to descriptions of symptoms or to details in the family or marital history should be noted and recorded. These and the mode of response to the questions are valuable in judging character, personality, and emotional state.

The patient's story may not be entirely correct or complete. He may not possess full or detailed information regarding his illness, may misinterpret his symptoms or give someone else's interpretation of them, wishfully alter or withhold information, or even deliberately prevaricate for some purpose. The patient may be a phlegmatic, insensitive individual who does not comprehend the significance of his symptoms, a garrulous person who cannot give a relevant or coherent story, or have multiple or vague complaints that cannot be readily articulated. Infants, young children, comatose or confused patients may be unable to give any history. Patients who are in pain or distress, have difficulty with speech or expression, are of low intelligence, or do not speak the examiner's language are often unable to give a satisfactory history for themselves. Patients with nondominant parietal lesions are often not fully aware of the extent of their deficit. It may be necessary to corroborate or supplement the history given by the patient by talking with an observer, relative, or friend, or even to obtain the entire history from someone else. Family members may be able to give important information about changes in behavior, memory, hearing, vision, speech, or coordination of which the patient may not be aware. It is frequently necessary to question both the patient and others in order to obtain a complete account of the illness. Family members and significant others sometimes accompany the patient during the interview. They can frequently provide important supplementary information. However, the family member must not be permitted to dominate the patient's account of the illness unless the patient is incapable of giving a history.

It is usually best to see the patient de novo with minimal prior review of the medical records. Too much information in advance of the patient encounter may bias one's opinion. If it later turns out that previous caregivers reached similar conclusions based on primary information, this reinforces the likelihood of a correct diagnosis. So, see the patient first, review old records later.

There are three approaches to utilizing information from past caregivers, whether from medical records or as relayed by the patient. In the first instance, the physician takes too much at face value and assumes that previous diagnoses must be correct. An opposite approach, actually used by some, is to assume all previous caregivers were incompetent, and their conclusions could not possibly be correct. This approach sometimes forces the extreme skeptic into a position of having to make some other diagnosis, even when the preponderance of the evidence indicates that previous physicians were correct. The logical middle ground is to make no assumptions regarding the opinions of previous caregivers. Use the information appropriately, matching it against what the patient relates and whatever other information is available. Do not unquestioningly believe it all, but do not perfunctorily dismiss it either. Discourage patients from grousing about their past medical care and avoid disparaging remarks about other physicians the patient may have seen. An accurate and detailed record of events in cases involving compensation and medicolegal problems is particularly important.

One efficient way to work is to combine reviewing past notes with talking directly with the patient. If the record contains a reasonably complete history, review it with the patient for accuracy. For instance, read from the record and say to the patient, "Dr. Payne says here that you have been having pain in the left leg for the past 6 months. Is that correct?" The patient might verify that information, or may say, "No, it's the right leg and it's more like 6 years." Such an approach can save considerable time when dealing with a patient who carries extensive previous records. A very useful method for summarizing a past workup is to make a table with two vertical columns, listing all tests which were done, with those that were normal in one column and those that were abnormal in the other column.

Many physicians find it useful to take notes during the interview. Contemporaneous note taking helps insure accuracy of the final report. A useful approach is simply to "take dictation" as the patient talks, particularly in the early stages of the encounter. A note sprinkled with patient quotations is often very illuminating. However, one must not be fixated on note taking. The trick is to interact with the patient, and take notes unobtrusively. The patient must not be left with the impression that the physician is paying attention to the note taking and not to them. Such notes are typically used for later transcription into some final format. Sometimes the patient comes armed with notes. The patient who has multiple complaints written on a scrap of paper is said to have *la maladie du petit papier;* tech savvy patients may come with computer printouts detailing their medical histories.

## THE PRESENTING COMPLAINT AND THE PRESENT ILLNESS

The neurologic history usually starts with obtaining the usual demographic data, but must also include handedness. The traditional approach to history taking begins with the chief complaint and present illness. In fact, many experienced clinicians begin with the *pertinent* past history, identifying major underlying past or chronic medical illnesses at the outset. This does not mean going into detail about unrelated past surgical procedures and the like. It does mean identifying major comorbidities which might have a direct or indirect bearing on the present illness. This technique helps to put the present illness in context and to prompt early consideration about whether the neurologic problem is a complication of some underlying condition or an independent process. It is inefficient to go through a long and laborious history in a patient with peripheral neuropathy, only to subsequently find out in the past history that the patient has known, long standing diabetes.

While a complete database is important, it is counterproductive to give short shrift to the details of the present illness. History taking should concentrate on the details of the presenting complaint. The majority of the time spent with a new patient should be devoted to the history and the majority of the history taking time should be devoted to the symptoms of the present illness. The answer most often lies in the details of the presenting problem. Begin with an open ended question, such as, "what sort of problems are you having?" Asking "what brought you here today?" often produces responses regarding a mode of transportation. And asking "what is wrong with you?" only invites wisecracks. After establishing the chief complaint or reason for the referral, make the patient start at the beginning of the story and go through more or less chronologically. Many patients will not do this unless so directed. The period of time leading up to the onset of symptoms should be dissected to uncover such things as the immunization that precipitated an episode of neuralgic amyotrophy, the diarrheal illness prior to an episode of Guillain-Barre syndrome, or the camping trip that lead to the tick bite. Patients are quick to assume that some recent event is the cause for their current difficulty. The physician must avoid the trap of assuming that temporal relationships prove etiologic relationships.

Record the chief complaint in the patient's own words. It is important to clarify important elements of the history that the patient is unlikely to spontaneously describe. Each symptom of the present illness should be analyzed systematically by asking the patient a series of questions to clear up any ambiguities. Determine exactly when the symptoms began, whether they are present constantly or intermittently, and if intermittently the character, duration, frequency, severity, and relationship to external factors. Determine the progression or regression of each symptom, whether there is any seasonal, diurnal, or nocturnal variability, and the response to treatment. In patients whose primary complaint is pain, determine the location; character or quality; severity; associated symptoms; and, if episodic, frequency, duration, and any specific precipitating or relieving factors. Some patients have difficulty describing such things as the character of a pain. Although spontaneous descriptions have more value, and leading questions should in general be avoided, it is perfectly permissible when necessary to offer possible choices, such as "dull like a toothache" or "sharp like a knife."

In neurologic patients, particular attention should be paid to determining the time course of the illness, as this is often instrumental in determining the etiology. An illness might be static, remittent, intermittent, progressive, or improving. Abrupt onset followed by improvement with variable degrees of recovery are characteristic of trauma and vascular events. Degenerative diseases have a gradual onset of symptoms and variable rate of progression. Tumors have a gradual onset and steady progression of symptoms, with the rate of progression depending on the tumor type. With some neoplasms hemorrhage or spontaneous necrosis may cause sudden onset or worsening. Multiple sclerosis is most often characterized by remissions and exacerbations, but with a progressive increase in the severity of symptoms; stationary, intermittent, and chronic progressive forms also occur. Infections usually have a relatively sudden, but not precipitous, onset followed by gradual improvement, and either complete or incomplete recovery. In many conditions symptoms appear some time before striking physical signs of disease are evident, and before neurodiagnostic testing detects significant abnormalities. It is important to know the major milestones of an illness: when the patient last considered himself to be well, when he had to stop work, when he began to use an assistive device, when he was forced to take to his bed. It is often useful to ascertain exactly how and how severely the patient considers himself disabled, as well as what crystallized the decision to seek medical care.

A careful history may uncover previous events which the patient may have forgotten or may not attach significance to. A history consistent with past vascular events, trauma or episodes of demyelination may shed entirely new light on the current symptoms. In the patient with symptoms of myelopathy, the episode of visual loss that occurred five years previously suddenly takes on a different meaning.

It is useful at some point to ask the patient what is worrying him. It occasionally turns out that the patient is very concerned over the possibility of some disorder that has not even occurred to the physician to consider. Patients with neurologic complaints are often apprehensive about having some dreadful disease, such as a brain tumor, ALS, multiple sclerosis, or muscular dystrophy. All these conditions are well known to the lay public, and patients or family members occasionally jump to outlandish conclusions about the cause of some symptom. Simple reassurance is occasionally all that is necessary.

## THE PAST MEDICAL HISTORY

The past history is important because neurologic symptoms may be related to systemic diseases. Relevant information includes a statement about general health; history of current, chronic, and past illnesses; hospitalizations; operations; accidents or injuries, particularly head trauma; infectious diseases; venereal diseases; congenital defects; diet; and sleeping patterns. Inquiry should be made about allergies and other drug reactions. Certain situations and comorbid conditions are of particular concern in the patient with neurologic symptomotology. The vegetarian or person with a history of gastric surgery or inflammatory bowel disease is at risk of developing vitamin $B_{12}$ deficiency, and the neurologic complications of connective tissue disorders, diabetes, thyroid disease, and sarcoidosis are protean. A history of cancer raises concern about metastatic disease as well as paraneoplastic syndromes. A history of valvular heart disease or recent myocardial infarction may be relevant in the patient with cerebrovascular disease. In some instances, even in an adult, a history of the patient's birth and early development is pertinent, including any complications of pregnancy, labor and delivery, birth trauma, birth weight, postnatal illness, health and development during childhood, convulsions with fever, learning ability and school performance,

A survey of current medications, both prescribed and over the counter, is always important. Many drugs have significant neurologic side effects. For example, confusion may develop in an elderly patient simply from the use of beta blocker ophthalmic solution; nonsteroidal anti-inflammatory drugs can cause aseptic meningitis; many drugs may cause dizziness, cramps, paresthesias, headache, weakness, and other side effects; and headaches are the most common side effect of proton pump inhibitors. Going over the details of the drug regimen may reveal that the patient is not taking a medication as intended. Pointed questions are often necessary to get at the issue of over the counter drugs, as many patients do not consider these as medicines. Occasional patients develop significant neurologic side effects from their well-intended vitamin regimen. Patients will take medicines from alternative health care practitioners or from a health food store, assuming these agents are safe because they are "natural," which is not always the case. Having the patient bring in all medication bottles, prescribed and over the counter, is occasionally fruitful.

## THE FAMILY HISTORY

The family history (FH) is essentially an inquiry into the possibility of heredofamilial disorders, and focuses on the patient's lineage; it is occasionally quite important in neurologic patients. Information about the nuclear family is also often relevant to the social history (see below). In addition to the usual questions about cancer, diabetes, hypertension, and cardiovascular disease, the FH is particularly relevant in patients with migraine, epilepsy, cerebrovascular disease, movement disorders, myopathy, and cerebellar disease, to list a few. In some patients, it is pertinent to inquire about a FH of alcoholism or other types of substance abuse. Family size is important. A negative FH is more reassuring in a patient with several siblings and a large extended family than in a patient with no siblings and few known relatives. It is not uncommon to encounter patients who were adopted and have no knowledge of their biological family.

There are traps, and a negative FH is not always really negative. Some diseases may be rampant in a kindred without any awareness of it by the affected individuals. With Charcot-Marie-Tooth disease, for example, so many family members may have the condition that the pes cavus and stork leg deformities are not recognized as abnormal. Chronic, disabling neurologic conditions in a family member may be attributed to another cause, such as "arthritis." Sometimes, family members deliberately withhold information about a known familial condition.

It is sometimes necessary to inquire about the relationship between the parents, exploring the possibility of consanguinity. In some situations, it is important to probe the patient's ethnic background, given the tendency of some neurologic disorders to occur in particular ethnic groups or in patients from certain geographic regions.

## SOCIAL HISTORY

The social history includes such things as the patient's marital status, educational level, occupation, and personal habits. The marital history should include the number of marriages, duration of present marriage, and health of the partner and children. At times it may be necessary to delve into marital adjustment and health of the relationship as well as the circumstances leading to any changes in marital status.

A question about the nature of the patient's work is routine. A detailed occupational history, occasionally necessary, should delve into both present and past occupations, with special reference to contact with neurotoxins, use of personal protective equipment, working environment, levels of exertion and repetitive motion activities, and co-worker illnesses. A record of frequent job changes or a poor work history may be important. If the patient is no longer working, determine when and why he stopped. In some situations, it is relevant to inquire about hobbies and avocations, particularly when toxin exposure or a repetitive motion injury is a diagnostic consideration. Previous residences, especially in the tropics or in areas where certain diseases are endemic, may be relevant.

A history of personal habits is important, with special reference to the use of alcohol, tobacco, drugs, coffee, tea, soft drinks and similar substances, or the reasons for abstinence. Patients are often not forthcoming about the use of alcohol and street drugs, especially those with something to hide. Answers may range from mildly disingenuous to bald-faced lies. Drugs and alcohol are sometimes a factor in the most seemingly unlikely circumstances. Patients notoriously underreport the amount of alcohol they consume; a commonly used heuristic is to double the admitted amount. To get a more realistic idea about the impact of alcohol on the patient's life the CAGE questionnaire is useful (Table 2.1). Even one positive response is suspicious; four are diagnostic of alcohol abuse. The HALT and BUMP are other similar question sets (Table 2.1). Some patients will not admit to drinking "alcohol" and will only confess when the examiner hits on their specific beverage of choice, e.g., gin. Always ask the patient who denies drinking at all some follow-up question: why he doesn't drink, if he ever drank, or when he quit. This may uncover a past or family history of substance abuse, or the patient may admit he quit only the week before. In the patient suspected of alcohol abuse, take a dietary history.

Patients are even more secretive about drug habits. Tactful opening questions might be to ask whether the patient has ever used drugs for other than medicinal purposes, ever abused prescription drugs, or ever ingested drugs other than by mouth. The vernacular is often necessary: patients understand "smoke crack" better than "inhale cocaine." It is useful to know the street names of commonly abused drugs, but these change frequently as both slang and drugs go in and out of fashion. A less refined type of substance abuse is to inhale common substances, such as spray

## TABLE 2.1

### Questions to Explore the Possibility of Alcohol Abuse

**CAGE questions**

Have you ever felt the need to Cut down on your drinking?

Have people Annoyed you by criticizing your drinking?

Have you ever felt Guilty about your drinking?

Have you ever had a morning "Eye-opener" to steady your nerves or get rid of a hangover?

**HALT questions**

Do you usually drink to get High?

Do you drink Alone?

Do you ever find yourself Looking forward to drinking?

Have you noticed that you are becoming Tolerant to alcohol?

**BUMP questions**

Have you ever had Blackouts?

Have you ever used alcohol in an Unplanned way (drank more than intended or continued to drink after having enough)?

Do you ever drink for Medicinal reasons (to control anxiety, depression or the "shakes")?

Do you find yourself Protecting your supply of alcohol (hoarding, buying extra)?

---

paint, airplane glue, paint thinner, and gasoline. It is astounding what some individuals will do. One patient was fond of smoking marijuana and inhaling gasoline, *leaded* specifically, so that he could hallucinate in color.

Determining if the patient has ever engaged in risky sexual behavior is sometimes important, and the subject always difficult to broach. Patients are often less reluctant to discuss the topic than the examiner. Useful opening gambits might include how often and with whom the patient has sex, whether the patient engages in unprotected sex, or whether the patient has ever had a sexually transmitted disease.

## REVIEW OF SYSTEMS

In primary care medicine the review of systems (ROS) is designed in part to detect health problems of which the patient may not complain, but which nevertheless require attention. In specialty practice, the ROS is done more to detect symptoms involving other systems of which the patient may not spontaneously complain but that provide clues to the diagnosis of the presenting complaint. Neurologic disease may cause dysfunction involving many different systems. In patients presenting with neurologic symptoms, a "neurologic review of systems" is useful after exploring the present illness to uncover relevant neurologic complaints. Some question areas worth probing into are summarized in Table 2.2. Symptoms of depression are often particularly relevant and are summarized in Table 2.3. A more general ROS may also reveal important information relevant to the present illness (Table 2.4). Occasional patients have a generally positive ROS, with complaints in multiple systems out of proportion to any evidence of organic disease. Patients with Briquet syndrome have a somatization disorder with multiple somatic complaints which they often describe in colorful, exaggerated terms.

The ROS is often done by questionnaire in outpatients. Another efficient method is to do the ROS during the physical examination, asking about symptoms related to each organ system as it is examined.

## TABLE 2.2

### A Neurologic System Review; Symptoms Worth Inquiring About in Patients Presenting with Neurologic Complaints

Any history of seizures or unexplained loss of consciousness
Headache
Vertigo or dizziness
Loss of vision
Diplopia
Difficulty hearing
Tinnitus
Difficulty with speech or swallowing
Weakness, difficulty moving, abnormal movements
Numbness, tingling
Tremor
Problems with gait, balance or coordination
Difficulty with sphincter control or sexual function
Difficulty with thinking or memory
Problems sleeping or excessive sleepiness
Depressive symptoms (Table 2.3)

Modified from: Campbell WW, Pridgeon RM. *Practical Primer of Clinical Neurology*. Philadelphia: Lippincott Williams and Wilkins, 2002.

## HISTORY IN SOME COMMON CONDITIONS

Some of the important historical features to explore in patients with some common neurologic complaints are summarized in Tables 2.5-2.13. There are too many potential neurologic presenting complaints to cover them all, so these tables should be regarded only as a starting point and an illustration of the process. Space does not permit an explanation of the differential diagnostic relevance of

## TABLE 2.3

### Some Symptoms Suggesting Depression

Depressed mood, sadness
Unexplained weight gain or loss
Increased or decreased appetite
Sleep disturbance
Lack of energy, tiredness, fatigue
Loss of interest in activities
Anhedonia
Feelings of guilt or worthlessness
Suicidal ideation
Psychomotor agitation or retardation
Sexual dysfunction
Difficulty concentrating or making decisions
Difficulty with memory

Modified from: Campbell WW, Pridgeon RM. *Practical Primer of Clinical Neurology*. Philadelphia: Lippincott Williams and Wilkins, 2002.

## TABLE 2.4

### Items in the Review of Systems of Possible Neurologic Relevance, with Examples of Potentially Related Neurologic Conditions in Parentheses

General
   Weight loss (depression, neoplasia)
   Decreased energy level (depression)
   Chills/fever (occult infection)
Head
   Headaches (many)
   Trauma (subdural hematoma)
Eyes
   Refractive status; lenses, refractive surgery
   Episodic visual loss (amaurosis fugax)
   Progressive visual loss (optic neuropathy)
   Diplopia (numerous)
   Ptosis (myasthenia gravis)
   Dry eyes (Sjögren syndrome)
   Photosensitivity (migraine)
   Eye pain (optic neuritis)
Ears
   Hearing loss (acoustic neuroma)
   Discharge (cholesteatoma)
   Tinnitus (Meniere disease)
   Vertigo (vestibulopathy)
   Vesicles *(H. zoster)*
Nose
   Anosmia (olfactory groove meningioma)
   Discharge (CSF rhinorrhea)
Mouth
   Sore tongue (nutritional deficiency)
Neck
   Pain (radiculopathy)
   Stiffness (meningitis)
Cardiovascular
   Heart disease (many)
   Claudication (neurogenic vs. vascular)
   Hypertension (cerebrovascular disease)
   Cardiac arrhythmia (cerebral embolism)
Respiratory
   Dyspnea (neuromuscular disease)
   Asthma (systemic vaculitis)
   Tuberculosis (meningitis)
Gastrointestinal
   Appetite change (hypothalamic lesion)

Excessive thirst (diabetes mellitus
or insipidus)
   Dysphagia (myasthenia)
   Constipation (dysautonomia, MNGIE)
   Vomiting (increased intracranial pressure)
   Hepatitis (vasculitis, cryoglobulinemia)
Genitourinary
   Urinary incontinence (neurogenic bladder)
   Urinary retention (neurogenic bladder)
   Impotence (dysautonomia)
   Polyuria (diabetes mellitus or insipidus)
   Spontaneous abortion (anticardiolipin
   syndrome)
   Sexually transmitted disease (neurosyphilis)
   Pigmenturia (porphyria, rhabdomyolysis)
Menstrual history
   Last menstrual period and contraception
   Oral contraceptive use (stroke)
   Hormone replacement therapy (migraine)
Endocrine
   Galactorrhea (pituitary tumor)
   Amenorrhea (pituitary insufficiency)
   Enlarging hands/feet (acromegaly)
   Thyroid disease (many)
Musculoskeletal
   Arthritis (connective tissue disease)
   Muscle cramps (ALS)
   Myalgias (myopathy)
Hematopoetic
   Anemia ($B_{12}$ deficiency)
   DVT (anti-cardiolipin syndrome)
Skin
   Rashes (Lyme disease, drug reactions)
   Insect bites (Lyme disease, rickettsial
   infection, tick paralysis)
   Birthmarks (phakamotoses)
Psychiatric
   Depression (many)
   Psychosis (CJD)
   Hallucination (Lewy body disease)
   Grandiosity (neurosyphilis)

CJD, Creutzfeldt-Jakob disease; DVT, deep venous thrombosis; MNGIE, mitochondrial neurogastrointestinal encephalomyopathy

## TABLE 2.5

**Important Historical Points in the Chronic Headache Patient; if the Patient Has More Than One Kind of Headache, Obtain the Information for Each Type**

Location of the pain (e.g., hemicranial, holocranial, occipitonuchal, bandlike)
Pain intensity/severity
Pain quality (e.g., steady, throbbing, stabbing)
Timing, duration, and frequency
Average daily caffeine intake
Average daily analgesic intake (including over-the-counter medications)
Precipitating factors (e.g., alcohol, sleep deprivation, oversleeping, foods, bright light)
Relieving factors (e.g., rest/quiet, dark room, activity, medications)
Response to treatment
Neurologic accompaniments (e.g., numbness, paresthesias, weakness, speech disturbance)
Visual accompaniments (e.g., scintillating scotoma, transient blindness)
Gastrointestinal accompaniments (e.g., nausea, vomiting, anorexia)
Associated symptoms (e.g., photophobia, phonophobia/sonophobia, tearing, nasal stuffiness)
Any history of head trauma

Modified from: Campbell WW, Pridgeon RM. *Practical Primer of Clinical Neurology*. Philadelphia: Lippincott Williams and Wilkins, 2002.

each of these elements of the history. Suffice it to say that each of these elements in the history has significance in ruling in or ruling out some diagnostic possibility. Such a "list" exists for every complaint in every patient. Learning and refining these lists is the challenge of medicine.

For example, Table 2.5 lists some of the specific important historical points helpful in evaluating the chronic headache patient. The following features are general rules and guidelines, not absolutes. Patients with migraine tend to have unilateral hemicranial or orbitofrontal throbbing pain associated with GI upset. Those suffering from migraine with aura (classical migraine) have visual or neurologic accompaniments. Patients usually seek relief by lying quietly in a dark, quiet environment. Patients with cluster headache tend to have unilateral nonpulsatile orbitofrontal pain with no visual, GI, or neurologic accompaniments and tend to get some relief by moving about. Patients with tension or muscle contraction headaches tend to have nonpulsatile pain which is bandlike or occipitonuchal in distribution, and unaccompanied by visual, neurological, or GI upset.

Table 2.6 lists some of the important elements in the history in patients with neck and arm pain. The primary differential diagnosis is usually between cervical radiculopathy and musculoskeletal conditions such as bursitis, tendinitis, impingement syndrome, and myofascial pain. Patients with a cervical disc usually have pain primarily in the neck, trapezius ridge, and upper shoulder region. Patients with cervical myofascial pain have pain in the same general distribution. Radiculopathy patients may have pain referred to the pectoral or periscapular regions, which is unusual in myofascial pain. Radiculopathy patients may have pain radiating in a radicular distribution down the arm. Pain radiating below the elbow usually means radiculopathy. Patients with radiculopathy have pain on movement of the neck; those with shoulder pathology have pain on movement of the shoulder. Patients with radiculopathy may have weakness or sensory symptoms in the involved extremity.

Tables 2.7 to 2.13 summarize some important historical particulars to consider in some of the other complaints frequently encountered in an outpatient setting.

## TABLE 2.6

**Important Historical Points in the Patient with Neck and Arm Pain; the Differential Diagnosis Is Most Often Between Radiculopathy and Musculoskeletal Pain**

Onset and duration (acute, subacute, chronic)
Pain intensity
Any history of injury
Any history of preceding viral infection or immunization
Any past history of disc herniation, disc surgery, or previous episodes of neck or arm pain
Location of the worst pain (e.g., neck, arm, shoulder)
Pain radiation pattern, if any (e.g., to shoulder, arm, pectoral region, periscapular region)
Relation of pain to neck movement
Relation of pain to arm and shoulder movement
Relieving factors
Any exacerbation with coughing, sneezing, straining at stool
Any weakness of the arm or hand
Any numbness, paresthesias, or dysesthesias of the arm or hand
Any associated leg weakness or bowel, bladder, or sexual dysfunction suggesting
    spinal cord compression

Modified from: Campbell WW, Pridgeon RM. *Practical Primer of Clinical Neurology*. Philadelphia: Lippincott Williams and Wilkins, 2002.

## TABLE 2.7

**Important Historical Points in the Patient with Back and Leg Pain; the Differential Diagnosis Is Most Often, as with Neck and Arm Pain, Between Radiculopathy and Musculoskeletal Pain**

Onset and duration (acute, subacute, chronic)
Pain intensity
Any history of injury
Any past history of disc herniation, disc surgery, or previous episodes of back/leg pain
Location of the worst pain (e.g., back, buttock, hip, leg)
Pain radiation pattern, if any (e.g., to buttock, thigh, leg, or foot)
Relation of pain to body position (e.g., standing, sitting, lying down)
Relation of pain to activity and movement (bending, stooping, leg motion)
Any exacerbation with coughing, sneezing, straining at stool
Any weakness of the leg, foot, or toes
Any numbness, paresthesias, or dysesthesias of the leg or foot
Relieving factors
Any associated bowel, bladder, or sexual dysfunction suggesting cauda equina compression
Any associated fever, weight loss, or morning stiffness

Modified from: Campbell WW, Pridgeon RM. *Practical Primer of Clinical Neurology*. Philadelphia: Lippincott Williams and Wilkins, 2002.

## TABLE 2.8

**Important Historical Points in the Dizzy Patient**

Patient's precise definition of dizziness
Nature of onset
Severity
Presence or absence of an illusion of motion
Symptoms present persistently or intermittently
If intermittently, frequency, duration, and timing of attacks
Relation of dizziness to body position (e.g., standing, sitting, lying)
Any precipitation of dizziness by head movement
Associated symptoms (e.g., nausea, vomiting, tinnitus, hearing loss,
weakness, numbness, diplopia, dysarthria, dysphagia, difficulty with gait or balance,
palpitations, shortness of breath, dry mouth,* chest pain)
Medications, especially antihypertensives or ototoxic drugs

*can be a clue to hyperventilation
Modified from: Campbell WW, Pridgeon RM. *Practical Primer of Clinical Neurology*. Philadelphia: Lippincott
    Williams and Wilkins, 2002.

## TABLE 2.9

**Important Historical Points in the Patient with Hand Numbness; the Primary
Considerations in the Differential Diagnosis Are Carpal Tunnel Syndrome and
Cervical Radiculopathy**

Symptoms constant or intermittent
If intermittent, timing, especially any relationship to time of day, especially any tendency
    for nocturnal symptoms, duration, and frequency
Relationship to activities (e.g., driving)
What part of hand most involved
Any involvement of arm, face, leg
Any problems with speech or vision associated with the hand numbness
Neck pain
Hand/arm pain
Hand/arm weakness
Any history of injury, especially old wrist injury
Any involvement of the opposite hand

Modified from: Campbell WW, Pridgeon RM. *Practical Primer of Clinical Neurology*. Philadelphia: Lippincott
    Williams and Wilkins, 2002.

## TABLE 2.10

**Important Historical Points in the Patient with a Suspected Transient Ischemic Attack; this Arises in Patients Who Have Had One or More Spells of Weakness or Numbness Involving One Side of the Body, Transient Loss of Vision, Symptoms of Vertebrobasilar Insufficiency, and Similar Problems**

Date of first spell and number of attacks
Frequency of attacks
Duration of attacks
Specific body parts and functions involved
Any associated difficulty with speech, vision, swallowing, etc.
Other associated symptoms (chest pain, shortness of breath, nausea and vomiting, headache)
Any history of hypertension, diabetes mellitus, hypercholesterolemia, coronary artery disease, peripheral vascular disease, drug abuse
Any past episodes suggestive of retinal, hemispheric, or vertebrobasilar TIA
Current medications especially aspirin, oral contraceptives, antihypertensives

Modified from: Campbell WW, Pridgeon RM. *Practical Primer of Clinical Neurology*. Philadelphia: Lippincott Williams and Wilkins, 2002.

## TABLE 2.11

**Important Historical Points in the Patient with Episodic Loss of Consciousness; the Differential Diagnosis of Syncope v. Seizure**

Timing of attacks (e.g., frequency, duration)
Patient's recollection of events
Circumstances of attack (e.g., in church, in the shower, after phlebotomy)
Events just prior to attack
Body position just prior to attack (e.g., supine, sitting, standing)
Presence of prodrome or aura
Any tonic or clonic activity
Any suggestion of focal onset
Any incontinence or tongue biting
Symptoms following the spell (e.g., sleeping, focal neurologic deficit)
Time to complete recovery
Witness description of attacks
Drug, alcohol, and medication exposure
Family history

Modified from: Campbell WW, Pridgeon RM. *Practical Primer of Clinical Neurology*. Philadelphia: Lippincott Williams and Wilkins, 2002.

TABLE 2.12

**Important Historical Points in the Patient with Numbness of the Feet; the Differential Diagnosis Is Usually Between Peripheral Neuropathy and Lumbosacral Radiculopathy; there Is a Further Extensive Differential Diagnosis of the Causes of Peripheral Neuropathy**

Whether symptoms are constant or intermittent
If intermittent, any relation to posture, activity, or movement
Any associated pain in the back, legs, or feet
Any weakness of the legs or feet
Any history of back injury, disc herniation, back surgery
Symmetry of symptoms
Any bowel, bladder, or sexual dysfunction
Any history of underlying systemic disease (e.g. diabetes mellitus, thyroid disease, anemia, low vitamin $B_{12}$ level)
Any weight loss
Drinking habits
Smoking history
Any history to suggest toxin exposure, vocational or recreational
Dietary history
Medication history, including vitamins
Family history of similar symptoms
Family history of diabetes, pernicious anemia, or peripheral neuropathy

Modified from: Campbell WW, Pridgeon RM. *Practical Primer of Clinical Neurology*. Philadelphia: Lippincott Williams and Wilkins, 2002.

TABLE 2.13

**Important Historical Points in the Patient Complaining of Memory Loss; the Primary Consideration Is to Distinguish Alzheimer Disease From Conditions (Especially Treatable Ones) that May Mimic It**

Duration of the problem
Getting worse, better, or staying the same
Examples of what is forgotten (minor things such as dates, anniversaries, etc. as compared to major things)
Does the patient still control the checkbook
Any tendency to get lost
Medication history, including OTC drugs
Drinking habits
Any headache
Any difficulty with the senses of smell or taste
Any difficulty with balance, walking, or bladder control
Any depressive symptoms (see Table 2.3)
Any recent head trauma
Past history of stroke or other vascular disease
Past history of thyroid disease, anemia, low $B_{12}$, any STD
Any risk factors for HIV
Family history of dementia or Alzheimer disease

Modified from: Campbell WW, Pridgeon RM. *Practical Primer of Clinical Neurology*. Philadelphia: Lippincott Williams and Wilkins, 2002.

# CHAPTER 3

# The General Physical Examination

**A**general physical examination (PE) usually accompanies a neurologic examination (NE). The extent of the general PE done depends on the circumstances and may range from minimal to extensive. The general PE in a neurologic patient need not be so detailed or painstaking as in a complicated internal medicine patient, but must be complete enough to reveal any relevant abnormalities. There are many excellent textbooks on physical diagnosis that provide an extensive discussion of general PE techniques.

Even the most compulsive internist doing a "complete physical" performs an NE the average neurologist would be consider cursory. In contrast, the neurologist performs a more complete NE, but only as much general PE as the circumstances dictate. Both are concerned about achieving the proper balance between efficiency and thoroughness. The internist or other primary care practitioner would like to learn how to incorporate the NE into the general PE; the neurologist would like to incorporate as much of the general PE as possible into the NE. In fact, any NE, even a cursory one, provides an opportunity to accomplish much of the general PE simply by observation and a few additional maneuvers.

The general examination begins with observation of the patient during the interview. Even the patient's voice may be relevant, as hoarseness, dysphonia, aphasia, dysarthria, confusion, and other things of neurologic significance may be apparent even at that early stage. An HEENT exam is a natural byproduct of an evaluation of the cranial nerves. When examining the pupils and extraocular movements, take the opportunity to note any abnormalities of the external eye and ocular adnexa, such as conjunctivitis, exophthalmos, lid retraction, lid lag, xanthelasma, or jaundice. When examining the mouth, as an extension of the general PE, search for any intraoral lesions, leukoplakia, or other abnormality. When examining the optic disc, also examine the retina for any evidence of diabetic or hypertensive retinopathy. While examining neurologic function in the upper extremities, there is ample opportunity to observe for the presence of clubbing, cyanosis, nail changes, hand deformity, arthropathy and so forth to complete the upper extremity examination portion of the general physical examination. Examining the legs and feet for strength, reflexes, sensation, and plantar responses provides an opportunity to coincidentally look at the skin and nails. Check for pretibial edema, leg length discrepancy, swollen or deformed knee or ankle joints, or any other abnormalities. Note the pattern of hair growth, any dystrophic changes in the nails, and feel the pulses in the feet. Do anything else necessary for the lower extremity portion of the general PE. An evaluation of gait and station provides a great deal of information about the musculoskeletal system. Note whether the patient has any orthopedic limitations, such as a varus deformity of the knee, genu recurvatum, or pelvic tilt. Gait testing also provides a convenient opportunity to examine the lumbosacral spine for tenderness and range of motion. After listening for carotid bruits, it requires little additional effort to palpate the neck for masses and thyromegaly.

The NE can thus serve as a core around which a general PE can be built. At the end of a good NE, one has only to listen to the heart and lungs and palpate the abdomen to have also done a fairly complete general PE. Sometimes it is not so important to do a skillful general PE as to be willing to do any at all, as some findings are obvious if one merely takes the trouble to look. Although there is virtually no part of the general PE that may not occasionally be noteworthy in a particular circumstance, some parts of the general PE are more often relevant and important in patients presenting with neurologic complaints. The general PE as particularly relevant for neurologic patients follows.

## VITAL SIGNS

Determining the blood pressure in both arms is useful in patients with suspected cerebrovascular disease, and measuring the blood pressure with the patient supine, seated, and upright may be necessary in some circumstances. The pulse rate and character are important, especially if increased intracranial pressure is suspected. A bounding pulse occurs in aortic regurgitation or hyperthyroidism and a small, slow pulse in aortic stenosis, all of which may have neurologic complications. Abnormalities of respiration, such as Cheyne-Stokes, Biot, or Kussmaul breathing may be seen in coma and other neurologic disorders. Either hyperpnea or periods of apnea may occur in increased intracranial pressure and in disturbances of the hypothalamus.

## GENERAL APPEARANCE

The general appearance of the patient may reveal evidence of acute or chronic illness; fever, pain, or distress; evidence of weight loss; abnormal posture of the trunk, head, or extremities; the general level of motor activity; unusual mannerisms; bizarre activities; restlessness; or immobility. Weight loss and evidence of malnutrition may indicate hyperthyroidism, Alzheimer disease, Whipple disease, celiac disease, or amyloidosis. The body fat level and distribution, together with the hair distribution and the secondary sexual development are important in the diagnosis of endocrinopathies and disorders of the hypothalamus. Note any outstanding deviations from normal development such as gigantism, dwarfism, gross deformities, amputations, contractures, and disproportion or asymmetries between body parts.

Specific abnormal postures may occur in diseases of the nervous system. Spastic hemiparesis causes flexion of the upper extremity with flexion and adduction at the shoulder, flexion at the elbow and wrist, and flexion and adduction of the fingers; in the lower extremity there is extension at the hip, knee, and ankle, with an equinus deformity of the foot. In Parkinson disease and related syndromes there is flexion of the neck, trunk, elbows, wrists, and knees, with stooping, rigidity, masking, slowness of movement, and tremors. In myopathies there may be lordosis, protrusion of the abdomen, a waddling gait, and hypertrophy of the calves. Peripheral nerve disease may cause wrist or foot drop or a claw hand. These neurogenic abnormalities may be confused with deformities due to such things as Dupuytren contracture, congenital pes cavus, changes due to trauma or arthritis, development abnormalities, habitual postures, and occupational factors.

### Head

The skull houses the brain and abnormalities of the head are common and often very important. Inspect the shape, symmetry, and size of the head, noting any apparent abnormalities or irregularities. Premature closure of cranial sutures can produce a wide variety of abnormally shaped skulls. Other deformities or developmental anomalies include hydrocephaly, macrocephaly, microcephaly, asymmetries or abnormalities of contour, disproportion between the facial and the cerebral portions, scars, and signs of recent trauma. In children, it is informative to measure the head circumference. Dilated veins, telangiectatic areas, or port-wine angiomas on the scalp or face may overlie a cerebral hemangioma, especially when such nevi are present in the trigeminal nerve distribution.

Palpation of the skull may disclose deformities due to old trauma, burr hole or craniotomy defects, tenderness, or scars. If there is a postoperative skull defect, note any bulging or tumefaction. The size and patency of the fontanelles is important in infants. Bulging of the fontanelles and suture separation can occur with increased intracranial pressure in children. Meningoceles and encephaloceles may cause palpable skull defects. Tumors may involve the scalp and skull. Palpable masses involving the scalp or skull may be metastatic carcinoma, lymphoma, leukemia, dermoid, or multiple myeloma. Neurofibromas of the scalp occur in von Recklinghausen disease. Localized swelling of the scalp may occur with osteomyelitis of the skull. Exostoses may indicate an underlying meningioma. Hydrocephalus that develops prior to suture closure often results in an enlarged, sometimes massive, head. Frontal bossing is another sign of hydrocephalus. Giant cell arteritis may cause induration and tenderness of the superficial temporal arteries. Transillumination may be useful in the diagnosis of hydrocephalus and hydranencephaly.

Percussion of the skull may disclose dullness on the side of a tumor or subdural hematoma, or a tympanitic percussion note in hydrocephalus and increased intracranial pressure in infants and children. Auscultatory percussion (percussion over the mid-frontal area while listening over various parts of the head with the stethoscope) may reveal relative dullness on the side of a mass lesion or subdural hematoma.

Auscultation of the head is sometimes useful. Bruits may be heard best over the temporal regions of the skull, the eyeballs, and the mastoids. Cephalic bruits may occur with angiomas, aneurysms, arteriovenous malformations, neoplasms that compress large arteries, and in the presence of atherosclerotic plaques that partially occlude cerebral or carotid arteries. They may also occur in the absence of disease. Ocular bruits usually signify occlusive intracranial cerebrovascular disease. A carotid bruit may be transmitted to the mastoid. An ocular bruit in a patient with an arteriovenous aneurysm may disappear on carotid compression. Murmurs may be transmitted from the heart or large vessels; systolic murmurs heard over the entire cranium in children are not always of pathologic significance.

An evaluation of the facies (the facial expression) may aid in neurologic diagnosis. Gross abnormalities are found in such conditions as acromegaly, cretinism, myxedema, hyperthyroidism, and Down syndrome. In some neurologic disorders there are characteristic changes in facial expression and mobility, such as the fixed ("masked") face of parkinsonism, the immobile face with precipitate laughter and crying seen in pseudobulbar palsy, the grimacing of athetosis and dystonia, and the ptosis and weakness of the facial muscles seen in some myopathies and myasthenia gravis.

## Eyes

Ophthalmologic abnormalities can provide many clues to the etiology of neurologic disease as well as to the presence of underlying systemic disease that may be causing neurologic symptomatology. Examples of findings of possible neurologic relevance include bilateral exophthalmos due to thyroid eye disease; unilateral proptosis due to thyroid eye disease, carotid-cavernous fistula, meningocele, encephalocele, or histiocytosis X; corneal clouding from mucopolysaccharidosis; Brushfield spots on the iris due to Down syndrome or Lisch nodules in neurofibromatosis; keratoconjunctivitis sicca due to Sjögren syndrome or other collagen vascular diseases; depositions of amyloid in the conjunctiva; herpes zoster ophthalmicus; pigmented pingueculae due to Gaucher disease; Kayser-Fleischer rings in Wilson disease; unilateral arcus senilis from carotid stenosis; tortuous conjunctival vessels in ataxia telangectasia; scleritis in Wegener granulomatosis; and nonsyphilitic interstitial keratitis in Cogan syndrome.

## Ears

Examination of the ears is particularly important in patients with hearing loss or vertigo. It is important to exclude a perforated tympanic membrane. Examination of the ear canal may reveal a glomus tumor in a patient with jugular foramen syndrome, vesicles due to herpes zoster infection, or evidence of a posterior fossa cholesteatoma. CSF otorrhea may cause a clear or bloody ear discharge. Before performing a caloric examination in a comatose patient it is important to be certain the ear canals are clear and the tympanic membranes intact.

## Nose, Mouth, and Throat

Perforation of the nasal septum may be a clue to cocaine abuse. A saddle nose may be a sign of congenital syphilis, evidence of bacterial infection a sign of cavernous sinus thrombosis, and watery drainage may be due to CSF rhinorrhea. In pernicious anemia the tongue is smooth and translucent with atrophy of the fungiform and filiform papillae, and associated redness and lack of coating (atrophic glossitis). In thiamine deficiency the tongue is smooth, shiny, atrophic, and reddened. A triple furrowed tongue is seen in myasthenia gravis; lingua plicata in Melkersson-Rosenthal syndrome; and macroglossia in amyloid, myxedema, and Down syndrome. Other potential findings include xerostomia in Sjögren syndrome, a lead line along the gums in lead toxicity, trismus in tetanus or polymyositis, and mucosal ulceration in Behcet disease. Notched teeth are a sign of congenital syphilis (Hutchinson teeth).

## Neck

Note any adenopathy, thyroid masses or enlargement, deformities, tenderness, rigidity, tilting, or other abnormalities of posture, asymmetries, changes in contour, or pain on movement. Normally the neck can be flexed so that the chin rests on the chest, and rotated from side to side without difficulty. Meningeal irritation may cause nuchal rigidity, head retraction, and opisthotonos. Neck movement may also be restricted with cervical spondylosis, cervical radiculopathy, and dystonias. In the Klippel-Feil syndrome, syringomyelia, and platybasia the neck may be short and broad, movement limited, and the hairline low. The carotid arteries should be cautiously and lightly palpated bilaterally, one at a time, and any abnormality or inequality noted, followed by auscultation for carotid bruits.

## Respiratory System and Thorax

Neurologic complications of pulmonary disease are common. Note the respiratory rate, rhythm, depth, and character of respirations. Pain on breathing, dyspnea, orthopnea, or shortness of breath on slight activity may be significant. Respiratory insufficiency is a frequent occurrence in neuromuscular disease. It may also be necessary to examine the breasts and search for axillary lymphadenopathy.

## Cardiovascular System

The cardiovascular examination is important because of the frequency of neurologic complications of hypertension, atherosclerosis, endocarditis, arrhythmias, and valvular disease. Evidence of atherosclerosis involving the peripheral blood vessels often correlates with cerebrovascular disease.

## Abdomen

Examination of the abdomen may reveal abnormal masses, enlarged viscera, abnormal pulsations or respiratory movements, or the presence of fluid. Hepatomegaly is common in cirrhosis, hepatitis, carcinoma, and amyloidosis; splenomegaly is common in mononucleosis, amyloidosis, and lymphoma. Ecchymosis of the flank may be evidence that a lumbosacral plexopathy is due to retroperitoneal hematoma. Ascites may be a clue to hepatic encephalopathy in a patient in a coma.

## Genitalia and Rectum

Examination of the genitalia, not often called for in neurologic patients, could reveal a chancre or the ulcerations of Behcet disease. The angiomas in Fabry disease are often found on the scrotum. A rectal examination is often necessary in patients with evidence of myelopathy or a cauda equina or conus medullaris syndrome.

## Spine

Examination of the spine is often important in neurologic patients. Note any deformity, abnormality of posture or motility, localized tenderness or muscle spasm. Tuberculosis and neoplasms of the spine may cause a marked kyphosis (gibbus); muscular dystrophy often results in an increased lumbar lordosis; and scoliosis is common in syringomyelia and Friedreich ataxia. Localized rigidity with a slight list or scoliosis and absence of the normal lordosis are frequent symptoms of lumbosacral radiculopathy. Dimpling of the skin or unusual hair growth over the sacrum suggest spinal dysraphism.

## Extremities

Note any limb deformities, contractures, edema, or color changes. Any variation from the normal in the size or shape of the hands, feet, or digits, as well as deformities, joint changes, contractures, pain or limitation of movement, localized tenderness, wasting, clubbed fingers, or ulcerations may be significant. Edema may be evidence of congestive heart failure or cardiomyopathy. Arthropathy may be a sign of connective tissue disease, sarcoidosis, or Whipple disease. Painless arthropathy (Charcot joint) occurs when a joint is deafferented. Decreased peripheral pulses occur in Takayasu disease as well as atherosclerosis. Acrocyanosis occurs in ergotism. Palmar erythema may be a clue to alcohol abuse. Diseases of the nervous system are found in association with such skeletal and developmental anomalies as syndactyly, polydactyly, and arachnodactyly.

## Skin

A careful examination of the skin can provide important evidence regarding the nature of a neurologic condition. Findings of possible neurologic relevance include: spider angiomas in alcohol abuse; erythema chronicum migrans in Lyme disease; purpura and petechiae in thrombotic thrombocytopenic purpura, meningococcemia, and Rocky Mountain spotted fever (all of which may have prominent neurologic manifestations); livedo reticularis in antiphospholipid syndrome and cryoglobulinemia; hyperpigmentation in Nelson syndrome, carotenemia, or Addison disease; and the numerous dermatologic manifestations of the neurocutaneous syndromes. Other important findings include signs of scleroderma; ichthyosis; scars, needle marks, or other evidence of intravenous substance abuse; bruises; and trophic changes. The degree of moisture or perspiration may be neurologically pertinent, and any localized or generalized increase or decrease in perspiration should be recorded. Skin changes may be of diagnostic significance in the endocrinopathies, diseases of the hypothalamus, and dysautonomia. In parkinsonism the skin may be greasy and seborrheic. Herpes zoster causes a vesicular eruption in the distribution of the involved root. Hemangiomas of the spinal cord may be accompanied by skin nevi in the same metamere. Symmetrically placed, painless, recurring, poorly healing lesions of the extremities may occur in syringomyelia and hereditary sensory neuropathy. Dermatomyositis causes characteristic skin lesions. Peripheral nerve disease, tabes dorsalis, and myelopathy may produce trophic changes in the skin. Skin changes may also be a manifestation of vitamin deficiency.

## Hair and Nails

Hair texture and distribution are important in the evaluation of endocrinopathies. Premature graying of the hair may be familial and of no clinical significance, but is frequently observed in pernicious anemia, and may occur in hypothalamic and other disorders. Poliosis occurs with Vogt-Kayanaga-Harada disease. Transverse discoloration of the nails (Mees lines) may occur with arsenic poisoning and debilitated states; clubbing of the nails occurs with bronchogenic carcinoma or heart disease. Abnormal nail bed capillary loops may be a sign of dermatomyositis.

## Nodes

Lymphadenopathy may occur in lymphoma, mononucleosis, HIV, Lyme disease, Niemann-Pick disease, Gaucher disease, phenytoin pseudolymphoma, sarcoidosis, Whipple disease, and in many other conditions that may also have neurologic manifestations.

# CHAPTER 4

# General Outline of the Neurologic Examination

The neurologic examination, as commonly done, includes the major categories listed in Table 4.1. Although the examination does not have to be performed in any particular sequence, and every physician develops his own routine for the examination, it is customary to record the neurologic examination in the general format outlined in Table 4.1, or with minor modifications.

The complete neurologic examination can be a complex and arduous undertaking. In fact, few neurologists do a truly complete exam on every patient. As with the general physical examination, the history focuses the neurologic examination so that certain aspects are emphasized in a given clinical situation. The exam done on a typical patient with headache is not the same as that done on a patient with low back pain, or dementia, or cerebrovascular disease. The examination should also be adapted for the circumstances. If the patient is in pain or apprehensive, it may initially focus on the area of complaint, followed later by a more thorough assessment. Only a brief examination may be possible for unstable or severely ill persons until their condition stabilizes. With comatose, combative or uncooperative patients, a compulsively complete examination is an impossibility. However, in each of these situations at least some maneuvers are employed to screen for neurologic dysfunction that is not necessarily suggested by the history. A rapid "screening" or "mini" neurologic examination may initially be adequate for persons with minor or intermittent symptoms. Every patient does not require every conceivable test, but all require a screening examination. The findings on such a screening examination determine the emphasis of a more searching subsequent examination. There are a number of ways to perform a screening examination. Table 4.2 details such an abbreviated examination from *DeJong's The Neurologic Examination.*

There are two basic ways to do a traditional neurologic examination, regional and systemic. A system approach evaluates the motor system, then the sensory system, and so on. A regional approach evaluates all the systems in a given region, such as the upper extremities, then the lower extremities. The screening exam outlined in Table 4.3 is an amalgam of the regional and system approaches geared for speed and efficiency. The concept is an examination that requires the nervous system to perform at a high level, relying heavily on sensitive signs, especially the flawless execution of complex functions. If the nervous system can perform a complex task perfectly, it is very unlikely there is significant pathology present, and going through a more extensive evaluation is not likely to prove productive. A neurologic examination that assesses complex functions and seeks signs that are sensitive indicators of pathology is efficient and not overly time consuming.

The examination begins with taking the medical history, which serves as a fair barometer of the mental status. Patients who can relate a logical, coherent, pertinent, and sensible narrative of

## TABLE 4.1

**Major Sections of the Neurologic Examination**

Mental status
Cranial nerves
Motor
Sensory
Reflexes
Cerebellar function, coordination
Gait and station
Other signs

their problem will seldom have abnormalities on more formal bedside mental status testing. On the other hand, a rambling, disjointed, incomplete history may be a clue to the presence of some cognitive impairment, even though there is no direct complaint of thinking or memory problems from the patient or the family. Similarly, psychiatric disease is sometimes betrayed by the patient's demeanor and style of history giving. If there is any suggestion of abnormality from the interaction with the patient during the history taking phase of the encounter, then a more detailed mental status examination should be carried out. Other reasons to do a formal mental status examination are discussed in Chapter 5. Simple observation is often useful. The patient's gait, voice, mannerisms, ability to dress and undress, and even handshake (grip myotonia) may suggest the diagnosis.

The Table 4.3 screening examination continues by doing everything that requires use of a penlight. Begin by noting the position of the eyelids and the width of the palpebral fissures bilaterally. Check the pupils for light reaction with the patient fixing at distance. If the pupillary light reaction is normal and equal in both eyes, checking the pupillary near reaction is not necessary. Continue by assessing extraocular movements in the six cardinal positions of gaze, having the patient follow the penlight. Be sure the patient has no diplopia or limitation of movement, and that ocular pursuit movements are smooth and fluid. With the eyes in primary and eccentric positions, look for any nystagmus. The eye examination is discussed in more detail in Chapters 9 and 10. With the light still in hand, prepare to examine the pharynx and oral cavity. Examination of trigeminal motor function is accomplished merely by watching the patient's jaw drop open prior to examining the mouth

## TABLE 4.2

**Components of a "Screening" Initial Neurologic Examination. Abnormalities or Specific Symptoms Should Lead to More Complete Evaluations**

1. Mentation and communication during conversation with examiner
2. Cranial nerves II, III, IV, VI: Visual acuity, gross fields, funduscopic, pupillary reactions, extraocular movements
3. Cranial nerves VII, VIII, IX, X, XII: Facial musculature and expression, gross hearing, voice, inspection of tongue
4. Muscle tone, strength, and bulk proximally and distally in all extremities; abnormal movements
5. Sensory: Pain or temperature medially and laterally in all extremities; vibration at ankles
6. Coordination: Rapid alternating movements of hands, finger-nose test, gait, station
7. Reflexes: Biceps, triceps, brachioradialis, quadriceps, Achilles, plantar, clonus

## TABLE 4.3

### Steps in a Screening Neurologic Examination

Mental status examination (during history taking or dispersed during the rest
of the examination)
Using a penlight
Pupils (at distance)
Extraocular movements
Pharynx and tongue (watch the jaw on mouth opening to be sure it drops vertically
to screen for trigeminal motor dysfunction)
Facial motor functions (grimace, close eyes tightly)
Visual fields
Fundi
Upper extremity formal strength examination—deltoid, triceps, wrist extensors,
and hand intrinsics
Examination for pronator drift, eyes closed
Examination of upper extremity stereognosis and upper and lower extremity double
simultaneous stimulation, while waiting for drift, eyes closed (evaluate fine motor control
during the patient's manipulation of the stereognosis test objects)
Examination of finger to nose coordination, eyes closed
Examination of arm and finger roll
Examination of lower extremity strength
Completion of the sensory assessment
Examination of deep tendon reflexes, upper and lower extremities
Elicitation of plantar responses
Examination of station and gait, heel and toe walking, hopping on each foot, tandem gait,
Romberg or eyes closed tandem

Modified from: Campbell WW, Pridgeon RM. *Practical Primer of Clinical Neurology.* Philadelphia: Lippincott
Williams and Wilkins, 2002.

and throat. When the pterygoids are unilaterally weak, the jaw invariably deviates toward the weak side on opening. This deviation, while subtle, is a sensitive indicator of trigeminal motor root pathology. Observe the tongue for atrophy or fasciculations. Have the patient phonate and be sure the median raphe of the palate elevates in the midline. There is little to be gained by checking the gag reflex if the patient has no complaints of dysphagia or dysarthria and there is no reason from the history to suspect a brainstem or cranial nerve lesion. Routine elicitation of the gag reflex is rarely informative and is unpleasant for the patient. Have the patient protrude the tongue and move it from side to side.

Functions requiring the use of the penlight completed, observe the nasolabial folds for depth and symmetry and compare the forehead wrinkles on both sides. Then have the patient grimace, vigorously baring the teeth, while closing the eyes tightly. Note the symmetry of the grimace, how many teeth are seen on each side, and the relative amplitude and velocity of the lower facial contraction, as well as the symmetry of the upper facial contraction. How completely the patient buries the eyelashes on the two sides is a sensitive indicator of orbicularis oculi strength.

If the patient has no complaints of hearing loss, tinnitus, vertigo, facial numbness or weakness and there is no specific reason suggested by the history to do so, routine examination of hearing is seldom productive. Examination of hearing is discussed further in Chapter 13. Complete the cranial nerve examination by checking the visual fields and fundi.

Screening examination of motor function, sensory function, and coordination in the upper extremities can be completed as one compound, multifaceted maneuver. In most clinical situations in which a screening examination is appropriate, the primary concern is to detect a lesion involving the corticospinal tract (CST). The CST preferentially innervates certain muscle groups, and these are the groups most likely to be weak because of an upper motor neuron lesion. In the upper extremity the CST innervated muscles are the finger extensors, wrist extensors, forearm supinators, external rotators of the shoulder, triceps, and deltoid. The cardinal CST muscles in the lower extremity are the hip flexors, the hamstrings, and the dorsiflexors of the foot and toes. In addition, one of the most important functions of the CST is to provide fine motor control to distal muscles. Fine motor control, including rapid alternating movements, would furthermore be impossible without normal cerebellar function. The screening examination focuses on detecting weakness in the CST distribution and impaired distal fine motor control. In the upper extremity, the best muscles for strength testing are the deltoid, triceps, wrist and finger extensors, and intrinsic hand muscles, especially the interossei. Although commonly done, it is very poor technique to use grip power to assess strength. The finger and wrist flexors are not corticospinal innervated, and are not likely to be weak with a mild corticospinal tract lesion. In addition, grip is a complex function with many different muscles involved, so it is insensitive to peripheral pathology as well. Although strength is the primary focus of the motor examination, it is important to note any changes in muscle bulk, e.g., atrophy, hypertrophy, or pseudohypertrophy; or muscle tone, e.g., rigidity, spasticity, or hypotonia; and to note any abnormal involuntary movements, e.g., tremor, fasciculations, or chorea.

When patients with mild CST lesions retain normal strength, ancillary maneuvers may detect the deficit. The most important of these is the examination for pronator drift. With the patient's upper extremities outstretched to the front, palms up, and with the eyes closed, observe the position of each extremity. Normally, the palms will remain flat, the elbows straight and the limbs horizontal. With a CST lesion, the strong muscles are the pronators, the biceps, and the internal rotators of the shoulder. As these overcome the weakened CST innervated muscles, the hand pronates, the elbow flexes, and the arm drifts downward.

A screening sensory examination assesses sensory function by tasking the nervous system with performing a complex and difficult function. If this function is executed flawlessly, the likelihood of finding clinically significant sensory loss through a more detailed examination is low. Testing for stereognosis and performing double simultaneous stimulation are efficient and sensitive screening tools. The period of time waiting for pronator drift to occur is a convenient time to begin examining upper extremity sensory functions. While the patient is still in "drift position"—arms outstretched in front, palms up, and eyes closed, ask him to indicate which side is touched, then lightly touch first one hand, then the other, then both, using minimal finger pressure, a cotton wisp, or a tissue. A set of stimuli to the lower extremities is also convenient at this point. Continue by testing for stereognosis. Place an object, such as a coin, a key, a safety pin, or a paper clip, into one of the patient's still upturned palms, and ask him to feel and identify it. Stereognosis is the ability to recognize and identify an object by feel; the inability to do so is astereognosis. Stereognosis can only be normal when all the peripheral sensory pathways and the parietal lobe association areas are intact; only when the primary sensory modalities are normal does astereognosis indicate a parietal lobe lesion. A patient with severe carpal tunnel syndrome and numb fingers may not be able to identify a small object by feel; this finding is NOT astereognosis. As a screening test, stereognosis is an excellent modality because it tests the entire sensory pathway, from the fingertips to the parietal lobe. If stereognosis is rapid and accurate, then all the sensory pathways must be functioning normally and detailed examination is not likely to be productive. If a deficit is found on this preliminary assessment, a detailed examination of sensory function is necessary to localize the site of the abnormality. Additional useful information can be gained by dropping the small stereognosis object more or less in the center of the palm. A patient with normal fine motor control will adroitly manipulate the object, move it to the fingertips, rub it between the thumb and opposed fingers, and announce the result. A patient with a mild corticospinal lesion, producing relatively subtle clinical signs without major weakness, may be clumsy in manipulating the object, and will occasionally drop it.

After testing double simultaneous stimulation and stereognosis, with the patient's eyes still closed, the hand and arm position is examined to determine if any drift has occurred. Then, eyes still closed, the patient is instructed to spread the fingers, then touch first one index finger and then the other to the tip of his nose. This is the finger-to-nose (FTN) test, which is used to look for intention tremor, incoordination, and past-pointing. Ordinarily, the FTN test is carried out with the patient's eyes open. For purposes of the screening exam, the more difficult maneuver of eyes closed FTN is performed first. If it is done perfectly, then neither cerebellar nor vestibular disease is likely. Complete the upper extremity examination by examining forearm roll, finger roll, and rapid alternating movements.

After completing examination of motor, sensory, and cerebellar function in the upper extremities, attention is turned to strength assessment of the lower extremities. The important muscles to examine are the CST innervated groups: hip flexors, knee flexors, and the dorsiflexors of the foot. Further sensory testing is convenient at this point, comparing primary modality sensibility on the two sides, comparing proximal to distal in the lower extremities if peripheral neuropathy is a diagnostic consideration, and examining vibratory sensation over the great toes.

Continue by eliciting the biceps, triceps, brachioradialis, knee, and ankle reflexes, then assess the plantar responses. Conclude the examination by checking station and gait. Excellent tests for gait and balance functions are tandem walking with eyes closed and hopping on either foot.

The rest of this book is devoted to the detailed assessment of the functions touched on in the screening examination.

# Mental Status Examination and Higher Cortical Functions

# CHAPTER 5

## The Mental Status Examination

The mental status examination is used to help determine if a patient has neurologic as opposed to psychiatric disease, to identify psychiatric disease which might be related to underlying neurologic disease, and to distinguish focal neurologic deficits from diffuse processes. Abnormalities of mental status could be due to a focal frontal lobe lesion such as a stroke or tumor, to diffuse disease such as metabolic encephalopathy, or to a degenerative process such as Alzheimer disease. Patients might have separate or comorbid psychiatric illness causing neurologic symptomatology, or psychiatric illness related to underlying neurologic disease, such as post stroke depression. The psychiatric mental status examination is longer and more involved than the neurologic mental status examination, as it explores elements of psychiatric function that are not usually included in a neurologic mental evaluation. One possible organization of the psychiatric interview and the elements of the structured mental status examination is shown in Table 5.1. The additional elements of the psychiatric mental status are listed in Table 5.2.

### MENTAL STATUS EXAMINATION

Careful observation of the patient during the history may aid in evaluating his emotional status, memory, intelligence, powers of observation, character, and personality. Observe the general appearance, attitude, and behavior of the patient, including whether he looks tidy, neat, and clean

## TABLE 5.1

**One Possible Organization of the Psychiatric Interview and the Mental Status Examination**

| Interview | Mental Status Examination |
| --- | --- |
| Appearance | Attention and concentration |
| Motoric behavior | Language |
| Mood and affect | Memory |
| Verbal output | Constructions |
| Thought | Calculation skills |
| Perception | Abstraction |
| | Insight and judgment |
| | Praxis |

or slovenly, dirty, and rumpled. Note the patient's manner, speech, and posture, and look for abnormalities of facial expression. There may be odd or unusual dress, gait, and mannerisms; prominent tattoos; excessive jewelry; or other evidence of eccentricity. Unkempt, disheveled patients or those dressed in multiple layers may have dementia, frontal lobe dysfunction, a confusional state, or schizophrenia. Depression, alcoholism, and substance abuse may lead to evidence of self-neglect. Flamboyant dress may suggest mania or hysteria. Patients with visuospatial disturbances or dressing apraxia due to a nondominant parietal lesion may not be able to get into their clothes properly.

The patient may show interest in the interview, understand the situation, and be in touch with the surroundings, or appear anxious, distracted, confused, absorbed, preoccupied, or inattentive. The patient may be engaged, cooperative, helpful, and pleasant or indifferent, irritable, hostile, or belligerent. He may be alert, even hypervigilant, or dull, somnolent, or stuporous. Patients who are disinhibited, aggressive, or overly familiar may have frontal lobe lesions. Patients who are jumpy

## TABLE 5.2

**Elements of the Psychiatric Mental Status Interview**

| | |
| --- | --- |
| Attitude | Cooperative, hostile, evasive, threatening, obsequious, belligerent |
| Affect | Range (expansive, flat); appropriateness; stability (labile, shallow); quality (silly, anxious) |
| Mood | Stated mood in response to question such as How are your spirits, How's your mood been? |
| Behavior | Psychomotor agitation or retardation |
| Speech | Rate (rapid, slow, pressured); volume (loud, soft, monotonous, histrionic); quality (fluent, neologisms, word salad) |
| Thought Process | Disorganized, illogical, loose associations, tangential, circumstantial, flight of ideas, perseveration, incoherent |
| Thought Content | Preoccupations, obsessions, ideas of reference, delusions, thought broadcasting, suicidal or homicidal ideation |
| Perception | Delusions, illusions, hallucinations (auditory, visual, other); spontaneously reported or in response to direct question, patient attending or responding to hallucination |

and hyperalert with autonomic hyperactivity (sweating, tachycardia) may be in drug withdrawal. Abnormal motor activity may include restlessness; repetitive, stereotypical movements; bizarre mannerisms; catatonia; and posturing. Inertia and psychomotor slowing suggest depression, dementia, or parkinsonism. Restlessness, agitation, and hyperactivity may occur with mania or drug ingestion. Note any tendency to emotional lability (pseudobulbar state) or apparent uncon-cern *(la belle indifference)*. The ability to establish rapport with the patient may give insight into the personality of both the patient and the physician. It is sometimes informative to observe patients when they are not aware of being watched.

If there is any suggestion of abnormality from the interaction with the patient during the his-tory taking phase of the encounter, then a more formal mental status examination (MSE) should be carried out. The formal MSE is a more structured process that expands on the information from the history. Detailed MSE should also be carried out if there is any complaint from the patient or family of memory difficulties, cognitive slippage, or a change in character, behavior, personality, or habits. For instance, formerly personable and affable patients who have become irascible and contentious may have early dementia. Other reasons to proceed further include symptoms that are vague and circumstantial, patients with known or suspected psychiatric disease or substance abuse, or when other aspects of the neurologic investigation indicate subtle or covert cognitive impairment could be present, such as anosmia suggesting a frontal lobe tumor.

A number of short screening mental status evaluation instruments have been developed for use at the bedside and in the clinic. The most widely used of these is the Folstein Mini-Mental State exam (MMSE), but there are others, including the Information-Memory-Concentration Test, Orientation-Memory-Concentration Test, Mental Status Questionnaire, Short Portable Mental Status Questionnaire (SPMSQ), Abbreviated Mental Test (AMT), Neurobehavioral Cognitive Status Examination, Short Test of Mental Status, Cambridge Cognitive Examination, and Cognistat (Table 5.3). The MMSE has a series of scored questions that provides a localization based overview of cognitive function, but does not assess any function in detail. The maximum score is 30. Minimum normal performance depends on age and educational level, but has been variously stated as between 24 and 27 (Table 5.4). The MMSE has limitations in both sensitivity and specificity, and should not be used as more than a screening instrument. It is affected not only by age and educa-tion, but by gender and cultural background. With a cutoff score of 24 the test is insensitive and will not detect mild cognitive impairment, especially in well educated or high functioning patients. A normal MMSE score does not reliably exclude dementia. There is also a relatively high false posi-tive rate. A comparison of the MMSE, AMT, and SPMSQ showed sensitivities of 80%, 77%, and 70% and specificities of 98%, 90%, and 89%, respectively. In patients where there is a question of

## TABLE 5.3

### The Short Orientation-Memory-Concentration Test for Cognitive Impairment

Ask the patient to
1. Name the month
2. Name the year
3. State the time of day
4. Remember the following memory phase: "John Brown, 42 Market Street, Chicago"
5. Count backwards 20 to 1
6. Name the months of the year in reverse
7. Recall the memory phrase

See Katzman R, Brown T, Fuld P, et al. Validation of a short orientation-memory-concentration test of cognitive impairment. *Am J Psychiat* 1983;140:734, for expected scores in various age groups.

## TABLE 5.4

**The Mean (Standard Deviation) Mini-Mental State Examination Scores Based on Age and Educational Level**

|  | 55–59 | 60–64 | 65–69 | 70–74 | 75–79 | 80–84 | >85 |
|---|---|---|---|---|---|---|---|
| 9 to 12 years or high school diploma | 28(2.2) | 28(2.2) | 28(2.2) | 27(1.6) | 27(1.5) | 25(2.3) | 26(2.0) |
| College experience or higher degree | 29(1.5) | 29(1.3) | 29(1.0) | 28(1.6) | 28(1.6) | 27(0.9) | 27(1.3) |

Adapted from Crum RM, Anthony JC, Sassett SS, et al. Population-based norms for the mini-mental state examination by age and educational level. *JAMA* 1993; 269:2386–2391.

cognitive impairment or a change in behavior and the MMSE or a similar instrument is normal, formal neuropsychological testing may provide more detail regarding the mental status.

Before making judgments about the patient's mental status, especially memory, the examiner should assure that the patient is alert, cooperative, attentive, and has no language impairment. Mental status cannot be adequately evaluated in a patient who is not alert or is aphasic. To avoid upsetting the patient, it is desirable, when possible, to examine the mental functions unobtrusively by asking questions that gently probe memory, intelligence, and other important functions without appearing to conduct an inquisition.

### Orientation and Attention

The formal mental status examination usually begins with an assessment of orientation. Normally, patients are said to be "oriented times three" if they know who they are, their location, and the date. Some examiners assess insight or the awareness of the situation as a fourth dimension of orientation. The details of orientation are sometimes telling. The patient may know the day of the week, but not the year. Orientation can be explored further when necessary by increasing or decreasing the difficulty level of the questions. Patients may know the season of the year if not the exact month; conversely, they may be oriented well enough to know their exact location down to the street address, hospital floor, and room number. Most patients can estimate the time within half an hour. Orientation questions can be used as a memory test for patients who are disoriented. If the patient is disoriented to time and place, they may be told the day, the month, the year, the city, etc., and implored to try to remember the information. Failure to remember this information by a patient who is attentive and has registered it suggests a severe memory deficit. Occasional patients cannot remember very basic information, such as the year, the city, or the name of the hospital, despite being repeatedly told, for more than a few seconds. In the presence of disease, orientation to time is impaired first, then orientation to place; only rarely is there disorientation to person.

Poor performance on complex tests of higher intellectual function cannot be attributed to cortical dysfunction if the patient is not attentive to the tasks. Defective attention taints all subsequent testing. Patients may appear grossly alert but are actually inattentive, distractable, and unable to concentrate. An early manifestation of toxic or metabolic encephalopathy is often a lack of attention and concentration in an apparently alert patient, which may progress to delirium or a confusional state. Confusion, inattention, and poor concentration may also be seen with frontal lobe dysfunction, posterior nondominant hemisphere lesions, and increased intracranial pressure. Lesions causing apathy or abulia also impair attention. Patients with dementing illnesses are not typically inattentive until the cognitive deficits are severe. The possibility of a CNS toxic or metabolic disturbance should be considered when the patient is inattentive.

Having the patient signal whenever the letter "A" is heard from a string of random letters dictated by the examiner, or having the patient cross out all the A's on a written sheet may reveal a lack of attention or task impersistence. In the line cancellation test, the patient is requested to bisect several lines randomly placed on a page. Inattentive, distractable patients may fail to complete the task. Patients with hemineglect may bisect all the lines off center, or ignore the lines on one side of the page.

Digit span forward is a good test of attention, concentration, and immediate memory. The examiner gives the patient a series of numbers of increasing length, beginning with 3 or 4, at a rate of about one per second, and the patient is asked to repeat them. The numbers should be random, not following any identifiable pattern, e.g., a phone number. Backward digit span, having the patient repeat a series of numbers in reverse order, is a more complex mental process that requires the ability to retain and manipulate the string of numbers. Expected performance is $7 \pm 2$ forward and $5 \pm 1$ backward. Reverse digit span should not be more than two digits fewer than the forward span. Forward digit span is also a test of repetition and may be impaired in aphasic patients. Another test of attention and concentration is a three step task. For instance, tear a piece of paper in half, then tear half of it in half and half in half again, so that there are three different sizes. Give the patient an instruction such as "give the large piece of paper to me, put the small piece on the bed, and you keep the other piece." Another multistep task might be, "stand up, face the door, and hold out your arms."

Attention has an important spatial component, and patients may fail to attend to one side of space (hemi-inattention or hemineglect). The nondominant (usually right) hemisphere has special responsibilities regarding attention. It seems to maintain attention in both right and left hemispace. The dominant hemisphere in contrast only attends to contralateral hemispace. Patients with right parietal lesions often have hemineglect for the left side of space. They may also ignore even a profound neurologic deficit involving the left side of the body (anosognosia). With dominant lesions, the nondominant hemisphere can attend well enough to both sides of space that hemineglect does not occur as a prominent feature. Bilateral lesions may be required to cause neglect of right hemispace. Neglect may also occur with thalamic lesions.

Mental control or concentration is a higher level function that requires the patient not only to attend to a complex task but to marshal other intellectual resources, such as the ability to mentally manipulate items. Tests of mental control include serial 7's or 3's, spelling *world* backwards (part of MMSE), and saying the days of the week or months of the year in reverse. Most normal adults can recite the months of the year backwards in less than 30 seconds. When underlying functions, e.g., calculation ability, are intact, defective mental control may indicate dorsolateral frontal lobe (executive) dysfunction, usually on the left.

## Memory

Memory has many facets and may be tested in different ways. Memory terminology is not used consistently, and a precise description of the task attempted is often more useful than describing the patient's "recent memory." A commonly used memory classification includes immediate (working memory), recent (short-term), and remote (long-term). Digit span is a test of attention and immediate memory, a very short term function in which the material is not actually committed to memory. A patient's fund of information reflects their remote memory. The fund of information includes basic school facts, such as state capitals, famous presidents, and important dates, as well as current information such as the sitting president, vice-president, governor, and similar public officials. The patient should also know personal information, such as their address, phone number, social security number, wedding anniversary date, and names of children. Mothers and grandmothers usually know the ages and birth dates of their children and grandchildren. These items are fertile ground for assessing remote memory and fund of information so long as there is some way to check the accuracy of responses. Judging the expected fund of information for patients with low educational attainment is often difficult, but any normal patient should be fluent with their personal information (except for the phone number, which many do not know, saying "I never call myself"). Asking directions is often useful, and tests both memory and spatial ability. Most patients are able to describe how to drive from their home to the place of the encounter, as well as the general direction and distance to major cities and local towns. Patients who work in very specialized fields and who have few outside interests are challenging to assess. Patients with major cognitive impairment may still recall some deeply ingrained, overlearned memories, e.g., days of the week, months of the year, nursery rhymes, and jingles.

Recent, or short term, memory is tested by giving the patient items to recall. The recall items may be simple objects, such as orange, umbrella, and automobile, or more complex, such as "John Brown, 42 Market St., Chicago." The items should be in different categories. After ensuring the patient has registered the items, proceed with other testing, and after approximately 5 minutes ask the patient to recall the items. Patients with severe memory deficits may not only fail to recall the items, they may fail to recall being asked to recall. Some patients may fail to remember the items, but can improve performance with hints or pick the items from a list. A distinction is made between retention and retrieval. Patients who are able to remember items with cueing or by picking from a list are able to retain the information, but not retrieve it. When cueing or picking do not improve performance, the defect is in retention. Patients with early dementing processes may have only a failure of retrieval. Another memory test is to ask the patient to remember the Babcock sentence ("One thing a nation must have to be rich and great is a large, secure supply of wood.") after 5 minutes. Normal patients can do this in three attempts. Tests of nonverbal memory include hiding objects in the patient's room as they watch, then having them remember where the objects are hidden, or asking them to remember shapes, colors, or figures.

## Calculations

Ability to count and calculate may be evaluated by asking the patient to count forward or backward, to count coins, or to make change. Dyscalculia is characteristic of lesions of the dominant parietal lobe, particularly the angular gyrus. Patients may be asked to select a certain amount from a handful of change presented by the examiner. Calculations may be more formally tested by having the patient perform simple arithmetic, mentally or on paper. The ability to calculate depends on the patient's native intelligence, their innate number sense or mathematical ability, and educational level. Basic calculations, such as $2 + 2$, are often rote, overlearned items from early schooling, and these test remote memory more than calculating ability. The average normal patient can perform mental calculations that involve two digit operations and require simple carrying and borrowing. If successful initially with very simple calculations, the patient should be pressed to at least a moderate level of difficulty, e.g., $12 \times 13$, $17 + 11$, $26 + 14$. Another test is to ask the patient to sequentially double a number until failure. Asking the patient to add or subtract a column of two or three digit numbers on paper further requires them to correctly align and manipulate a column of numbers and gives insight not only into calculating skill, but into their visuospatial ability, which may be particularly impaired with nondominant parietal lesions. Simple mathematical problems may be presented, e.g., if apples are a quarter apiece, how many can you buy for a dollar? how many quarters are in $1.50? if a loaf of bread cost 89 cents and you paid with a dollar, what change would you get back? A commonly used calculation task is subtracting serial 7's from 100 (failing that, serial 3's). This function also requires attention and concentration. Counting to 20 is more of a remote memory test and counting backward from 20 more of an attentional task. There is little difference in calculating ability across age groups, and little impairment in early Alzheimer disease, but advancing disease dramatically alters calculation ability.

Aphasic patients may have difficulty with calculations because they make paraphasic errors involving the numbers. Impaired calculating ability may occur with posterior dominant hemisphere lesions, either as an isolated defect or as part of Gerstmann syndrome. These patients have a true anarithmetria, a primary disturbance of calculating ability.

## Abstract Thinking

The ability to think abstractly is typically tested by asking the patient to describe similarities and differences and to interpret proverbs and aphorisms. The patient may be asked what is alike about an apple and a banana, a car and an airplane, a watch and a ruler, or a poem and a statue; or to tell the difference between a lie and a mistake, between laziness and idleness, or between a cable and a chain. The patient may be unable to interpret a proverb, or may interpret it concretely or literally. For "Don't cry over spilt milk," the patient thinking concretely will talk about accidents, milk, spillage, cleanup, and other things which miss the point. The usefulness of proverb interpretation has been questioned. It seems many examiners are not precisely sure themselves what some of the proverbs mean. Some commonly used proverbs include: a rolling stone gathers no moss, a stitch in time saves nine, Rome wasn't built in a day, and people who live in glass houses shouldn't throw stones. Bizarre, peculiar proverb interpretations may be given by patients with psychiatric disease, or normal people not familiar with the idiomatic usage. It may be useful to throw in a concatenated, mixed, and confused proverb or saying such as "the hand that rocks the cradle shouldn't throw stones," to test both the patient's abstraction ability and sense of humor. Impaired abstraction occurs in many conditions, but is particularly common with frontal lobe disorders.

## Insight and Judgment

Common insight and judgment questions, such as asking the patient what they would do if they found a sealed, addressed, stamped letter on the sidewalk, or smelled smoke in a crowded theater may be less useful than determining if the patient has insight into his illness and the implications of any functional impairment. Historical information from family members about the patient's actual judgment in real life situations may be more enlightening than these artificial constructs. Patients with no concern about their illness have impaired judgment. Patients with poor judgment may behave impulsively or inappropriately during the examination. Many neurologic conditions may impair judgment, particularly processes that affect the orbitofrontal regions. Lack of insight into the illness, to the point of denial of any disability, may occur with nondominant parietal lesions.

## Frontal Lobe Function

Frontal lobe dysfunction may be subtle. The usual methods of bedside testing, including formal neuropsychological assessment, may fail to detect even significant frontal lobe dysfunction. Comparison with the patient's premorbid personality and behavior are often more telling than assessment based on population derived reference information. In addition to the standard tests of abstract thinking and proverb interpretation, special techniques designed to evaluate frontal lobe function may be useful. Tests helpful for evaluating frontal lobe function include verbal fluency by word list generation, assessment of the ability to alternate tasks or switch between tests, abstraction ability, and tests for perseveration, apathy, and impulsivity,

Patients who do not have anomia when tested by other methods may not be able to generate word lists. The Wisconsin Card Sort test is used by neuropsychologists to determine if the patient can shift between tasks (shift sets). The formal test requires the patient to discover through trial and error the expected sorting of cards by color, shape, or number, then to recognize and adapt to a change in the scheme. A bedside variation is to ask the patient to detect a pattern when the examiner switches a coin between hands behind his back, e.g., twice in the right hand, once in the left, then to change the pattern and see if the patient detects the new scheme. Perseveration is the abnormal, inappropriate repetition of words or actions. Patients with frontal lesions, especially those involving the dominant dorsolateral prefrontal cortex, have difficulty abandoning the initial pattern of responses, and tend to perseverate. In trail making tests the patient is required to connect in sequence either letters or numbers scattered around a page (Trails A), or to alternate connecting letters and numbers, e.g., A-1-B-2-C-3 (Trails B). In another test of alternating ability, the patient writes a string of M's and N's, all connected. In Luria's fist-edge-palm test, the patient is asked to repetitively place the hand down in a series of motions: fist, edge of hand, palm, over and over. There is a tendency to perseveration and difficulty accurately executing the sequences of hand positions, particularly with frontal lobe lesions. In copying tasks involving drawing simple figures with multiple loops, patients with perseveration may insert extra loops.

The Stroop test assesses the patient's ability to inhibit automatic responses. In the "little-big" test the words little and big are printed on separate cards in both upper and lower case letters, and the patient required to respond aloud "big" if the print is upper case, even in response to the word "little," or vice versa. A variation is to write several color names in nonmatching colors, e.g., write the word blue with a red marker, then ask the patient to read the cards by stating the color of the print not the written name of the color. Patients with frontal lobe dysfunction have trouble inhibiting the tendency to read the color name. The antisaccade task is another measure of the ability to inhibit automatic responses.

Lhermitte first described "utilization behavior" and "imitation behavior" in patients with frontal lobe damage. Patients with utilization behavior will reach out and use objects in the environment in an automatic manner, and are not able to inhibit this response. Similarly, patients with imitation behavior will imitate the examiner's gestures, even if specifically told to refrain.

## Other Mental Status Tests

Other procedures used to evaluate cognitive function include assessment of visuospatial and constructional ability, praxis, language disturbances, recognition (visual, tactile, and auditory), right-left orientation, and finger identification. These are discussed in subsequent chapters.

# CHAPTER 6

# Disorders of Speech
# and Language

**P**honation, strictly defined, is the production of vocal sounds without word formation; it is entirely a function of the larynx. Howls of rage, the squeals of little girls, and singing a note with the mouth open are phonation. A vocalization is the sound made by the vibration of the vocal folds, modified by workings of the vocal tract. Speech consists of words, articulate vocal sounds that symbolize and communicate ideas. Articulation is the enunciation of words and phrases; it is a function of organs and muscles innervated by the brainstem. Language is a mechanism for expressing thoughts and ideas: by speech (auditory symbols), by writing (graphic symbols), or by gestures and pantomime (motor symbols). Language may be regarded as any means of expressing or communicating feeling or thought using a system of symbols. Grammar (or syntax) is the set of rules for organizing the symbols to enhance their meaning.

Language is a function of the cerebral cortex. Language and speech are uniquely human attributes. Linguistic communication requires not only the motor acts necessary for execution, but also the reception and interpretation of these acts when they are carried out by others, along with the retention, recall, and visualization of the symbols. Speech is as dependent upon the interpretation of the auditory and visual images, and the association of these images with the motor centers that control expression, as upon the motor elements of expression.

In neurologic patients, the speech abnormalities most often encountered are dysarthria and aphasia. The essential difference is that aphasia is a disorder of language and dysarthria is a disorder of the motor production or articulation of speech. The common vernacular phrase "slurred speech," could be due to either. Aphasia usually affects other language functions such as reading and writing. Dysarthria is defective articulation of sounds or words of neurologic origin. In dysarthria, language functions are normal and the patient speaks with proper syntax, but pronunciation is faulty because of a breakdown in performing the coordinated muscular movements necessary for speech production. A good general rule is that no matter how garbled the speech, if the patient is speaking in correct sentences, using grammar and vocabulary commensurate with their dialect and education, they have dysarthria and not aphasia. In dysarthria there are often other accompanying bulbar abnormalities, such as dysphagia, and a brainstem lesion is usually a prominent clinical consideration. Dysarthria is a problem with articulation of speech, aphasia is a problem with language function. The implications of these two conditions are quite different. Disturbed language function is always due to brain disease, but dysfunction limited to the speech mechanisms may occur with many conditions, neurologic and nonneurologic.

## ANATOMY AND PHYSIOLOGY OF ARTICULATION

Sounds are produced by expired air passing through the vocal cords. Properly articulated speech requires coordination between the respiratory muscles and the muscles of the larynx, pharynx, soft palate, tongue, and lips. All these components are referred to as the vocal (oral) tract. Respiratory movements determine the strength and rhythm of the voice. Variations in pitch are produced by alterations in the tension and length of the vocal cords and the rate and character of the vibrations transmitted to the column of air that passes between them. Modifications in sound are produced by changes in the size and shape of the glottis, pharynx, and mouth, and by changes in the position of the tongue, soft palate, and lips. The oropharynx, nasopharynx, and mouth act as resonating chambers and further influence the timbre and character of the voice. Speech may be possible in the absence of vocal cords, and whispered speech may be possible in inspiration as well as expiration. An electrolarynx produces electromechanical vibrations in the oral tract that are then articulated into speech. Whispered sounds are also entirely articulatory.

Articulation is one of the vital bulbar functions. Several cranial nerves are involved in speech production, and an adequate appraisal of speech requires evaluating the function of each. The trigeminal nerves control the muscles of mastication and open and close the mouth. The facial nerves control the muscles of facial expression, especially the branches to the orbicularis oris and other smaller muscles about the mouth that control lip movement. The vagus nerves and glossopharyngeal nerves control the soft palate, pharynx, and larynx, and the hypoglossal nerves control tongue movements. The upper cervical nerves, which communicate with the lower cranial nerves and in part supply the infrahyoid and suprahyoid muscles, the cervical sympathetic nerves that contribute to the pharyngeal plexus, and the phrenic and intercostal nerves also contribute to normal speech.

## TYPES OF SPEECH SOUNDS

Voiced sounds are produced by narrowing the glottis so that the vocal cords are approximated. Voiceless sounds are made with the glottis open. Either type of sound may be modulated by adjusting the size and shape of the vocal cavities. Vowels are largely of laryngeal origin, but are modified by the resonance of the vocal cavities. Certain vowel sounds such as i, a, and y are modified by the soft palate. Consonants may be either voiced or voiceless; they are enunciated by constriction or closure at one or more points along the vocal tract. A fricative is a sound articulated through a not quite closed glottis that creates turbulence in the airflow causing a frictional rustling of the breath, e.g., f, soft s.

Speech sounds may be placed in different categories related to the place of articulation, e.g., labiodental, interdental, alveolar, palatal, alveopalatal, velar, and uvular. From an anatomic and neurologic viewpoint it is more important to recognize how various sounds are produced. Articulated labials (b, p, m, and w) are formed principally by the lips. Modified labials (o and u, and to a lesser extent i, e, and a) are altered by lip contraction. Labiodentals (f and v) are formed by placing the teeth against the lower lip. Linguals are sounds formed with tongue action. T, d, l, r, and n are tongue-point, or alveolar, sounds, formed by touching the tip of the tongue to the upper alveolar ridge. S, z, sh, zh, ch, and j are dentals, or tongue-blade sounds. To hear distorted linguals, place the tip of your tongue against the back of your bottom teeth, hold it there and say "top dog," "go jump," and "train." To hear distorted labials, hold your upper lip between the thumb and forefinger of one hand and your bottom lip similarly with the other and say "my baby." Gutturals (velars, or tongue-back sounds such as k, g, and ng) are articulated between the back of the tongue and the soft palate. Palatals (German ch and g, and the French gn) are formed when the dorsum of the tongue approximates the hard palate.

Normal articulation depends on proper function and neuromuscular control of the vocal tract. Normal development of the tongue, larynx, and soft palate, and adequate hearing are essential to proper pronunciation. The cultural and emotional background of the individual are also important in appraising speech. No two individuals possess the same speech patterns. This is true not only for pitch and timbre, but also for the quality, duration, and intensity of tones and sounds, and for the ability to pronounce certain words and syllables. Normal variations in enunciation and articulation result from regional variations in speech patterns ("accents") evident in the pronunciation of vowels and many of the consonants. Education and training are important factors. The uneducated, illiterate, and mentally deficient may mispronounce letters and syllables despite normal powers of articulation. Some individuals are never able to make certain sounds. Those who learned another language before English may never master the pronunciation of certain English sounds. Adult native English speakers may never be able to accurately pronounce some of the guttural and palatal sounds that are part of some languages.

## EXAMINATION OF ARTICULATION

Examination of articulation begins with noting the patient's spontaneous speech in normal conversation, usually during taking of the history. The accuracy of pronunciation, rate of speech, resonance, and prosody (variations in pitch, rhythm, and stress of pronunciation) are noted. Abnormalities of articulation include tremulousness, stuttering, slurring or sliding of letters or words, scanning, explosiveness, and difficulties with specific sound formations. Some difficult to enunciate phrases have been traditionally used to test articulation. These require the pronunciation of labials, linguals, and, to a lesser extent, velars. The nonsense phrase "puhtuhkuh" or "pataka" tests all three: labials (puh/pa), linguals (tuh/ta), and velars (kuh/ka). Traditional phrases have been selected to test primarily the labials and linguals, such letters as l, r, b, p, t, and d. As the patient repeats these phrases, various aspects of the dysarthria may become more evident. These phrases are time-honored, perhaps above their actual value, and are to a certain extent colloquial. Nonetheless, they are often useful. Pronouncing r's requires a facile tongue, and many of the test phrases are loaded with this letter. The best test words and phrases have the significant consonants and vowels placed in the initial, middle, and final positions. Commonly used words and phrases include: third riding artillery brigade, Methodist Episcopal, West Register Street, liquid electricity, truly rural, voluntary retribution, baby hippopotamus, and irretrievable ball. Phrases such as "my baby ate a cupcake on the train" contain all the pertinent elements.

Have the patient repeat a syllable such as "puh" over and over as rapidly as possible. Normally the syllable can be pronounced accurately at a rate of 5-7 Hz. Similarly for "tuh" and "kuh." Listen for abnormally slow or rapid repetition, regularity and evenness, uniform loudness, or tremulousness.

Weakness and fatigueability of articulation, such as might occur in myasthenia gravis, may be brought out by having the patient count to 100 at about one number per second, enunciating each number clearly. Listen for the voice to become hoarse, hypernasal, slurred, or breathy. Disturbances of laryngeal function and of speech rhythm may be elicited by having the patient attempt prolonged phonation, such as by singing and holding a high "a" or "e" or "ah" sound. Assess loudness, pitch, quality (hoarseness, breathiness), steadiness, nasality, and duration. The voice may break, waver, or flutter excessively, particularly when there is cerebellar dysfunction. Note whether the pitch of the voice is appropriate for the patient's age and sex.

Normal coughing requires normal vocal cord movement. A normal cough indicates that vocal cord innervation is intact. Dysphonia with a normal cough suggests laryngeal disease or a nonorganic speech disturbance. The glottal coup (glottic click, coup de glotte) is the sharp sound at the beginning of a cough. The intensity of the glottic click reflects the power of vocal cord adduction. The glottic click may also be elicited by asking the patient to say "oh-oh," or make a sharp, forceful grunting sound. A cough without a glottal coup (bovine cough) suggests vocal cord palsy.

Resonance is an important voice quality. Normal resonance depends on an adequate seal between the oropharynx and nasopharynx (velopharyngeal competence). When palatal weakness causes an inadequate seal on pronouncing sounds that require high oral pressure, the voice has a "nasal" quality. An audible nasal emission is nasal air escape that causes a snorting sound.

Hypernasality is more noticeable when the head is tipped forward; it is less evident when the patient lies with his head back, because the weakened soft palate falls back by its own weight and closes off the nasopharynx. Velopharyngeal incompetence is common in patients with cleft palate.

## DISORDERS OF ARTICULATION

Lesions of the nervous system may cause various abnormalities of sound production and word formulation (Table 6.1). Laryngeal disorders may alter the volume, quality, or pitch of the voice (dysphonia). Laryngitis causes dysphonia. Aphonia is complete voice loss. A central or peripheral disturbance of the innervation of the articulatory muscles may cause dysarthria. Lesions may involve the peripheral nerves, brainstem nuclei, or the central corticobulbar, extrapyramidal, or cerebellar pathways. Anarthria is a total inability to articulate because of a defect in the control of the peripheral speech musculature.

Lesions of the cerebral centers and connections that subserve language function may cause aphasia, an abnormality of language, even though the articulation mechanisms may be intact. Mutism is a total inability to speak; usually the patient appears to make no attempt to speak or make sounds. Mutism is usually of psychogenic origin if present in an apparently otherwise normal patient, but may occur with lesions of the cerebrum, brainstem, and cerebellum (especially in children).

## TABLE 6.1

**Differential Diagnosis of Abnormal Speech in the Absence of Obvious Oral Abnormality**

Speech abnormal
    Language functions (syntax, naming, comprehension, etc.) abnormal → aphasia
    Language functions normal
        Voice volume, pitch, timbre abnormal
            Dysphonia
                High-pitched, strained, choking → adductor spasmodic dysphonia
                Hoarse, whispery, mute
                    Cough abnormal → vocal cord palsy
                    Cough normal
                        Abductor spasmodic dysphonia
                        Local laryngeal disease
                        Nonorganic dysphonia
      Voice volume and pitch normal
        Speech rhythm, prosody abnormal
            Speech slurred, drunken sounding → cerebellar dysfunction v. intoxication
            Speech flat, monotonous, without normal inflection or emotionality
            → Extrapyramidal dysfunction v. right frontal lobe lesion
        Speech rhythm, prosody normal
            Speech hypernasal
                Palatal weakness
            Abnormal labials (puh, papa, mama, baby hippopotamus)
                Facial weakness
            Abnormal linguals (tuh, daddy, darn it)
                Anterior tongue weakness
             Abnormal velars (kuh, cupcake, coke)
                Palatal or posterior tongue weakness

Abnormalities of articulation may be caused by many different pathologic conditions. Disturbances in the respiratory rhythm interfere with speech, and respiratory muscle weakness causes a feeble voice with abnormalities in regularity and rhythm. Laryngeal disease may cause severe speech impairment, but whispered speech may still be possible. In children, articulation disturbances may be developmental and are often temporary. Structural abnormalities of the vocal tract, such as congenital craniofacial defects (cleft palate, cleft lip), ankyloglossia (abnormal shortness of the frenulum of the tongue; "tongue-tie"), adenoidal hypertrophy, vocal cord edema or nodules, nasal obstruction, or perforated nasal septum may cause abnormalities in sound production. The importance of the teeth in articulation is apparent in the speech of edentulous patients.

Neurologic disturbances of articulation may be caused by primary muscle diseases affecting the tongue, larynx, and pharynx; neuromuscular junction disorders; lower motor neuron disease involving either the cranial nerve nuclei or the peripheral nerves that supply the muscles of articulation; cerebellar dysfunction, basal ganglia disease, or disturbances of the upper motor neuron control of vocalization. Lesions of the hypoglossal nerve or nucleus, or local disorders of the tongue such as ankyloglossia, may cause impairment of all enunciation, but with special difficulty pronouncing lingual sounds. The speech is lisping in character and is clumsy and indistinct. Paralysis of the laryngeal musculature causes hoarseness, and the patient may not be able to speak above a whisper; there is particular difficulty pronouncing vowels. Similar changes occur in laryngitis and in tumors of the larynx. With unilateral laryngeal muscle weakness, such as in recurrent laryngeal nerve lesions, the voice is usually low-pitched and hoarse, but occasionally severe unilateral vocal cord weakness may be present without much effect on speech because the normal vocal cord is able to adduct across the midline and approximate the abnormal cord. Hoarseness due to slight vocal cord weakness may be brought out by having the patient talk with the head turned to one side. With paralysis of the cricothyroid, the voice is hoarse and deep and fatigues quickly. In bilateral abductor paralysis, speech is moderately affected, but in bilateral total paralysis it is lost.

Paralysis limited to the pharynx causes little detectable impairment of articulation. Weakness of the soft palate results in nasal speech, caused by inability to seal off the nasal from the oral cavity. Voice sounds have an added abnormal resonance. There is special difficulty with the velar sounds, but labials and linguals are also affected, as much of the air necessary for their production escapes through the nose. The speech resembles that of a patient with a cleft palate. Characteristically, b becomes m, d becomes n, and k becomes ng. Amyotrophic lateral sclerosis and myasthenia gravis are common causes of this type of speech difficulty.

Seventh nerve paralysis causes difficulty in pronouncing labials and labiodentals. Dysarthria is noticeable only in peripheral facial palsy; the facial weakness in the central type of facial palsy is usually too mild to interfere with articulation. Bell palsy occasionally causes marked dysarthria because of inability to close the mouth, purse the lips, and distend the cheeks. Similar articulatory defects are found in myopathies involving the labial muscles (e.g., facioscapulohumeral or oculopharyngeal dystrophy), in cleft lip, and with wounds of the lips. There is little impairment of articulation in trigeminal nerve lesions unless the involvement is bilateral; in such cases there are usually other characteristics of bulbar speech. Trismus may affect speech because the patient is unable to open the mouth normally.

Lower motor neuron disorders causing difficulty in articulation may occur in cranial neuropathies. Lesions of the ninth and eleventh nerves usually do not affect articulation. A unilateral lesion of CN X causes hypernasality. Lesions involving the vagus bilaterally distal to the origin of the superior laryngeal nerve may leave the vocal cords paralyzed in adduction, resulting in a weak voice with stridor. With more proximal lesions, there is no stridor but the voice and cough are weak.

Neuromuscular disorders, particularly neuromuscular junction disorders, often interfere with speech. In myasthenia gravis (MG), prolonged speaking, such as counting, may cause progressive weakness of the voice with a decrease in volume and at times the development of a bulbar or nasal quality, which may even proceed to anarthria. As the voice fatigues, the speech of a patient with bulbar myasthenia may be reduced to an incoherent whisper. An occasional myasthenic patient must hold the jaw closed with the hand in order to enunciate.

In progressive bulbar palsy, dysarthria results from weakness of the tongue, pharynx, larynx, soft palate, and, to a lesser extent, the facial muscles, lips, and muscles of mastication. Both articulation and phonation may be affected; speech is slow and hesitant with failure of correct enunciation, and all sounds and syllables may be indistinct. The patient talks as though his mouth were full of mashed potatoes. Supranuclear lesions involving the corticobulbar pathways may also cause dysarthria. Unilateral cortical lesions do not usually affect speech unless they are in the dominant hemisphere and cause aphasia. Occasionally some dysarthria accompanies aphasia. Rarely, lesions in the cortical motor areas for articulation may cause severe dysarthria without aphasia. Both dysarthria and dysprosody, or a defect in rhythm, melody, and pitch, have been described with localized frontal lobe lesions; these may be due to an apraxia of speech.

Bilateral supranuclear lesions involving the cortex, corona radiata, internal capsule, cerebral peduncles, pons, or upper medulla may cause pseudobulbar palsy with spastic dysarthria. The muscles which govern articulation are both weak and spastic. Phonation is typically strained-strangled, and articulation and diadochokinesis are slow.

Lesions of the basal ganglia may affect speech. Athetotic grimaces of the face and tongue may interfere with speech. Irregular spasmodic contractions of the diaphragm and other respiratory muscles, together with spasms of the tongue and pharynx, may give the speech a curious jerky and groaning character. In addition, there may be a pseudobulbar element with slurred, indistinct, spastic speech. When chorea is present, the violent movements of the face, tongue, and respiratory muscles may make the speech jerky, irregular, and hesitant. The patient may be unable to maintain phonation and occasionally there is loss of the ability to speak.

Speech in parkinsonism is often mumbled, hesitant, rapid, and soft (hypophonic). There may sometimes be bradylalia, with feeble, slow, slurred speech because of muscular rigidity and immobility of the lips and tongue. There is dysprosody and the speech lacks inflections, accents, and modulation. The patient speaks in a monotone, and the words are slurred and run into one another. The voice becomes increasingly weak as the patient talks, and he may become unable to speak above a whisper; as the speech becomes more indistinct it may become inaudible or practically disappear. Words may be chopped off. There may be sudden blocks and hesitations, or speech may stop abruptly. There may be pathologic repetition of syllables, words, or phrases (palilalia). Like the parkinsonian gait, the speech may show festination, with a tendency to hurry toward the end of sentences or long words.

Voice tremor produces rhythmic alterations in loudness and pitch. There may be associated tremor of the extremities or head, or other signs of neurologic dysfunction. Voice tremor may further complicate the other speech disturbances of parkinsonism. Voice tremor occurs commonly in essential tremor, a frequently familial syndrome which most often affects the hands. Fine voice tremors are characteristic of essential tremor; coarse tremors are more commensurate with cerebellar disease. Voice tremor is a common manifestation of anxiety. Lip and chin tremors, when severe, may interfere with speech. In habit spasms, Tourette syndrome, and obsessive-compulsive states, there may be articulatory tics causing grunts, groans, or barking sounds. In Tourette syndrome, palilalia may also occur.

Cerebellar dysfunction causes a defect of articulatory coordination (scanning speech, ataxic dysarthria, or speech asynergy). There is a lack of smooth coordination of the tongue, lips, pharynx, and diaphragm. Ataxic speech is slow, slurred, irregular, labored, and jerky. Words are pronounced with irregular force and speed, with involuntary variations in loudness and pitch lending an explosive quality. There are unintentional pauses causing words and syllables to be erratically broken, with excessive separation of syllables and skipped sounds in words producing a disconnected, disjointed, faltering, staccato articulation (scanning speech). The speech pattern is reminiscent of a person who is sobbing or breathing hard from exertion. The unusual spacing of sounds with perceptible pauses between words and irregular accenting of syllables may cause a jerky, sing-song cadence that resembles the reading of poetry. Ataxic speech is particularly characteristic of multiple sclerosis. It may be accompanied by grimaces and irregular respirations. Ataxia of the voice and scanning speech may be more apparent when the patient repeats a fairly long sentence.

Spasmodic dysphonia is a focal dystonia characterized by a striking abnormality of voice production. In adductor dysphonia, irregular involuntary spasms of the vocal muscles causes erratic adduction of the cords. As the patient strains to speak through the narrowed vocal tract, the voice takes on a high pitched, choked quality that varies markedly during the course of a sentence. It is most marked in stressed vowels.

Secondary speech disturbances may also occur without abnormalities or specific dysfunction of the articulatory apparatus, as seen in individuals with hearing defects, delayed physical development, mental retardation, and psychogenic disturbances.

## NONORGANIC SPEECH DISORDERS

Emotional and psychogenic factors influence articulation. Speech, but not language, disorders may occur on a nonorganic basis. Nonorganic voice disorders can take many different forms and can be caused by a variety of factors. The most common nonorganic voice disorders are dysphonia and aphonia. Onset is often abrupt, perhaps in association with emotional trauma; there may be periods of remission, and the condition may suddenly disappear. The speech defect may vary in type from time to time. It is often bizarre, and does not correspond to any organic pattern. The patient may fail to articulate and speak only by whispering. Speech may be lost but the patient is able to sing, whistle, and cough. There may be associated dysphagia and globus hystericus. In anxiety and agitation the speech may be broken, tremulous, high-pitched, uneven, and breathless. Stuttering and stammering are common.

## APHASIA

When focal brain disease affects primary cortex, the resulting deficit reflects the area involved, e.g., hemiparesis with conditions affecting the posterior frontal lobe, or visual field defects with conditions affecting the occipital lobe. When disease affects association cortex or areas of the brain which subserve high level integrative function, a variety of abnormalities of "higher cortical function" may result. Aphasia refers to a disorder of language, including various combinations of impairment in the ability to spontaneously produce, understand, and repeat speech, as well as defects in the ability to read and write. A deficit affecting only speech is usually dysarthria, due to cerebellar disease or weakness or spasticity of the speech producing musculature.

A simple definition of aphasia is a disorder of previously intact language abilities due to brain damage. A more comprehensive definition considers it a defect in (dysphasia) or loss of (aphasia) the power of expression by speech, writing, or gestures or a defect in or loss of the ability to comprehend spoken or written language or to interpret gestures, due to brain damage. Aphasia implies that the language disorder is not due to paralysis or disability of the organs of speech or of muscles governing other forms of expression. The term dysphasia is not helpful and easily confused with dysphagia, and has fallen into disuse.

There are three cortical levels involved in language comprehension. The first is the level of "arrival," a function of the primary cortical reception areas; at this level language symbols are perceived, seen, or heard, without further differentiation of the impulses. The second level is that of "knowing," or gnostic function, concerned with the recognition of impulses, formulation of engrams for recall of stimuli, and revisualization. The third level, the one of greatest importance in aphasia, has to do with recognition of symbols in the form of words, or the higher elaboration and association of learned symbols as a function of language. There are also three levels of motor speech function. In aphasia, the most elementary of these is least frequently affected, and the most complex most often involved. Most primitive is the emotional level; the patient may respond to a painful stimulus with an "ouch," even though other language functions are entirely absent. Emotional language may be preserved when all other language functions are lost. Next is the automatic level, that concerned with casual, automatic speech; the patient may be able to answer questions with words such as "yes" and "no," count, or recite the days of the week, even though other elements of speech are severely impaired. The highest level is propositional, volitional, symbolic, or intellectualized language, which is most easily disrupted and most difficult to repair. Language requires the use of symbols (sounds, marks, gestures) for communication. Propositional language is the communication of thoughts, ideas, feelings, and judgments using words, syntax, semantics, and rules of conversation. A normal individual is able to understand complex sentences and make statements that require thought and concentration.

## ANATOMY OF THE LANGUAGE CENTERS

The language centers are located in the perisylvian areas of the language dominant hemisphere (Fig. 6.1). The language areas form a C shaped mass of tissue around the lips of the Sylvian fissure extending from Broca area to Wernicke area. The central sulcus intersects the Sylvian fissure near its posterior ramus. The posterior inferior frontal (PIF) language areas lie in front of the central sulcus in the frontal lobe and are referred to as anterior or prerolandic. The posterior superior temporal (PST) areas lie posterior to the central sulcus and are referred to as posterior or postrolandic. The anterior speech areas subserve the motor, or expressive, aspects and the posterior areas the sensory, or perceptive, aspects of language. Broca speech area lies in the inferior frontal gyrus. It is essentially the motor association cortex, the executive area for language function, that lies just anterior to the primary motor areas for the lips, tongue, and face. The region of the left precentral gyrus of the insula, a cortical area beneath the frontal and temporal lobes, seems to be important in the motor planning of speech. Wernicke speech area lies in the superior temporal gyrus. It is essentially the sensory association cortex that lies just posterior to the primary auditory cortex. The arcuate fasciculus is a deep white matter tract that arches from Wernicke area around the posterior end of the Sylvian fissure and through the subcortical white matter of the insula to Broca area. Other tracts in the subcortical white matter of the insula provide additional connections between the PIF and PST areas. The angular gyrus is part of the inferior parietal lobule; it caps the posterior ramus of the Sylvian fissure and lies between Wernicke area and the visual cortex. The angular gyrus is important for reading

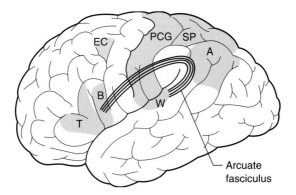

*FIGURE 6.1* ● Centers important in language. A, Angular gyrus; B, Broca area; EC, Exner writing center; SP, Superior parietal lobule, which with the PCG (postcentral gyrus) is important in tactile recognition; T, Pars triangularis; W, Wernicke area.

and similar nonverbal language functions. The supramarginal gyrus also lies between the visual cortex and the posterior perisylvian language areas and is involved with visual language functions.

## EXAMINATION OF THE PATIENT WITH APHASIA

Initial appraisal of language function takes place during the taking of the history. Obvious deficits require exploration, but there may be language deficits that are not readily apparent during history taking, such as the inability to repeat that is the essential characteristic of conduction aphasia, so some degree of formal assessment is usually prudent. In evaluating aphasia it is important to know about the patient's handedness (and sometimes the familial tendencies toward handedness), cultural background, native language and other languages spoken, vocabulary, educational level, intellectual capacity, and vocation.

About 90% to 95% of the population is right handed. The left cerebral hemisphere is dominant for language in 99% of right handers, and 60% to 70% of left handers. Of the remaining left handers, about half are right hemisphere dominant and about half have mixed dominance. Since clinical abnormalities of higher cortical function, especially language, are heavily influenced by dominance, determination of the patient's handedness and dominance status is paramount. Cerebral dominance and handedness are at least in part hereditary. In right handed patients, aphasia will be due to a left hemisphere lesion in 99% of the cases; the other 1% are "crossed aphasics." In left handers the situation is much more variable.

There are six separate components of language function that are typically tested in the clinical arena: spontaneous (conversational) speech, auditory comprehension, naming, reading, writing, and the ability to repeat. It is often useful to assess these components individually before trying to synthesize the findings into a diagnostic entity.

### Spontaneous Speech

In addition to high level propositional speech, spontaneous utterances may include the lower level functions of emotional and automatic speech. Emotional speech is spontaneous speech prompted by a high emotional charge. Some patients with aphasia, primarily non-fluent aphasia, even when severe, may swear and curse eloquently when angry, often to the shock and surprise of friends and family. Automatic speech refers to the recitation of simple overlearned items from early childhood, or to a specific retained speech fragment which an aphasic patient is still capable of saying even in the presence of severe non-fluency. Even when unable to produce propositional speech, an aphasic patient may be able to automatically count, say the days of the week or months of the year, repeat the alphabet, say his name, or recite nursery rhymes. Some aphasic patients are able to sing simple overlearned songs, such as Happy Birthday, even when they are unable to speak. A retained fragment that an aphasic patient repeats over and over has been referred to as a monophasia (recurring utterance, verbal stereotypy, verbal automatism, verbigeration). In monophasia, the individual's vocabulary is limited to a single word, phrase, or sentence, such as "do-do-do" or "Oh, God." Verbal automatisms occur most often in global aphasia. The recurrent utterance may be a real word or a neologism. Sometimes the monophasia is an outrageous expletive that bursts from an otherwise dignified and respectable patient under socially awkward circumstances.

A paraphasia is a speech error in which the patient substitutes a wrong word or sound for the intended word or sound. Paraphasic errors are common in aphasic patients. In a phonemic (phonologic, literal) paraphasia, there is the addition, deletion, or substitution of a phoneme but the word is recognizable and may be clearly pronounced. Substitution of the wrong phoneme would cause the patient to say "blotch" instead of watch, or "thumbness" instead of numbness. Technically, a literal paraphasia is a single letter substitution. Phonemic paraphasia is the preferable term since a single letter substitution also changes the phoneme and the brain thinks in phonemes, not letters. Illiterate patients commit phonemic paraphasias despite their ignorance of letters. In a semantic (verbal) paraphasia, the patient substitutes the wrong word. A semantic paraphasia would cause the patient to say "ring" instead of watch. Paraphasias are similar to the malapropisms, spoonerisms, and sniglets everyone occasionally utters, but aphasic patients make them more often and may not recognize them as wrong. A neologism is a novel utterance, a non-word made up on the spot. The patient might call a watch a "woshap." Phonemic paraphasias are more typical of anterior, and semantic paraphasias more typical of posterior, perisylvian lesions.

In evaluating propositional speech, note pronunciation, word and sentence formation, fluency, cadence, rhythm, prosody, omission or transposition of syllables or words, misuse of words, circumlocutions, repetition, perseveration, paraphasias, jargon, and the use of neologisms. Aphasic patients may use unusual synonyms or circumlocutions in order to avoid the use of a word that cannot be recalled. There may be omissions of words, hesitations and inappropriate pauses, perseveration, difficulty understanding the implication of words, verbal automatisms, agrammatism, jargon or gibberish. When the patient is having difficulty with fluency, it is difficult to evaluate propositional spontaneous speech. Fluency refers to the volume of speech output. Normal speech is 100 to 115 words per minute. Speech output is often as low as 10 to 15 words per minute, sometimes less, in patients with nonfluent aphasia. If the maximum sentence length is <7 words, the patient is nonfluent. Patients are usually aware of nonfluency and frustrated by it. Their speech may tend toward the laconic, answering questions but trying to speak no more than necessary. Patience and open ended questions are the best approaches in persuading the patient to converse. Patients unable to express themselves through speech may use pantomime or gesture, shaking or nodding the head, shrugging the shoulders, or demonstrating visible emotional reactions. In severe aphasia the patient may be unable to utter a single word.

## COMPREHENSION

The patient's responses to verbal requests and commands and to everyday questions and comments give information about his ability to understand speech. Comprehension may be tested by having the patient follow verbal commands ("show me your teeth," "stick out your tongue," "close your eyes," or "point to the ceiling"). Comprehension can be judged reasonably intact if the patient follows a complicated, multi-step command, but failure to follow a command, even a simple one, does not necessarily prove that comprehension is impaired. A patient may not comply because of apraxia. A patient with a left hemisphere lesion may even have apraxia for functions of their non-paretic left hand. They may be unable to salute, wave goodbye, or perform other simple functions on command using the left hand because of involvement of fibers that transmit information from the language areas on the left to the motor areas on the right (sympathetic apraxia). When the patient does not follow simple commands, establish whether he can say or shake his head "yes" and "no." Then ask ridiculous, simple questions, such as "are you from the planet Jupiter," "did you have nails for breakfast," "are you riding in a taxicab," or "are you a man (or a woman)." The answers to the ridiculously simple questions should be known. The responses may be nonverbal. An elderly woman who laughs when asked "are you pregnant" has understood the question. More complex yes-no questions might include "is a mother older than her daughter," "do you have dinner before breakfast," "can you fly in a car," "did the sun come up this morning," or "do you have feet on the ends of your legs." Since the chance of a correct response is 50%, it is important to ask enough questions to exclude lucky answers. The patient may have more difficulty with polysyllabic words and long sentences than with simple words and short sentences. Compound sentences and double or complex commands may be used to see if comprehension is more than superficial. The aphasia examination begins to overlap with the mental status examination with commands such as "place one coin on the table, give me the second, and keep the third in your hand" or "here is a piece of paper; tear it in four parts and place one on the table, give one to me, and keep two for yourself." Both comprehension and retention are evaluated by telling a short story and then asking questions about it. Patients with impaired comprehension have particular difficulty with passive constructions ("the lion was killed by the tiger, which animal is dead?" or "the boy was slapped by the girl, who got hit?") and possessives (is my wife's brother a man or a woman?).

Patients who are unable to comprehend spoken or written language may understand pantomime, gestures, and symbols. They may imitate the examiner in placing a finger to the nose or putting out the tongue. Imitation, however, is a lower level function than comprehension.

Many aphasic patients have difficulty with right-left orientation, especially with posterior lesions. Right-left confusion is part of Gerstmann syndrome. Testing right-left orientation might include such commands as "show me your right thumb" or "touch your right ear with your left thumb." It is important to determine baseline function before concluding a patient has right-left confusion.

## NAMING

Testing naming ability is an important part of the aphasia examination. Naming is a delicate function, and most aphasic patients have some difficulty with it. However, naming defects are nonspecific. In anomic aphasia, an inability to name is an isolated defect, but more often misnaming occurs as part of some other aphasic, or even non-aphasic, syndrome. In confrontation naming, the patient is asked to name simple objects such as a key, pencil, coin, watch, parts of the body (nose, ear, chin, fingernail, knuckle), or to name colors. When lost for the name of an object, the patient may describe it or tell its use. The patient may be able to name an object, such as a watch, but be unable to identify the component parts, such as the band or buckle. Some caution is necessary, as there are age, cultural, and even gender influences at work. When unable to retrieve a name, an aphasic patient may be able to select the correct name from a list. Another naming test is to have the patient point to something named by the examiner, e.g., the telephone, the window.

A sensitive method of testing spontaneous naming ability is word list generation. The patient is asked to name as many items as possible in a certain category in one minute. Animals are a common category for testing spontaneous naming. The patient may name any type of animals (farm, zoo, etc.), but groups should not be suggested ahead of time since there may be an inability to shift groups. It is wise to check more than one item category; other useful categories include tools, foods, countries, and modes of transportation. Spontaneous naming ability also depends on age and educational level. Normal patients should name a minimum of 12 items in a category; some adjustment may be necessary for poorly educated and older patients. Another measure of spontaneous naming is to ask the patient to list all the words they can think of that begin with a certain letter. The "F-A-S" test is popular. The patient thinks of words beginning with one of these letters, excluding proper nouns or morphological variants. For FAS, a person of average education should produce 12 or more words per letter in 1 minute, or 36 words with all three letters in three minutes. Standardization and reference values for testing naming are imperfect. Language competence depends on education, dialect, experience, and other factors. Often the reference population does not include less well educated people, nor every dialect. Poor word list generation may also occur with dementia, depression, parkinsonism, and prefrontal lesions. Responsive naming is also useful, and uses audition rather than vision. The patient may be asked for nouns ("where do teachers work"), verbs ("what do you do with a cup") or adjectives ("how does sugar taste").

## REPETITION

The ability to repeat may be selectively involved or paradoxically preserved in certain aphasic syndromes. Most often the inability to repeat is proportional to the defect in comprehension or fluency, and repetition is a good screening test for aphasia. The patient is asked to repeat words or phrases back to the examiner. A patient's repetition span, the number of words he can repeat, is usually two more than his digit span. Simple repetition tasks might include counting, avoiding numbers that might be repeated by automatic speech, or single words. More complex tasks include polysyllabic words, such as "catastrophe," phrases, such as "if he were here, I would go away," or tongue twisters such as "Popocatepetl" (po-poh-cah-teh-petl, a volcano in Mexico). The stock phrases used to test for dysarthria work for this purpose as well. A popular phrase for testing repetition in aphasia is "no ifs, ands, or buts." Omitting the s's may not be an error in some dialects of English. A better repetition test is "they heard him speak on the radio last night" (modified from the Boston Diagnostic Aphasia Examination). Patients with impaired repetition may omit words, change the word order, or commit paraphasic errors. Repetition is preserved in anomic, transcortical, and some cases of subcortical aphasia.

## WRITING

The patient's ability to use written language should also be assessed. It may be disturbed in conjunction with abnormalities of spoken language, or separately. Patients who are aphasic in speech are also aphasic in writing, but writing may be preserved in patients with dysarthria or verbal apraxia. In all aphasias, reading and writing are typically worse than understanding and speaking, probably because they are secondarily acquired skills. The patient may be asked to write spontaneously or to dictation. A spontaneous writing sample might include a few words, a sentence, or a paragraph. The writing sample usually reveals the same sorts of naming difficulties and paraphasias evident in the patient's speech. Patients may be able to write elementary, overlearned things such as name, address, days of the week, and months of the year, but unable to write more complex material. There may be a difference in the patient's ability to print and to write in cursive.

## READING

The patient's ability to comprehend written language symbols can be tested by having him read. Written language is perceived by the visual system and the information conveyed to the perisylvian language centers. Dysfunction of the language centers or interruption of the connections with the visual system may cause an inability to read (alexia). Reading difficulty due to acquired alexia is unrelated to the developmental (congenital) dyslexia seen most often in school-age boys that may cause severe reading disability. Patients may have alexia without any accompanying inability to comprehend speech—the syndrome of pure word blindness. Alexia may occur with or without a hemianopia. Alexia may occur with or without accompanying agraphia. Most patients with alexia also have difficulty with writing (alexia with agraphia). Some patients have alexia without agraphia, a disconnection syndrome. Judging reading ability by having the patient follow a written command such as "close your eyes" involves a praxis element and should be interpreted with caution. For patients unable to read aloud, use questions that can be answered by "yes" or "no," or by gestures. It is also important to determine whether the patient is able to read his own writing. Reading aloud is a different task from reading comprehension, and may be preserved despite impaired reading comprehension.

## CLASSIFICATION OF THE APHASIAS

Classification of the aphasias is problematic. These disorders vary in severity, even with a lesion in the same location, and are frequently mixed in type. There have been many attempts at classification from anatomic, physiologic, and psychological points of view. None is entirely satisfactory. A strictly anatomic classification does not apply in all instances, for a small lesion may cause severe impairment of both fluency and comprehension, while an extensive lesion sometimes causes an isolated defect. Lesions similar in size and location on imaging studies may be associated with different aphasic syndromes even in persons with identical cerebral dominance for speech, and lesions in different locations and of variable size may produce similar aphasic syndromes. Nevertheless, some general relationships exist between anatomic sites and the type of aphasia.

One common classification divides aphasias into expressive and receptive types. In expressive aphasia, the patient has difficulty with speech output and struggles to talk (nonfluent); in receptive aphasia the primary difficulty is with understanding language, while speech output is unaffected (fluent). A major problem with the expressive-receptive classification of aphasia is that all aphasic patients have difficulty expressing themselves. This causes difficulty, particularly for trainees and non-neurologists. There is a tendency to classify almost all aphasias as expressive,

## TABLE 6.2

**The Major Aphasia Syndromes**

| | Aphasia Classification | | | | | |
|---|---|---|---|---|---|---|
| | Relative Severities | | | | | |
| | Fluency | Auditory Comprehension | Repetition | Naming | Reading | Writing |
| Broca | − | + | − | − | − | − |
| Global | − | − | − | − | − | − |
| Wernicke | + | − | − | − | − | − |
| Conduction | + | + | − | +/− | + | + |
| Anomic | + | + | + | − | + | − |
| Transcortical, mixed | − | − | + | − | − | − |
| Transcortical, motor | − | + | + | − | − | − |
| Transcortical, sensory | + | − | + | − | − | − |
| Verbal apraxia | − | + | − | − | − | + |

+, function is relatively intact. −, function is abnormal. +/−, involvement is mild or impairment equivocal.
Modified from Campbell WW, Pridgeon RP. *Practical Primer of Clinical Neurology.* Philadelphia: Lippincott Williams & Wilkins, 2002.

even when they are flagrantly receptive. It requires some clinical experience to recognize that a patient may be having difficulty expressing himself linguistically because of a defect in the reception (comprehension) of spoken language.

The Broca-Wernicke-Lichtheim model was further described and popularized by Benson, Geschwind, and others at the Boston Aphasia Research Center. It divides aphasias into fluent and nonfluent varieties (Tables 6.2 and 6.3). If speech output is high and articulation facile, the aphasia is referred to as fluent; if speech output is sparse and effortful the aphasia is classified as nonfluent. Nonfluency occurs when a lesion involves the anterior speech areas in the region of Broca area in the frontal lobe. When these areas are relatively spared fluency is preserved. Broca is a type of nonfluent aphasia. When the posterior speech areas in the region of Wernicke area in the temporal lobe are involved, auditory comprehension is impaired. When this area is spared, comprehension is relatively preserved. The most common fluent aphasia is Wernicke. In global or total aphasia there is both nonfluency and impaired comprehension; the lesion may involve both anterior and posterior speech areas. Other types of aphasia include conduction, anomic, and transcortical. Difficulty arises because not all patients can be satisfactorily placed into one of these categories. The clinical features of aphasia evolve over time. For example, global aphasia can occur with a purely anterior lesion, but usually evolves into a Broca. If seen acutely, about 60% to 80% of aphasic patients fit into the anterior-nonfluent/posterior-fluent classification.

### Broca Aphasia (Nonfluent, Expressive, Motor, Anterior, Prerolandic, Executive)

Broca aphasia is a nonfluent type of aphasia due to a lesion involving the anterior perisylvian speech areas in the PIF region (Fig. 6.2). Patients have nonfluent spontaneous speech with a

## TABLE 6.3

**Organization of Common Aphasia Syndromes (According to Whether Spontaneous Speech Is Fluent or Nonfluent and Whether Auditory Comprehension and Repetition Are Good or Poor)**

Nonfluent
  Good comprehension
    Good repetition                  Transcortical motor
    Poor repetition
      Aphasic writing             Broca
      Writing intact              Verbal apraxia
  Poor comprehension
    Good repetition                  Mixed transcortical
    Poor repetition                  Global
Fluent
  Good comprehension
    Good repetition                  Anomic
    Poor repetition                  Conduction
  Poor comprehension
    Good repetition                  Transcortical sensory
    Poor repetition
      Poor reading
      comprehension            Wernicke
      Intact reading
      comprehension            Pure word deafness

decreased amount of linguistic output: few words, short sentences, and poor grammar. Any degree of nonfluency is possible, as long as fluency is impaired compared to comprehension. In severe Broca aphasia the speech consists of nouns and substantive verbs produced with great effort. Patients are aware of and frustrated by their difficulty speaking. There is a tendency to leave out nonessential words such as adjectives, adverbs, and functor words (articles, pronouns, conjunctions,

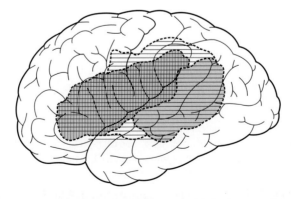

**FIGURE 6.2** ● The extent of the lesion classically causing global aphasia is indicated by the dashed outer line, the lesion causing Broca aphasia by the crosshatched lines, and the lesion causing Wernicke aphasia by the horizontal lined area.

and prepositions that serve primarily to provide sentence structure rather than convey meaning). Such parsimonious use of language is sometimes referred to as telegraphic speech. The patient knows what he wishes to say, but is unable to say it, or to say it correctly. The ability to comprehend speech is relatively unimpaired. Because of the severe nonfluency, patients are unable to repeat what they hear and unable to read aloud. The patient can identify objects but not name them. Although the patient is nonfluent for propositional speech, there may be preservation of emotional and automatic speech, and the patient may be able to sing. Occasionally speech is reduced to monophasia or recurrent utterances. The patient is aphasic in writing as in speech, even when using the non-paretic, usually left, hand. Preservation of writing suggests verbal apraxia (see below). Patients with Broca aphasia classically have a contralateral hemiparesis or faciobrachial paresis, but no visual field deficit.

Occasionally, lesions affect areas of the brain that control speech but not language. The patient may have difficulty with speech, but comprehension is perfect and writing is not affected. Emotional and automatic speech functions are preserved. The problem is essentially an isolated apraxia for speech, which may or may not be accompanied by other evidence of buccofacial apraxia. The lesion is these cases may be confined to Broca area, while in the more typical case of Broca aphasia the lesion is usually more extensive. This condition has been called apraxia of speech (AOS; verbal apraxia, cortical dysarthria, acquired apraxia of speech, Broca area aphasia, mini-Broca, or baby-Broca). Patients with AOS appear to have forgotten how to make the sounds of speech. There is speech sound distortion as their articulatory muscles grope for the right position. There is defective control but no weakness of the vocal tract. Prosody may be impaired and speech may have a stuttering quality. The speech pattern may change so that the patient sounds as though he has developed a foreign accent.

### Wernicke Aphasia (Fluent, Receptive, Sensory, Posterior, Postrolandic)

Wernicke aphasia is due to a lesion in the PST region which involves the auditory association cortex and the angular and supramarginal gyri (Fig. 6.2). Patients are unable to understand speech (word deafness). They are relatively fluent, with a normal or even increased word output (logorrhea), but there is loss of the ability to comprehend the significance of spoken words or recall their meaning. Speech production is effortless; phrase and sentence length and prosody are normal. Although speech is abundant, it is devoid of meaningful content. The patient can still hear and can recognize voices, but not the words they utter. Paraphasic errors are frequent, resulting in incorrect or unintelligible words, unconventional and gibberish sounds, and senseless combinations. The speech abounds in neologisms. There is an inability to use proper syntax, so that sentence structure is defective (paragrammatism). The resultant misuse of words and defective syntax is termed agrammatism. There may be circumlocution and an excess of small filler words. Speech may be fluent but the patient cannot understand his own speech; he is not aware of, and does not correct, his errors in speaking. The frequent paraphasias and neologisms, combined with agrammatism, along with the high word output, may lead to completely unintelligible speech, termed jargon aphasia or word salad. Hughlings-Jackson described this type of aphasia as "plentiful words wrongly used." Naming and repetition deficits arise from poor comprehension. Patients with Wernicke aphasia often have a visual field deficit but no hemiparesis. When due to vascular disease, the ischemia is usually in the distribution of the inferior division of the MCA.

### Global (Total, Expressive-Receptive, Complete) Aphasia

In global aphasia, a large lesion has destroyed the entire perisylvian language center or separate lesions have destroyed both the PIF and PST regions (Fig. 6.2). Grossly nonfluent speech is combined with a severe comprehension deficit and inability to name or repeat. Typically there is both a hemiplegia and a visual field cut. Global aphasia is usually due to internal carotid or proximal MCA occlusion. In some patients, comprehension improves, leaving a deficit resembling Broca aphasia.

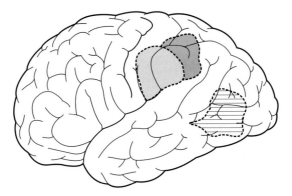

**FIGURE 6.3** ● The lesion classically causing conduction aphasia is indicated by the lightly shaded area, the lesion causing anomic aphasia by horizontal lines, and the lesion causing the angular gyrus syndrome by the darkly shaded area.

## Conduction (Associative, Commissural, Central, Deep) Aphasia

Conduction aphasia is due to a lesion that interrupts the conduction of impulses between Wernicke and Broca areas. The characteristic deficit is poor repetition with preservation of other language functions. The patient is fluent and comprehension is unaffected; naming is variable. The lesion most often lies in the deep white matter in the region of the supramarginal gyrus and involves the arcuate fasciculus and other fiber tracts that run from the posterior to the anterior language areas (Fig. 6.3). The etiology is most often an embolic occlusion of a terminal branch of the MCA. Because it disconnects the anterior from the posterior perisylvian language areas, conduction aphasia represents one of the disconnection syndromes.

## Anomic (Amnesic, Amnestic, Nominal) Aphasia

In anomic aphasia, there is a deficit in naming ability with preservation of other language functions. The patients are fluent, have good comprehension, and are able to repeat. Anomic aphasia is the most common but least specific type of aphasia. Anomia occurs with every type of aphasia. Patients with any aphasia type as it develops or recovers may pass through a stage in which anomia is the primary finding, and it may be the most persistent deficit. Only when anomia occurs as an isolated deficit throughout the course of the illness is the designation anomic aphasia appropriate. When anomic aphasia is accompanied by all four elements of Gerstmann syndrome, the lesion virtually always lies in the dominant angular gyrus (Fig. 6.3).

## Transcortical Aphasia

The transcortical aphasias are syndromes in which the perisylvian language area is preserved but disconnected from the rest of the brain (Fig. 6.4). The usual etiology is a watershed (border zone) infarction. Because the PIF and PST areas and the connecting arcuate fasciculus are intact, the patients are aphasic but have a paradoxical preservation of the ability to repeat. Repetition can be so well preserved that the patients display echolalia, repeating everything they hear. When the condition is severe and the entire perisylvian language complex is separated from the rest of the brain, the patients are not fluent in spontaneous speech and are unable to comprehend. This syndrome has been termed isolation of the speech area, or mixed transcortical aphasia. When the lesion is primarily anterior the syndrome resembles Broca aphasia with nonfluency in spontaneous speech but intact comprehension. Repetition is better then spontaneous speech. This is the syndrome of transcortical motor aphasia (anterior isolation syndrome). The supplementary motor area and dorsolateral

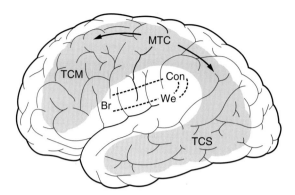

**FIGURE 6.4** ● Areas typically involved in transcortical aphasias; these correspond to the watershed zones between major arterial distributions. Br, Broca; We, Wernicke; Con, conduction; TCM, transcortical motor; TCS, transcortical sensory; MTC, mixed transcortical. (From Benson DF, Geschwind N. The aphasias and related disturbances. In: Joynt RJ, ed. *Clinical Neurology*. Philadelphia: J.B. Lippincott, 1990;1–34.)

prefrontal cortex, which are responsible for the planning and initiation of speech, are isolated from the PIF region. In transcortical sensory aphasia (posterior isolation syndrome) there is greater involvement of the posterior language areas. The PST region is isolated from the surrounding parietal, occipital, and temporal cortex that store word associations. The patients are fluent, but have difficulty with comprehension; repetition is better than spontaneous speech. The transcortical aphasias are more common than is often appreciated.

### Subcortical Aphasia

Subcortical aphasia refers to language disorders that arise not from damage to the perisylvian language areas, but from lesions, usually vascular, involving the thalamus, caudate, putamen, or internal capsule of the language dominant hemisphere. The speech disorder is difficult to categorize in the Broca-Wernicke scheme and may most reasonably be a transcortical aphasia.

## NONDOMINANT HEMISPHERE LANGUAGE DISTURBANCES

How much language function resides in the nondominant hemisphere remains a matter of debate. Non-right-handers, particularly, are thought to have some speech function in the nondominant hemisphere. Some of the recovery from aphasia and the persistence of emotional and automatic speech suggest some language function may be present in the minor hemisphere. Lesions of the nondominant hemisphere cause speech disturbances that affect the nonlinguistic elements of language. There is loss or impairment of the rhythm and emotional elements of language. Prosody refers to the melodic aspects of speech; the modulation of pitch, volume, intonation, and inflection that conveys nuances of meaning and emotional content. Hyperprosody is exaggeration, hypoprosody a decrease, and aprosody an absence of the prosodic component of speech. Dysprosody, typically hypoprosody or aprosody, may occur with right hemisphere lesions. Patients lose the ability to convey emotion in speech or to detect the emotion expressed by others.

## ALEXIA AND AGRAPHIA

A lesion of the primary visual cortex causes loss of visual perception. With a lesion involving the visual association cortex, visual perception is intact but there may be impairment of the ability to recognize and interpret visual stimuli. The region of the angular gyrus and the adjacent cortex in the dominant hemisphere (Fig. 6.1) is important for the recognition and interpretation of symbols in the form of letters and words. Connections between the visual cortex and the dominant angular gyrus are vital for visual recognition of language symbols. Geschwind said the angular gyrus, "turns written language into spoken language and vice versa." Loss of the ability to read in the absence of actual loss of vision is alexia (word blindness). A lesion of the angular gyrus, or its connections to the visual cortex, causes alexia. There is loss of the ability to recognize, interpret, and recall the meaning of visual language symbols. Printed words have no meaning, although the patient may talk without difficulty and understand what is said to him.

Loss of the ability to write not due to weakness, incoordination, or other neurologic dysfunction of the arm or hand is called agraphia. Milder involvement may be referred to as dysgraphia. There are three types of agraphia: aphasic, constructional, and apractic. Agraphia is seen in all types of aphasia except pure word blindness and pure word mutism. Although agraphia typically accompanies aphasia, it may occur as an isolated finding and as part of other syndromes in which the patient is not aphasic. Agraphia without alexia is a feature of Gerstmann syndrome. Agraphia may be manifested as contraction of words, omission of letters or syllables, transposition of words, or mirror writing. Having the patient write spontaneously will usually bring out all the errors present in speech as well as spelling and letter formation errors. Patients with constructional apraxia may also have difficulty writing. The visuospatial deficit interferes with the proper alignment and orientation of the text. Apractic agraphia is due to inability to properly use the writing hand in the absence of other deficits.

# CHAPTER 7

# Agnosia, Apraxia, and Related Disorders of Higher Cortical Function

Gnosia (Gr. *gnosis*, knowledge) refers to the higher synthesis of sensory impulses, with resulting perception, appreciation, and recognition of stimuli. Agnosia refers to the loss or impairment of the ability to know or recognize the meaning or import of a sensory stimulus, even though it has been perceived. Agnosia occurs in the absence of any impairment of cognition, attention, or alertness. The patients are not aphasic and do not have word finding or a generalized naming impairment. Hughlings-Jackson saw agnosia as a non-language form of aphasia. Agnosias are usually specific for a given sensory modality and can occur with any type of sensory stimulus. Agnosias that involve the primary sensory modalities may represent disconnection syndromes that disrupt communication between a specific cortical sensory area and the language areas, causing a restricted anomia. Tactile agnosia refers to the inability to recognize stimuli by feel, visual agnosia the inability to recognize visually, and auditory (acoustic) agnosia the inability to know or recognize by audition. Body-image agnosia (autotopagnosia) is loss or impairment of the ability to name and recognize body parts. Finger agnosia is a type of autotopagnosia involving the fingers. Auditory agnosia is the loss of recognition of sounds; phonagnosia is the loss of recognition of familiar voices. Time agnosia refers to loss of time sense without disorientation in other spheres. Visuospatial agnosia is loss or impairment in the ability to judge direction, distance, and motion and to understand three dimensional spatial relationships. Because of the impaired spatial judgment and visual disorientation, the patient cannot find his way in familiar surroundings. Multimodal agnosias may occur with dysfunction of the association areas in the parietal and temporal lobes that assimilate sensory information from more than one domain.

Astereognosis (stereoanesthesia) is loss of the ability to recognize and identify an object by touch despite intact primary sensory modalities. There is no loss of perceptual ability. The patient can feel the object, sensing its dimensions, texture, and other relevant information. However, he is unable to synthesize this information and correlate it with past experience and stored information about similar objects in order to recognize and identify it. Stereognosis is tested by asking the patient to identify, with eyes closed, common objects placed into their hand (coin, key, button, safety pin, paper clip). The most convincing deficit is when the patient is able to identify with the other hand an object they were unable to identify with the tested hand. When primary sensory modalities in the hand are impaired, as by radiculopathy or neuropathy, failure to identify an object by touch is not astereognosis. Astereognosis usually indicates a lesion involving the contralateral parietal lobe. Rarely, a lesion of either parietal lobe can produce astereognosis bilaterally. It has also been reported to occur with lesions involving the anterior corpus callosum and the thalamic radiations. If there is hand weakness, the examiner may hold and move the object between the patient's fingers. It is striking to see a patient with a paralyzed hand from a pure motor capsular stroke demonstrate exquisitely intact stereognosis when tested in this fashion. In tactile agnosia, the patient is unable to identify the object with either hand, but can identify it visually. Graphesthesia is a similar function. It is tested by writing numbers on the patient's palm or fingertips. The inability to recognize the numbers is referred to as agraphesthesia; in the presence of intact primary sensory modalities, it usually indicates a lesion involving the contralateral parietal lobe.

Finger agnosia refers to the loss or impairment of the ability to recognize, name, or select individual fingers of the patient's own hands or the hands of the examiner. The patient loses the ability to name individual fingers, point to fingers named by the examiner, or move named fingers on request, in the absence of any other naming deficit. Testing for finger agnosia may be conveniently combined with assessment of right-left orientation. The simplest test of right-left orientation is to ask the patient to raise a specific hand. More challenging is to have the patient touch a body part on one side, e.g., the right ear, with a specific digit of the other side, e.g., the left thumb. Even more strenuous is when the examiner faces the patient, crosses his forearms with hands and fingers extended, and requests the patient to touch one of the examiner's fingers on a specific side, e.g, the left index. A very challenging test is to ask the patient to touch a specific finger as the examiner faces away from the patient with forearms crossed behind his back, using a confusing syntax, e.g., "with your left hand touch my right index finger." Finger agnosia and right-left confusion, along with agraphia and acalculia, make up Gerstmann syndrome. Finger agnosia alone is not highly localizing, but when all components of the syndrome are present the lesion is likely to lie in the region of the dominant angular gyrus.

In the visual agnosias, there is loss or impairment of the ability to recognize things visually, despite intact vision (psychic blindness or mindblindness). Areas 18 and 19 are particularly important for visual gnostic functions. Visual agnosia is not a sensory defect but a problem in recognition. There is impairment in the higher visual association processes necessary for recognition and naming, not explicable by any deficit in visual perception. Patients can see but cannot make sense of the visual world. Teuber said visual agnosia was a "percept stripped of its meaning." Oliver Sacks provided an entertaining and informative description of the clinical picture of visual agnosia in *The Man Who Mistook His Wife For a Hat* (Touchstone Books, 1985).

Some occipital lobe lesions, particularly of the primary visual cortex, cause color blindness (central achromatopsia). Lesions of the association areas may cause color agnosia. In color agnosia, the patient cannot name or identify colors, although he is not color blind and can discern the numbers on color plates. Patients may not be able to remember the color of common things, e.g., the sky. In prosopagnosia (face or facial agnosia, face blindness), there is an inability to recognize familiar faces. The patient may not be able to identify people by looking at their faces, even close family members, but may immediately identify the person by the sound of their voice. The patient may recognize a face as a face but cannot associate it with a particular individual. They learn to identify people using other cues. In extreme examples, the patient is unable to recognize himself in a mirror or photograph. Patients with prosopagnosia, and other visual agnosias, usually have bilateral lesions of the occipitotemporal area involving the lingual, fusiform, and parahippocampal gyri. Prosopagnosia can occur with unilateral right posterior hemispheric lesions.

Apraxia (Gr. *praxis,* action) is the inability to carry out on request a high-level, familiar, purposeful motor act in the absence of any weakness, sensory loss, or other deficit involving the affected part. The patient must have intact comprehension and be cooperative and attentive to the task. Another definition of apraxia is the inability to perform an act on command that the patient is able to perform spontaneously. There are many varieties of apraxia. The ones seen most often are ideomotor, buccofacial, constructional, and dressing apraxia. Some of the other apraxias include apraxia of eyelid opening, eyelid closure, gaze, and gait.

The simplest form is limb kinetic apraxia. This category probably should not exist. These patients have difficulty with fine motor control. They typically have very mild lesions involving the corticospinal tract that are not severe enough to cause detectable weakness, but are severe enough to impair coordination and dexterity. Limb kinetic apraxia is due to dysfunction of the primary motor pathways. In other forms of apraxia the primary motor and sensory cortical areas are intact.

In ideomotor (motor) apraxia, the patient is unable to perform a complex command (salute, wave goodbye, snap the fingers, make a fist, show how to hitchhike) with the involved extremity, sometimes with either extremity. The patient may be unable to pantomime how to use common implements (hammer, toothbrush, comb) or how to kick or throw a ball. They may substitute a hand or finger for the imagined object, e.g., raking the fingers through the hair instead of showing how to use a comb, snapping fingers together as the blades when asked to show how to use scissors. The patient may be unable to carry out the act on command but be able to imitate it. Rarely, the patient may be unable to carry out an act on command or imitation, such as showing how to use a comb, but be able to use the actual object. In ideomotor apraxia, there may be a disconnection between the language or visual centers that understand the command and the motor areas tasked with carrying it out. Patients may have apraxia for whole body movements. They are unable to, on command, do such things as stand up, take a bow, or stand like a boxer.

Sympathetic apraxia is the inability of a patient to perform a complex motor act with the nonparetic limb in the presence of a unilateral dominant hemisphere lesion. For instance, a patient with a left hemisphere lesion causing Broca aphasia may be unable to show how to wave goodbye using the left hand. This is because the fibers connecting the language areas of the left hemisphere with the motor areas of the right hemisphere are disrupted. The patient understands the request, has no weakness of the left hand, but is unable to execute because the right hemisphere never receives the command.

In ideational (conceptual) apraxia, the patient is able to carry out individual components of a complex motor act, but cannot perform the entire sequence properly. Patients may perform each step correctly, but in attempting the sequence they omit steps or get the steps out of order. Ideational apraxia seems to be an impairment in conceptualizing the overall goal of the activity sequence or an inability to plan the series of steps. For instance, in showing how to drive a car, the patient might try to put the car in drive before starting the engine. When asked to demonstrate how to mail a letter, the patient may seal the envelope before inserting the letter, or mail the letter before affixing the stamp. Ideational apraxia may occur with damage to the left posterior temporoparietal junction or in patients with generalized cognitive impairment.

In buccofacial apraxia, patients are unable to execute on request complex acts involving the lips, mouth, and face, such as whistling, coughing, pursing the lips, sticking out the tongue, or blowing a kiss or pantomime blowing out a match or sniffing a flower. There is no weakness of the mouth, lips, or face, but the patient is unable to make the requested movement. The patient may spontaneously lick his lips, but is unable to do so on command. Apraxia of such midline functions is common in patients with lesions involving either hemisphere. Failure to execute such acts should not necessarily be construed as evidence of impaired comprehension in aphasic patients.

Other common types of apraxia include dressing and constructional. Constructional or dressing apraxia may occur with parietal lobe lesions which interfere with the patient's ability to comprehend spatial relationships. In constructional apraxia, the patient is unable to copy geometric forms of any complexity because of impaired visuospatial skills. They may be able to draw a square but not a three dimensional cube. They may be able to draw individual shapes, but cannot synthesize them into a more complex geometric figure, e.g., a square with a triangle perched on its upper right corner and a circle attached to the lower right corner, all touching. The patient may also be asked to draw actual things, such as a three dimensional house with a roof and chimney, a clock, or a daisy. Patients with hemineglect may fail to put petals on one side of the daisy. A test

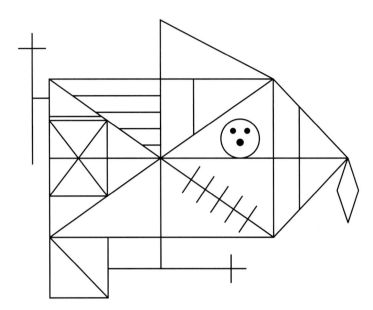

*FIGURE 7.1* ●     The Rey-Osterrieth Complex Figure for evaluating constructional ability.

for both praxis and cognition is to have the patient draw a clock face, insert the numbers, and draw the hands at a specific time, e.g., 3:10, or "10 minutes past 3)." Patients with hemineglect may fail to put the numbers on one side of the clock. Patients with frontal lobe dysfunction or a confusional state may have a disorganized and confused approach to the task, making multiple errors. A patient with cognitive impairment may forget the proper arrangement of numbers or how to indicate a specific time. Some patients cannot interpret 3:10 and will put one hand on the 10 and the other on the 3, indicating 2:50 or 10:15. The Rey-Osterrieth figure is very complex and can bring out subtle constructional apraxia (Fig. 7.1). Constructional tasks are particularly useful for differentiating psychiatric from neurologic disease. Impaired constructional ability is a sensitive indicator of lesions involving various parts of the brain, but in patients with psychiatric disease constructional ability is preserved.

In dressing apraxia, the patient loses the ability to don clothing correctly. There is loss of the ability to manipulate the clothing in space and to understand its three dimensional relationships. Patients with hemineglect may fail to dress one side of the body. A useful test for dressing apraxia is to turn one sleeve of the hospital gown or robe inside out, then have the patient try to put it on. Patients with dressing apraxia are often baffled. Dressing apraxia can be particularly disabling, as the patient struggles for a long period of time each morning simply to get dressed. Constructional apraxia would be very disabling for a patient who was an artist or craftsman.

## DISCONNECTION SYNDROMES

Disconnection syndromes are disorders in which the fiber tracts that interconnect primary cortical areas are disrupted, with preservation of the cortical areas of origin. Neurologic dysfunction occurs not because of destruction of cortex but because of defects in intrahemispheric or interhemispheric communication. Some of the disconnection syndromes include alexia without agraphia, ideomotor apraxia, sympathetic apraxia, pure word deafness, conduction aphasia, and the transcortical aphasias. The modality specific agnosias may be disconnection syndromes in which the primary sensory area for a given modality is disconnected from the language and memory areas of the brain that are responsible for recognition and naming. Disconnection syndromes may result from any process that disrupts subcortical white matter, including infarction, hemorrhage, neoplasm, and trauma.

## ATTENTIONAL DEFICITS

In addition to the generalized defects in attention seen in patients with altered mental status and other diffuse cerebral disturbances, there may be selective defects of attention in patients with focal cerebral lesions. These are seen primarily in right handed patients with right (non-dominant) hemisphere lesions, especially those that involve the inferior parietal lobule. A variety of terms have been used to describe the phenomenon: extinction, neglect, hemi-neglect, hemi-inattention, denial, spatial inattention. Hemi-attention may be modality specific. The mildest manifestation of a right parietal lesion is extinction of the contralateral stimulus with double simultaneous stimulation on visual field or somatosensory testing. Although primary sensory modalities are intact, when touched simultaneously on both sides the patient fails to appreciate the stimulus on the involved side or fails to see the stimulus in the involved visual hemifield. Patients with multimodal hemineglect may extinguish all types of contralesional stimuli, and may completely ignore the left side of space. On the line bisection test they fail to see the left half of the line. They bisect the right half, drawing their vertical tick about one-quarter of the way down the line from the right. If lines are drawn all over the page, the patient may fail to bisect any of the lines on the left. When presented with a complex drawing, such as the cookie theft picture, they may describe what is taking place on the right side of the picture, but fail to notice the cookie theft happening on the left. In motor neglect (hemiakinesia), all of the patient's motor activities are directed to one side of space.

Babinski introduced the cumbersome term anosognosia to refer to a patient's lack of awareness of their neurologic deficit. It occurs particularly in patients with non-dominant parietal lesions. It is not uncommon to see patients with a right parietal infarction on imaging studies but no clinical history of the event, in part due to this lack of recognition of deficits involving the left side of the body. Occasional patients with severe left hemiplegia may deny there is anything wrong with the involved limbs. Even when the examiner dangles the patient's paralyzed left hand before his face and asks if there is anything wrong with this hand, the patient may deny it. The most severe form of anosognosia is when the patient denies owning the hand (asomatognosia). Occasional patients become belligerent in denying that the hand dangling before them is theirs. They commonly say the hand belongs to the examiner. Patients with anosognosia may refuse to remain in the bed with this "other person."

Patients with persistent anosognosia typically have large right hemisphere strokes causing severe left hemisensory loss and left spatial neglect. Anosognosia for the hemiplegia may result from impaired proprioceptive mechanisms that leave the patient unaware of the position and movement of the affected limbs. Anosognosia for hemiplegia has also been reported with pontine lesions. Patients may deny or neglect other neurologic deficits as well, particularly loss of vision due to bilateral occipital lobe lesions (cortical blindness, Anton syndrome).

# The Cranial Nerves

# CHAPTER 8

# The Olfactory Nerve

The olfactory nerve is a sensory nerve with but one function, smell. Only volatile substances soluble in lipids or water are perceived as odors. In true anosmia there is loss of ability to perceive or recognize not only scents but also flavors, for much of what is interpreted as taste involves smell. Flavor is a synthesis of sensations derived from the olfactory nerves, taste buds, and other sensory end-organs. A patient with olfactory impairment may complain of loss of taste rather than of smell. Patients with unilateral anosmia may be unaware of any impairment. Olfaction is a phylogenetically ancient sensation. In lower mammals where olfaction is extremely important, the olfactory cortex constitutes a large part of the cerebral hemispheres. In higher primates and man, the area of the uncus and anterior hippocampal gyrus is likely the primary olfactory cortex. The connections between the olfactory system, hypothalamus, certain brainstem nuclei, and autonomic centers is pertinent to the understanding of many visceral functions. Olfaction is the only sensation not directly processed in the thalamus.

Important historical points to address in a patient with a smell or taste disturbance include past head injury; smoking; recent upper-respiratory infection; systemic illness; nutrition; and exposure to toxins, medications, or illicit drugs. Changes in the flavor of coffee may be particularly informative. Unilateral loss of smell is more significant than bilateral, which may be caused by many conditions, primarily conductive (Table 8.1). Impairments due to anosmia are not trivial. The problem is not merely that patients with disturbances of smell sensation miss out on some of life's pleasures; they may also miss olfactory danger signals, such as spoiled food, smoke, and leaking gas. As with hearing, olfactory deficits are sometimes divided into (a) conductive deficits, due to processes interfering with the ability of odorants to contact the olfactory epithelium, such as nasal

## TABLE 8.1

**Some Causes of Persistent Loss of Smell**

| | |
|---|---|
| Olfactory groove meningioma | Smoking |
| Frontal lobe tumor, especially glioma | Chronic rhinitis |
| Sellar/parasellar tumor | Deviated nasal septum |
| Neuro-olfactory tumor (esthesioneuroblastoma) | Nasal polyps |
| Korsakoff syndrome | Intranasal tumors (e.g., epidermoid carcinoma) |
| Vitamin deficiency ($B_6$, $B_{12}$, A) | Postviral |
| Zinc or copper deficiency | General anesthesia |
| Craniocerebral trauma, including surgery | Dental trauma |
| Alzheimer disease | Chemical burns of the olfactory epithelium |
| Parkinson disease | Normal aging |
| Multiple sclerosis | Pregnancy |
| Congenital anosmia | Meningitis |
| Arhinencephaly | Chemotherapeutic agents |
| Olfactory dysgenesis | Cadmium toxicity |
| Kallmann syndrome (hereditary hypogonadism with anosmia) | Antihistamines |
| | Propylthiouracil |
| Dysautonornia | Antibiotics |
| Refsum syndrome | Levodopa |
| Psychiatric conditions (depression, conversion disorder, schizophrenia) | Cocaine |
| | Amphetamines |
| Chronic sinus disease | Radiation therapy |

polyps; and (b) sensorineural or neurogenic deficits, due to dysfunction of the receptors or their central connections.

Before evaluating smell, ensure that the nasal passages are open. Most cases of impaired smell are due to intranasal obstructions. Acute or chronic rhinitis and chronic sinusitis may seriously interfere with olfaction. Smell is tested using nonirritating stimuli. Avoid substances such as ammonia that may stimulate the trigeminal nerve instead of the olfactory nerve, causing a response that can be confused with olfaction. The nasal passages are richly innervated by free nerve endings from the trigeminal system, which respond to many substances. Some patients with impaired taste and smell enjoy spicy food because of its stimulation of the trigeminal system.

Examine each nostril separately while occluding the other. With the patient's eyes closed and one nostril occluded, bring the test substance near the open one. Ask the patient to sniff and indicate whether she smells something and, if so, to identify it. Repeat for the other nostril and compare the two sides. The side that might be abnormal should be examined first. Many substances can be used to test smell (e.g., wintergreen, cloves, coffee, and cinnamon). At the bedside or in the clinic one can use mouthwash, toothpaste, alcohol, soap, and similar substances. Commercial scratch-and-sniff strips are available.

The perception of odor is more important than accurate identification. Perceiving the presence of an odor indicates continuity of the olfactory pathways; identification of the odor indicates intact cortical function as well. Since there is bilateral innervation, a lesion central to the decussation of the olfactory pathways never causes loss of smell, and a lesion of the olfactory cortex does not produce anosmia. The appreciation of the presence of a smell, even without recognition, excludes anosmia.

## DISORDERS OF OLFACTORY FUNCTION

Loss of smell may occur in a variety of conditions (Table 8.1). It may be congenital or acquired. The top four causes of anosmia are upper-respiratory tract infection (URI), trauma, nasal and sinus disease, and idiopathic. Persistent olfactory loss following a URI is the most common etiology, accounting for 15% to 25% of cases. Some definitions regarding disorders of smell are reviewed in Table 8.2.

Few instances of disturbed smell are of neurologic origin. Lesions involving the orbital surface of the brain may cause unilateral anosmia. Meningiomas of the sphenoidal ridge or olfactory groove and gliomas of the frontal lobe may damage the olfactory bulbs or tracts. A typical clinical picture with sphenoidal ridge meningioma consists of unilateral optic atrophy or papilledema and exophthalmos, and ipsilateral anosmia. In meningiomas of the olfactory groove or cribriform plate area, unilateral anosmia occurs early, progressing to bilateral anosmia, often accompanied by optic neuropathy. Anosmia may also occur with other frontal lobe tumors, and with parasellar and pituitary lesions.

The Foster Kennedy syndrome consists of anosmia accompanied by unilateral ipsilateral optic atrophy and contralateral papilledema, classically due to a large tumor involving the orbitofrontal region, such as an olfactory groove meningioma. The anosmia and optic atrophy are due to direct compression; the contralateral papilledema occurs late when intracranial pressure increases. The atrophic optic disc cannot swell and the unusual picture of optic atrophy in one eye and papilledema in the fellow eye develops. This ophthalmologic picture, without the anosmia, is more often due to anterior optic nerve ischemia, sometimes termed the pseudo-Foster Kennedy syndrome. A mass causing asymmetric compression of both optic nerves may cause a similar picture.

Chronic intranasal cocaine use may cause anosmia. Rarely, toxins such as cadmium or toluene may cause anosmia, usually accompanied by other neurologic abnormalities. Disturbances of taste and smell may result from deficiency of vitamin $B_{12}$, $B_6$, or A, and from the effects of some drugs. Decreased sense of smell has been often attributed to abnormalities in zinc metabolism. Anosmia may accompany some degenerative dementias, especially Alzheimer disease.

Craniocerebral trauma may result in damage to the olfactory nerves at the cribriform plate due to coup or contrecoup forces. Anosmia complicates 5% to 20% of major head injuries, sometimes in isolation and sometimes with other sequellae such as diabetes insipidus and cerebrospinal fluid (CSF) rhinorrhea. The incidence of anosmia may be as high as 80% in patients with CSF rhinorrhea.

## TABLE 8.2

### Terms and Definitions Related to Olfactory Abnormalities

| | |
|---|---|
| Anosmia | No sense of smell |
| Hyposmia | A decrease in the sense of smell |
| Hyperosmia | An overly acute sense of smell |
| Dysosmia | Impairment or defect in the sense of smell |
| Parosmia | Perversion or distortion of smell |
| Phantosmia | Perception of an odor that is not real |
| Presbyosmia | Decrease in the sense of smell due to aging |
| Cacosmia | Inappropriately disagreeable odors |
| Coprosmia | Cacosmia with a fecal scent |
| Olfactory agnosia | Inability to identify or interpret detected odors |

Disorders of smell other than hyposmia or anosmia occasionally occur. Hyperosmia is usually functional, but it can occur with certain types of substance abuse and in migraine. Parosmia and cacosmia are often due to psychiatric disease but occasionally follow head trauma and may accompany conductive dysosmia. Olfactory hallucinations are most often due to psychosis, but they can result from a lesion of the central olfactory system, usually neoplastic or vascular, or as a manifestation of seizure. So-called uncinate fits are complex partial or temporal lobe seizures preceded by an olfactory or gustatory aura, usually disagreeable, and often accompanied, as the patient loses awareness, by smacking of the lips or chewing movements. Such attacks are typically due to a seizure focus involving medial temporal lobe structures. There is never objective loss of smell interictally.

# CHAPTER 9

# The Optic Nerve

Optic nerve function is tested by examining the various modalities of vision: the visual acuity, the visual fields (VFs), and special components of vision, such as color vision and day and night vision. The optic nerve is the one cranial nerve that can be visualized directly, and no neurologic, or indeed general, physical examination is complete without an ophthalmoscopic inspection of the optic disc and the retina.

Ideally, the eyes are examined individually. When testing acuity and color vision it is important to occlude the eye not being tested. Before performing the optic nerve examination, look for local ocular abnormalities such as cataract, conjunctival irritation, corneal scarring or opacity, iritis, foreign bodies, photophobia, arcus senilis, glaucoma, or an ocular prosthesis. The presence of a unilateral arcus corneae with ipsilateral carotid disease has been reported. In Wilson disease (hepatolenticular degeneration) a yellowish-orange brown coloration 1 mm to 3 mm wide (Kayser-Fleischer ring) may be seen around the rim of the cornea, more easily in light-eyed individuals. It is due to copper deposition in the posterior stroma and in Descemet's membrane. It is best seen with a slit lamp. Cataracts may be present in patients with myotonic dystrophy, certain rare hereditary conditions with disturbed lipid or amino acid metabolism, and in many other conditions.

## VISUAL ACUITY

Visual acuity charts, such as the Snellen chart, consist of letters, numbers, or figures that get progressively smaller, and can be read at distances from 10 ft to 200 ft by normal individuals (Figure 9.1). The difference between near and distance vision and between vision with and without correction are points of primarily ophthalmological interest. For neurologic purposes, only the patient's best-corrected visual acuity is pertinent. Refractive errors, media opacities, and similar optometric problems are irrelevant. Acuity is always measured using the patient's accustomed correction.

For distance vision measurement in the United States, a Snellen chart is placed 20 ft from the patient; at that distance there is relaxation of accommodation, and the light rays are nearly parallel. The eyes are tested separately. In countries using the metric system, the distance is usually given as 6 m. The ability to resolve test characters (optotypes) approximately 1-in high at 20 ft is normal (20/20 or 6/6) visual acuity. These characters subtend 5 minutes of visual arc at the eye; the components of the characters (e.g., the crossbar on the A) subtend 1 minute of arc. The acuity is the line where more than half of the characters are accurately read. If the patient can read the 20/30 line and two characters on the 20/25 line, the notation is 20/30 + 2. By conventional notation, the distance from the test chart, 20 or 6, is the numerator, and the distance at which the smallest type read by

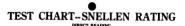

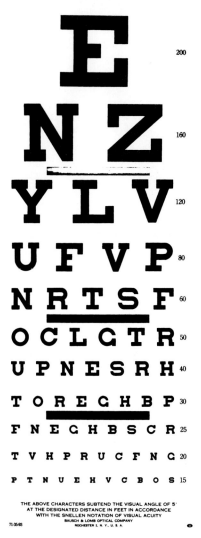

FIGURE 9.1  ●  Snellen test chart.

the patient should be seen by a person with normal acuity is the denominator. An acuity of 20/40 (6/12) means the individual must move in to 20 ft to read letters a normal person can read at 40 ft. This does not mean the patient's acuity is one half of normal. In fact, an individual with a distance acuity of 20/40 has only a 16.4% loss of vision.

Since few neurology clinics, offices, or hospital rooms have 20-ft eye lanes, testing is commonly done at a closer distance. Neurologists frequently assess vision with a near card (see Toolkit). Though examination of distance vision is preferable, the requisite devices are generally not at hand. There are pocket cards designed for testing at 6 ft, a convenient distance that usually eliminates the need for presbyopic correction (see Toolkit). Near vision is tested with a near card, such as the Rosenbaum pocket vision screening card, held at the near point (14 in or 35.5 cm). Good lighting is essential. A penlight shone directly on the line being read is useful for bedside testing.

If the patient cannot read the 20/200 line at 20 ft, the distance may be shortened and the fraction adjusted. Ability to read the line at 5 ft is vision of 5/200, equivalent to 20/800. Vision worse than the measurable 20/800 is described as counts fingers (CF), hand motion (HM), light perception (LP), or no light perception (NLP). The average finger is approximately the same size as the 20/200 character, so ability to count fingers at 5 ft is equivalent to an acuity of 20/800.

When a patient has impaired vision, an attempt should be made to exclude refractive error by any available means. If the patient has corrective lenses, they should be worn. In the absence of correction, improvement of vision by looking through a pinhole suggests impairment related to a refractive error. Commercial multi-pinhole devices are available. A crude pinhole is included in the Toolkit. A substitute can be made by making three or four holes with a pin in a 3 X 5 card in a circle about the size of a quarter. The multiple pinholes help the patient locate one. The patient should then attempt to read further down the acuity card through the pinhole. The pinhole permits only central light rays to enter the eye. These are less likely to be disrupted by refractive errors such as presbyopia and astigmatism. If a pinhole was used, make some notation, such as 20/20 (ph). If the visual impairment is due to a neurologic process, such as optic neuritis (ON), vision will not improve with a pinhole. Under some circumstances, such as with opacities in the media (e.g., cataract), vision may get worse with pinhole.

## COLOR VISION

Color blindness (achromatopsia) is an X-linked condition present in about 3% to 4% of males. Disturbances of color vision may also occur in neurologic conditions. Loss of color vision may precede other visual deficits. Color deficits may be partial or total. Color plates or pseudoisochromatic plates (Ishihara, Hardy-Ritter-Rand, or similar) formally and quantitatively assess color vision. Having the patient identify the colors in a fabric, such as a tie or a dress, can provide a crude estimate. The Toolkit contains some screening plates for color vision.

In neurologic disease, red perception is usually lost first. Desaturation to red, or red washout, describes a graying down or loss of intensity of red. The bright red cap on a bottle of mydriatic drops is a common test object. The patient compares the brightness or redness in right versus left hemifields, temporal versus nasal hemifields, or central versus peripheral fields. No right/left or temporal/nasal desaturation to red occurs normally. Red does normally look brighter in the center of the visual field than off center; reversal of this pattern suggests impairment of central vision. Patients may also compare the brightness or intensity of an examining light in one eye versus the other. A diminution of brightness on one side suggests optic nerve dysfunction; its significance is the same as for red desaturation.

## THE VISUAL FIELDS

The VF examination is a very important and, unfortunately, often omitted part of the neurologic examination. The VF is the limit of peripheral vision, the area in which an object can be seen while the eye remains fixed. Macular vision is sharp. Peripheral images are not as distinct, and objects are more visible if they are moving. The normal VF extends to 90 degrees to 100 degrees temporally, about 60 degrees nasally, 50 degrees to 60 degrees superiorly, and 60 degrees to 75 degrees inferiorly. The field is wider in the inferior and temporal quadrants than in the superior and nasal quadrants (Figure 9.2). With binocular vision, the VFs of the two eyes overlap except for the unpaired temporal crescent extending from 60 degrees to 90 degrees on the horizontal meridian, which is seen by one eye only. The monocular temporal crescent exists because of the anatomy of the retina. The nasal retina extends farther forward, more peripherally, than the temporal. This is the true reason that the temporal VF is more expansive, not because the nose is blocking the nasal field.

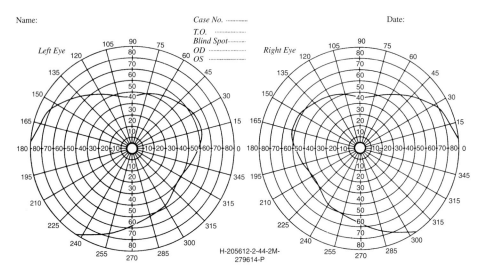

**FIGURE 9.2** ● The normal visual fields.

   Visual field examination results are most accurate in an individual who is alert and cooperative and will maintain fixation. Wandering of the eye impairs the evaluation. Crude assessment is
possible even in uncooperative patients if the target is interesting enough (e.g., food or paper
money). Fatigue and weakness may lengthen the latency between perception of the test object and
the response to it, giving a false impression of VF deficit. Close cooperation, good fixation, and
adequate illumination are essential for mapping of the blind spot and delineation of scotomas.
   Clinicians use several different methods for visual field evaluation. The time and energy
expended on bedside confrontation testing depends on the patient's history and on the facilities
available for formal field testing with tangent screen (central 30 degrees) or perimetry (entire
field). Even sophisticated confrontation testing cannot approach the accuracy of formal fields.
   The confrontation visual field exam can be tailored to the circumstances and done as superficially or as thoroughly as the situation requires. Sophisticated bedside techniques can explore the
VFs in detail if circumstances warrant. If the patient has no specific visual complaint, and if other
aspects of the history and examination do not suggest a field defect is likely, then a screening
exam is appropriate. This can be accomplished rapidly and with great sensitivity using small
amplitude finger movements in the far periphery of the VF. Recall that the VFs extend temporally
to 90+ degrees. Extending elbows and index fingers, the examiner should position the fingers
nearly directly lateral to the lateral canthus at a distance of about 24 in. Superficially, this appears
to be a binocular examination, but, properly placed, the finger targets are actually in the unpaired
monocular temporal crescent part of the visual field. With the targets positioned, make a small
amplitude flexion movement with the tip of one index finger, perhaps 2 cm in amplitude. Have the
patient "point to the finger that moves." This language is more efficient than attempting a right-
left verbal description where the patient's and examiner's rights and lefts are reversed. Stimuli
should be delivered in each upper quadrant individually, then both together, and then similarly for
the lower quadrants. Including bilateral simultaneous stimuli is necessary to detect subtle defects,
which may be manifested only by extinction of one stimulus on double simultaneous stimulation.
This technique of small finger movements in the far periphery in both upper and lower quadrants
is an excellent screen; when properly done, even binocularly, this technique misses few VF defects.
Always bear in mind that primary ophthalmological disorders such as glaucoma, diabetic retinopathy, and retinal detachment can also alter the visual fields.

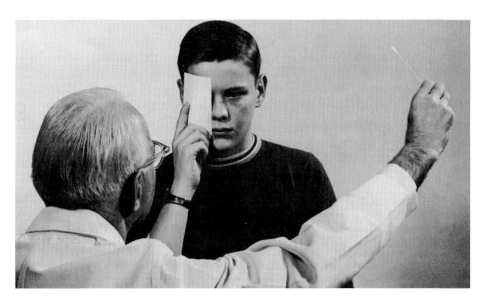

**FIGURE 9.3** ● Confrontation method of testing the visual fields.

With any hint of abnormality, or if the patient has or could be expected to have a visual problem, higher-level testing is in order. Examining monocularly, techniques include having the patient assess the brightness and clarity of the examiner's hands as they are held in the right and left hemifields, in both upper and lower quadrants, or having the patient count fingers fleetingly presented in various parts of the field.

More exacting techniques compare the patient's field dimensions with the examiner's, using various targets—still or moving fingers, the head of a cotton swab, colored pinheads, or similar objects. Positioning the patient and examiner at the same eye level, and gazing eyeball to eyeball over an 18- to 24-in span, targets introduced midway between and brought into the VF along various meridians should appear to both people simultaneously in all parts of the field except temporally, where the examiner must simply develop a feel for the extent of a normal field (Figure 9.3).

For obtunded, uncooperative, or aphasic patients, paper money (the larger the denomination the better) makes a compelling target. Even if the examiner has only a $1 bill, suggest to the patient that it might be $100. The patient who can see will glance at or reach for the object. Children may respond to keys (no jingling), candy, or other visually interesting objects. Infants may turn the head and eyes toward a diffuse light within a few days after birth. Moving a penlight into the VF and noting when the patient blinks is sometimes useful. Checking for blink to threat—the menace reflex—provides a crude last-resort method. The examiner's hand or fingers are brought in rapidly from the side, as if to strike the patient or poke him in the eye. The patient may wince, draw back, or blink. The threatening movement should be deliberate enough to avoid stimulating the cornea with an induced air current.

Testing central fields can include having the patient gaze at the examiner's face and report any defects, such as a missing or blurred nose. Having the patient survey a gridwork (Amsler grid) while fixing on a central point is a sensitive method to detect scotomas (see Toolkit). Probing the central field with a small white or red object may detect moderate or large scotomas. With a cooperative patient, one can estimate the size of the blind spot.

By convention, visual fields are depicted as seen by the patient (i.e., right eye drawn on the right). This convention is backwards from most things in clinical medicine, and violations of the rule occur sufficiently often that labeling notations are prudent. When confrontation fields are not adequate for the clinical circumstances, formal fields are done. These might include tangent screen examination, kinetic perimetry, or computerized automated static perimetry.

## VISUAL FIELD ABNORMALITIES

For neurologic purposes, visual field abnormalities can be divided into scotomas, hemianopias, altitudinal defects, and concentric constriction or contraction of the fields. Figure 9.4 depicts some examples of different types of field defects. Because of the anatomy and organization of the visual system, neurologic disorders tend to produce straight-edged defects that respect either the horizontal or vertical meridian, or have a characteristic shape because of the arrangement of the nerve fiber layer (NFL). Respect of the horizontal meridian may occur because of the horizontal temporal raphe and the arching sweep of NFL axons above and below the macula. This pattern is characteristic of optic nerve, optic disc, and NFL lesions. The vascular supply of the retina consists of superior and inferior branches of the central retinal artery, which supply the upper and lower retina, respectively. Vascular disease characteristically causes altitudinal field defects that are sharply demarcated horizontally. The calcarine cortex is organized into a superior and an inferior bank, and lesions involving only one bank may produce VF defects that respect the horizontal meridian. The vertical meridian is respected because of the division into nasal and temporal hemiretinas that occurs at the chiasmal decussation and is maintained through the retrochiasmal visual pathways.

### Scotomas

A scotoma is an area of impaired vision in the field, with normal surrounding vision. With an absolute scotoma, there is no visual function within the scotoma to testing with all sizes and colors of objects. With a relative scotoma, visual function is depressed but not absent; smaller objects and colored objects are more likely to detect the abnormality. A positive scotoma causes blackness or a sense of blockage of vision, as though an object were interposed; it suggests disease of the retina, especially the macula or choroid. Positive scotomas are often due to exudate or hemorrhage involving the retina or opacity in the media. A negative scotoma is an absence of vision, a blank spot as if part of the field had been erased; it suggests optic nerve disease but can occur with lesions more posteriorly. With a negative scotoma the defect may not be perceived until a VF examination is done.

A scotoma can often be demonstrated on confrontation VF testing using small objects and carefully exploring the central fields, but they are best demonstrated by the use of the tangent screen. The physiologic blind spot is a scotoma corresponding to the optic nerve head, which contains no rods or cones and is blind to all visual impressions. The physiologic blind spot is situated 15 degrees lateral to and just below the center of fixation because the disc lies nasal to the macula and the blind spot is projected into the temporal field. The blind spot is enlarged in papilledema and ON.

Scotomas are described by their location or their shape. A central scotoma involves the fixation point and is seen in macular or optic nerve disease. It is typical for ON but can occur in vascular and compressive lesions (Figure 9.4A). A paracentral scotoma involves the areas adjacent to the fixation point, and it has the same implications as for a central scotoma. A cecocentral scotoma extends from the blind spot to fixation. It is usually accompanied by loss of all central vision with preservation of a small amount of peripheral vision, and it strongly suggests optic nerve disease (Figure 9.4B and Figure 9.5). Central, paracentral, and cecocentral scotomas are all suggestive of a process involving the papillomacular bundle. Any scotoma involving the blind spot implies optic neuropathy.

An arcuate scotoma is a crescent defect arching out of the blind spot, usually due to optic neuropathy with the brunt of damage falling on the fibers forming the superior and inferior nerve fiber layer arcades. A junctional scotoma is an optic nerve defect in one eye (central, paracentral, or cecocentral scotoma) and a superior temporal defect in the opposite eye. This is due to a lesion (usually a mass) that involves one optic nerve close to the chiasm, which damages the inferior nasal fibers from the opposite eye (Wilbrand's knee) as they loop forward into the proximal optic

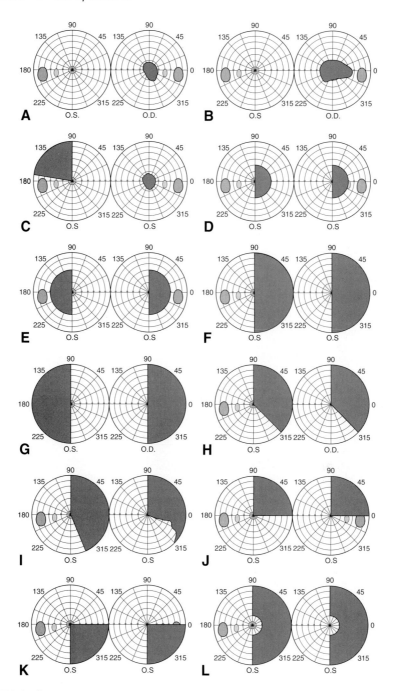

*FIGURE 9.4* ● Types of visual field defects. **A.** Central scotoma **B.** Cecocentral scotoma **C.** Junctional scotoma **D.** Homonymous scotomas **E.** Heteronymous scotomas **F.** Right homonymous hemianopia **G.** Bitemporal hemianopia **H.** Congruous right homonymous hemianopia **I.** Incongruous right homonymous hemianopia **J.** Right superior quadrantopia ("pie in the sky") **K.** Right inferior quadrantopia **L.** Macular-sparing right homonymous hemianopia.

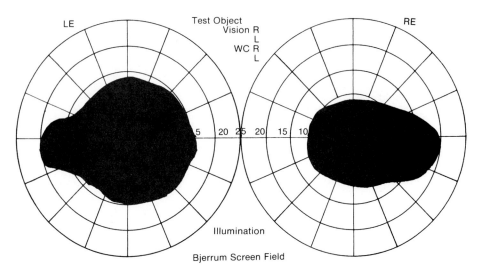

**FIGURE 9.5** ● Bilateral cecocentral scotomas in a patient with bilateral optic neuritis.

nerve on the side of the lesion (Figure 9.6 and Figure 9.4C). The temporal VF defect in the contralateral eye may be subtle and easily missed.

Although scotomas most often result from disease of the retina or optic nerve, they may also be caused by cerebral lesions. Occipital pole lesions primarily affecting the macular area can produce contralateral homonymous hemianopic scotomas (Figure 9.4D). Since the bulk of fibers in the chiasm come from the macula, early compression may preferentially affect central vision producing bitemporal heteronymous paracentral scotomas (Figure 9.4E); with progression of the lesion, a full blown bitemporal hemianopia will appear (Figure 9.4G).

## Hemianopia

Hemianopia is impaired vision in half the visual field of each eye; hemianopic defects do not cross the vertical meridian. Hemianopias may be homonymous or heteronymous. A homonymous hemianopia causes impaired vision in corresponding halves of each eye (e.g., a right homonymous hemianopia is a defect in the right half of each eye). Homonymous hemianopias are caused by lesions posterior to the optic chiasm, with interruption of the fibers from the temporal half of the ipsilateral retina and the nasal half of the contralateral retina. Vision is lost in the ipsilateral nasal field and the contralateral temporal field (Figure 9.7). A heteronymous hemianopia is impaired

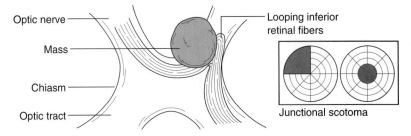

**FIGURE 9.6** ● A mass impinging on the optic nerve at its junction with the chiasm, producing a junctional scotoma.

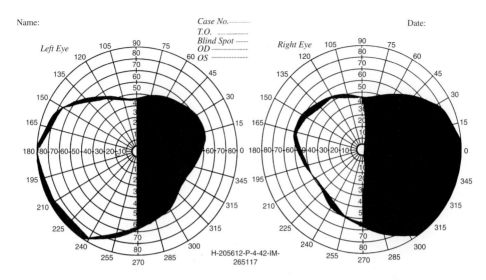

**FIGURE 9.7** ● Macular splitting right homonymous hemianopia in a patient with a neoplasm of the left occipital lobe.

vision in opposite halves of each eye (e.g., the right half in one eye and the left half in the other). Unilateral homonymous hemianopias, even those with macular splitting, do not affect visual acuity. Patients can read normally with the preserved half of the macula, but those with left-sided hemianopias may have trouble finding the line to be read. Occasionally patients with homonymous hemianopia will read only half of the line on the acuity chart.

A homonymous hemianopia may be complete or incomplete. If incomplete it may be congruous or incongruous. A congruous hemianopia shows similarly shaped defects in each eye (Figure 9.4H). The closer the optic radiations get to the occipital lobe, the closer lie corresponding visual fibers from the two eyes. The more congruous the field defect, the more posterior the lesion is likely to be. An incongruous hemianopia is differently shaped defects in the two eyes (Figure 9.4I). The more incongruous the defect, the more anterior the lesion. The most incongruous hemianopias occur with optic tract and lateral geniculate lesions. With a complete hemianopia, congruity cannot be assessed; the only localization possible is to identify the lesion as contralateral and retrochiasmal. A superior quadrantopsia implies a lesion in the temporal lobe affecting Meyer's loop (inferior retinal fibers): "pie in the sky" (Figure 9.4J). An inferior quadrantopsia implies a parietal lobe lesion affecting superior retinal fibers (Figure 9.4K). A macular-sparing hemianopia is one that spares the area immediately around fixation; it implies an occipital lobe lesion (Figure 9.4L). The explanation for macular sparing remains unclear.

Incomplete homonymous VF defects are common. These include partial or irregular defects in one or both of the hemifields, relative rather than absolute loss of vision, an inability to localize the visual stimulus, and hemianopia only for objects of a certain color (hemiachromatopsia). Extinction (visual inattention) is hemianopic suppression of the visual stimulus in the involved hemifield when bilateral simultaneous stimuli are delivered. Visual extinction is most characteristic of lesions involving the nondominant parietal lobe.

Heteronymous hemianopias are usually bitemporal; only rarely are they binasal. A bitemporal hemianopia is usually due to chiasmatic disease, such as a pituitary tumor growing up out of the sella tursica and pressing on the underside of the chiasm (Figure 9.8). Bitemporal field defects can usually be detected earliest by demonstrating bitemporal desaturation to red. Because of the anterior inferior position of decussating inferior nasal fibers, lesions impinging from below produce

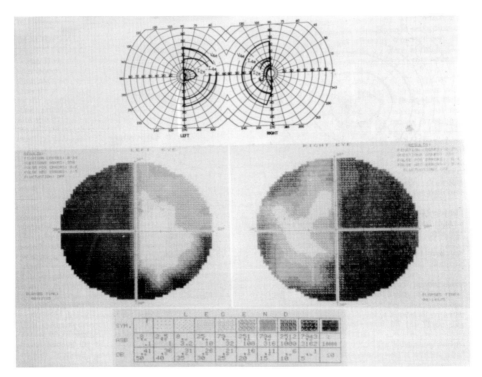

**FIGURE 9.8**  ●  (Top) Visual field performed on a Goldmann perimeter in a patient with a chiasmal lesion. (Bottom) Humphrey perimeter field in the same patient. (From Beck RW, Bergstrom TJ, Lichter PR. A clinical comparison of visual field testing with a new automated perimeter, the Humphrey Field Analyzer, and the Goldmann perimeter. *Ophthalmology* 1985; 92:77–82. Used with permission.)

upper temporal field defects, which evolve into a bitemporal hemianopia (Figure 9.9). Lesions encroaching from above tend to cause inferior temporal defects initially. The defect will be first and worst in the upper quadrants with infrachiasmatic masses (e.g., pituitary adenoma), and it will be first and worst in the lower quadrants with suprachiasmatic masses (e.g., craniopharyngioma). The most common cause of bitemporal hemianopia is a pituitary adenoma; occasionally it results from other parasellar or suprasellar lesions such as meningioma and craniopharyngioma, as well as glioma of the optic chiasm, aneurysms, trauma, and hydrocephalus.

An altitudinal visual field defect is one involving the upper or lower half of vision, usually in one eye, and usually due to retinal vascular disease (central retinal artery or branch occlusion or anterior ischemic optic neuropathy). A partial altitudinal defect may approximate a quadrantopsia. Altitudinal defects do not cross the horizontal meridian.

Constriction of the VFs is characterized by a narrowing of the range of vision, which may affect one or all parts of the periphery. Constriction may be regular or irregular, concentric or eccentric, temporal or nasal, and upper or lower. Symmetric concentric contraction is most frequent and is characterized by a more or less even, progressive reduction in field diameter through all meridians. Concentric constriction of the VFs may occur with optic atrophy, especially secondary to papilledema or late glaucoma, or with retinal disease, especially retinitis pigmentosa. Diffuse depression is the static perimeter equivalent of constriction on kinetic perimetry. Concentric constriction of the fields is sometimes seen in hysteria. A suspicious finding is when the fields fail to enlarge as expected with testing at increasing distance (tubular fields).

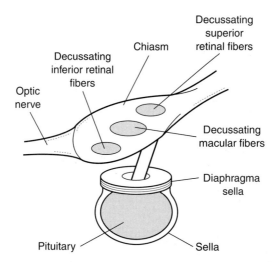

*FIGURE 9.9* ● The macular fibers decussate as a separate compact bundle, inferior retinal (superior visual field) fibers cross inferiorly, and superior retinal (inferior visual field) fibers superiorly. Masses imping-ing from below (e.g., pituitary adenoma) tend to cause early defects in the superior temporal fields; masses impinging from above (e.g., craniopharyngioma) tend to cause early defects in the inferior temporal fields.

## THE OPHTHALMOSCOPIC EXAMINATION

The physician using a direct ophthalmoscope is like a one-eyed Eskimo peering into a dark igloo from the entryway with a flashlight. Only a narrow sector of the posterior pole is visible, and there is no stereopsis. Pupil dilation significantly increases the field of view. Indirect ophthalmoscopy, used by ophthalmologists, can stereoscopically view almost the entire vista of the fundus. New PanOptic direct ophthalmoscopes (Welch-Allyn) give the advantage of a broader view but still reveal only the posterior pole. In the neurologic examination, the areas of primary concern are the disc, the macula, and the arteries. The disc is normally round or a vertically oriented slight oval. The nasal margin is normally slightly blurred compared to the temporal. The disc consists of a peripheral neuroretinal rim and a central cup. The neuroretinal rim consists of axons streaming from the retina to enter the optic nerve. The physiologic cup is a slight depression in the center of the disc that is less pinkish than the rim and shows a faint latticework due to the underlying lam-ina cribrosa. The rim is elevated slightly above the cup. To locate the disc, a helpful technique is to find a retinal blood vessel, focus on it, and then follow it to the disc. The myelinated axons mak-ing up its substance render the normal optic disc yellowish white. It is paler temporally where the papillomacular bundle enters. The normal disc lies flat and well demarcated against the surround-ing retina, with arteries and veins crossing the margins and capillaries staining the surface a faint pink. Varying amounts of pigmentation are present in the retina near the temporal border of the disc, especially in dark-skinned persons. At times a pigment ring may completely surround the disc. The macula is a dark area that lies about 2 disc diameters temporal to and slightly below the disc.

## LOCALIZATION AND DISORDERS OF VISUAL FUNCTION

Disorders of the afferent visual system can be divided into prechiasmal, chiasmal, and retrochiasmal. Disease in each of these locations has characteristic features that usually permit its localization. The etiologic processes affecting these different segments of the afferent visual system are quite different. As a generalization, prechiasmal lesions cause monocular visual loss; impaired color perception; a central, paracentral, or cecocentral VF defect; and an afferent pupillary defect (APD).

The disc may or may not appear abnormal depending on the exact location of the lesion. Chiasmal lesions cause heteronymous VF defects, most often bitemporal hemianopia, with preservation of visual acuity and color perception and a normal appearing optic disc. Retrochiasmal lesions cause a contralateral homonymous hemianopia and have no effect on acuity or disc appearance. There is usually no effect on color vision, but some central lesions may cause achromatopsia. A summary of the features of disease involving the macula, optic nerve, chiasm, optic tract, lateral geniculate body (LGB), optic radiations, and calcarine cortex can be found in Table 9.1.

## Prechiasmal Lesions

Prechiasmal disorders affect the optic nerve. Disorders can be divided into those that affect the disc (papillopathy) and those that affect the retrobulbar segment between the globe and the chiasm. The macula gives rise to the majority of the fibers in the optic nerve, and disease of the macula itself can cause a clinical picture that is at times difficult to distinguish from optic neuropathy. Common causes of maculopathy include age-related macular degeneration and central serous retinopathy (Table 9.1).

## Disorders of the Optic Disc

The color and appearance of the disc may change in a variety of circumstances. The disc may change color—to abnormally pale in optic atrophy or to abnormally red with disc edema. The margins may become obscured because of disc edema or the presence of anomalies. Edema of the disc is nonspecific. It may reflect increased intracranial pressure, or it may occur because of optic nerve inflammation, ischemia, or other local processes. By convention, disc swelling due to increased intracranial pressure is referred to as papilledema; under all other circumstances, the noncommittal terms disc edema or disc swelling are preferred. Visual function provides a critical clue to the nature of disc abnormalities. Patients with acute papilledema and those with disc anomalies have normal visual acuity, visual fields, and color perception. Impairment of these functions is the rule in patients suffering from optic neuropathies of any etiology. The first step in evaluating a questionably abnormal disc is therefore a careful assessment of vision.

## Papilledema

Increased intracranial pressure exerts pressure on the optic nerves, which impairs axoplasmic flow and produces axonal edema and an increased volume of axoplasm at the disc. The swollen axons impair venous return from the retina, engorging first the capillaries on the disc surface, then the retinal veins, and ultimately causing splinter- and flame-shaped hemorrhages as well as cotton wool exudates in the retinal nerve fiber layer. Further axonal swelling eventually leads to elevation of the disc above the retinal surface.

The four stages of papilledema are early, fully developed, chronic, and atrophic. Fully developed papilledema is obvious, with elevation of the disc surface, humping of vessels crossing the disc margin, obliteration of disc margins, peripapillary hemorrhages, cotton wool exudates, engorged and tortuous retinal veins, and marked disc hyperemia. The recognition of early papilledema is much more problematic (Figure 9.10). Occasionally, the only way to resolve the question of early papilledema is by serial observation. The earliest change is loss of previously observed spontaneous venous pulsations (SVP). The presence of SVPs indicates an intracranial pressure less than approximately 200 mm $H_2O$. However, since they are absent in 10% to 20% of normals, only the disappearance of previously observed SVPs is clearly pathologic.

As papilledema develops, increased venous back pressure dilates the capillaries on the disc surface, transforming its normal yellowish-pink color to fiery red. Blurring of the superior and inferior margins evolves soon after. However, since these margins are normally the least distinct areas of the disc, blurry margins alone are not enough to diagnose papilledema. There is no alteration of the physiologic cup with early papilledema. With further evolution, the patient with early papilledema will

TABLE 9.1

**Clinical Characteristics of Acute Lesions Involving Different Parts of the Afferent Visual Pathway**

| | Visual Acuity | Color Vision | Visual Field Defect | Pupillary Function | Disc Appearance | Comment |
|---|---|---|---|---|---|---|
| Macula | Decr | Decr | Ipsilateral central scotoma | Possible mild APD | Normal | May have metamorphosia; macula may be abnormal on ophthalmoscopy; common etiologies: age-related macular degeneration, central serous retinopathy, hole, cystoid macular edema, trauma, toxic retinopathy |
| *Optic Nerve* Papillopathy | Decr | Decr | Ipsilateral central, paracentral, or cecocentral scotoma | APD | Edema | With ON may have pain on eye movement; common etiologies: idiopathic ON, MS, AION, postviral, sarcoid, LHON, collagen vascular disease, neurosyphilis, diabetes, papillophlebitis |
| Retrobulbar neuropathy | Decr | Decr | Same as papillopathy | APD | Normal | May have proptosis; common etiologies: ON, MS, optic nerve compression, glioma, infiltrative lesions, trauma, sarcoid, toxins, collagen vascular disease, infection, posterior ischemic optic neuropathy |
| Distal optic nerve, near chiasm | Decr | Decr | Junctional scotoma | APD | Normal | May have evidence of a sellar/parasellar mass; common etiology: mass lesion |
| Chiasm | Normal | Normal | Bitemporal hemianopia | Normal | Normal | May develop bowtie atrophy; APD can occur in eye with greatest VF loss; common etiologies: tumor (e.g., pituitary adenoma, suprasellar meningioma), demyelination, trauma, radionecrosis, aneurysm, ischemia, chiasmal glioma, sarcoid, optochiasmatic arachnoiditis |

*(continued)*

**TABLE 9.1** (*Continued*)

Clinical Characteristics of Acute Lesions Involving Different Parts of the Afferent Visual Pathway

| | Visual Acuity | Color Vision | Visual Field Defect | Pupillary Function | Disc Appearance | Comment |
|---|---|---|---|---|---|---|
| Optic tract | Normal | Normal | Contralateral incongruous homonymous hemianopia | Mild APD in contra-lateral eye | Normal | May be involved with disease involving the posterior chiasm; common etiologies: demyelinating disease, trauma, mass lesion, stroke |
| Lateral geniculate body | Normal | Normal | Contralateral incongruous homonymous hemianopia | Normal | Normal | Common etiologies: ischemia, trauma, mass lesion |
| *Optic Radiations* | | | | | | |
| Temporal lobe | Normal | Normal | Contralateral superior quadrantopia | Normal | Normal | May have visual hallucinations in the affected hemifield; common etiologies: tumor, stroke, hematoma, trauma, mass lesion |
| Parietal lobe | Normal | Normal | Contralateral inferior quadrantopia | Normal | Normal | May have asymmetric OKN; patient may be unaware of the deficit, especially with nondominant hemisphere lesions; common etiologies: tumor, stroke, trauma, hematoma |
| Calcarine cortex | Normal | Normal | Contralateral congruous homonymous hemianopia | Normal | Normal | Macula sparing frequent; common etiologies: stroke, trauma, tumor, demyelinating disease |

AION, anterior ischemic optic neuropathy; APD, afferent papillary defect; decr, decreased; LHON, Leber hereditary optic neuropathy; MS, multiple sclerosis; OKN, optokinetic nystagmus; ON, optic neuritis.

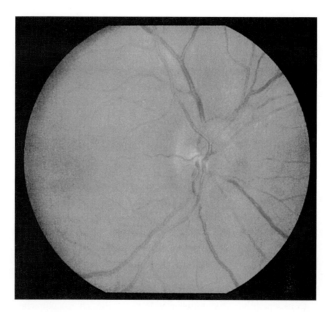

*FIGURE 9.10* ● Early papilledema.

develop diffuse disc edema, cup obscuration, hemorrhages, exudates, and venous engorgement. Frank disc elevation then ensues as the fundus ripens into fully developed papilledema (Figure 9.11). In chronic papilledema, hemorrhages and exudates resolve and leave a markedly swollen "champagne cork" disc bulging up from the plane of the retina. If unrelieved, impaired axoplasmic flow eventually leads to death of axons and visual impairment, which evolves into the stage of atrophic papilledema, or secondary optic atrophy. Papilledema ordinarily develops over days to weeks. With acutely increased intracranial pressure due to subarachnoid or intracranial hemorrhage, it may develop within hours. Measuring diopters of disc elevation ophthalmoscopically has little utility.

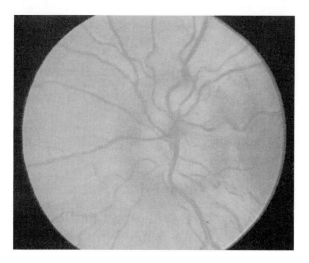

*FIGURE 9.11* ● Severe papilledema.

## TABLE 9.2

### Some Causes of Unilateral Disc Edema

Optic neuritis
Anterior ischemic optic neuropathy
Compression of the optic nerve in the orbit
Central retinal vein occlusion
Optic nerve infiltration
Diabetic papillopathy
Syphilis
Leber hereditary optic neuropathy
Increased intracranial pressure (rare)

Acute papilledema causes no impairment of visual acuity or color vision. The blind spot may be enlarged, but VF testing is otherwise normal. In patients who develop optic atrophy following papilledema, the visual morbidity can be severe and may include blindness.

### Other Causes of Disc Edema

Changes ophthalmoscopically indistinguishable from papilledema occur when conditions primarily affecting the optic nerve papilla cause disc edema. Papilledema is usually bilateral; other causes of disc edema are often unilateral (Table 9.2). Optic neuropathies generally cause marked visual impairment, including loss of acuity, central or cecocentral scotoma, loss of color perception, and an APD. Disease of the optic nerve head is usually due to demyelination, ischemia, inflammation, or compression. There are many causes of optic neuropathy; some of the more common conditions are listed in Table 9.3.

### Pseudopapilledema

Some conditions affecting the nerve head cause striking disc changes of little or no clinical import. This circumstance arises frequently when routine ophthalmoscopy unexpectedly reveals an abnormal appearing disc in a patient with migraine or some seemingly benign neurologic complaint. Such

## TABLE 9.3

### Some Causes of Optic Neuropathy

Optic neuritis
Ischemic optic neuropathy
Optic nerve compression
Papillophlebitis
Optic nerve infiltration (carcinomatous, lymphomatous)
Sarcoidosis
Diabetic papillopathy
Tobacco-alcohol amblyopia
Nutritional deficiency, especially vitamin $B_{12}$
Drugs
Toxins
Hereditary optic neuropathy (Leber, Kjer)
Glaucoma

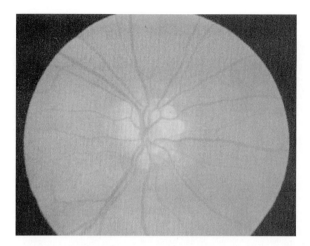

**FIGURE 9.12**  ●  Drusen of the optic nerve head simulating papilledema.

patients generally have normal vision and no visual complaints. Common causes of pseudopapilledema include optic nerve drusen and myelinated nerve fibers (Figures 9.12 and 9.13). Distinguishing pseudopapilledema from acquired disc edema can be difficult.

## Optic Atrophy

In optic atrophy, the disc is paler than normal and more sharply demarcated from the surrounding retina, sometimes having a punched-out appearance (Figure 9.14). The disc margins stand out distinctly; the physiologic cup may be abnormally prominent and extend to the margin of the disc. Loss of myeli-

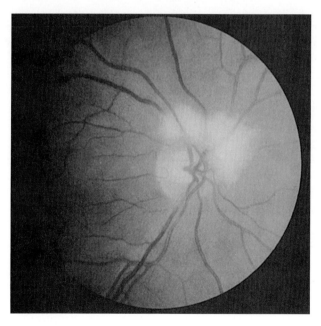

**FIGURE 9.13**  ●  Medullated nerve fibers.

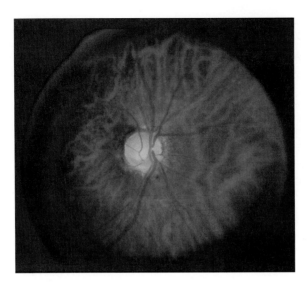

**FIGURE 9.14**   ●   Primary optic atrophy.

nated axons and their supporting capillaries with replacement by gliotic scar produce the lack of color, which may vary from a dirty gray to a blue-white color to stark white. An atrophic disc may appear perceptibly smaller. Pallor of the temporal portion of the disc—a classical finding in MS—may precede definite atrophy, but normal physiologic temporal pallor makes this finding often equivocal.

Optic atrophy may follow some other condition (ON, anterior ischemic optic neuropathy, or papilledema) and is then referred to as secondary or consecutive optic atrophy. Primary optic atrophy, appearing de novo, occurs as a heredofamilial condition (e.g., Leber hereditary optic neuropathy) or after toxic, metabolic, nutritional, compressive, or glaucomatous insult to the nerve. Some causes of optic atrophy are listed in Table 9.4. A patient may have disc edema in one eye and optic atrophy in the other eye (Foster Kennedy syndrome).

## TABLE 9.4

### Some Causes of Optic Atrophy

Optic neuritis
Glaucoma
Trauma
Chronic papilledema
Ischemic optic neuropathy
Leber hereditary optic neuropathy
Drugs
Toxins
Optic nerve compression
Deficiency states
Central nervous system syphilis

## Retrobulbar Optic Neuropathy

The retrobulbar portion of the nerve may be affected by most of the diseases that affect the optic disc. The clinical picture is similar except that there is no disc edema acutely, but optic atrophy may follow later. When ON strikes the retrobulbar portion of the nerve, marked visual impairment occurs but the disc appearance remains normal, since the pathology is posterior to the papilla. Optic papillopathy thus causes impaired vision and an abnormal disc; retrobulbar optic neuropathy causes impaired vision and a normal disc; and papilledema causes an abnormal disc but does not affect vision acutely. A major difference between retrobulbar neuropathy and papillopathy is the increased incidence of compression as an etiology in the former.

## Chiasmal Lesions

Pituitary tumors, craniopharyngiomas, meningiomas, gliomas, and carotid aneurysms are the lesions that commonly involve the chiasm. Because the chiasm lies about a centimeter above the diaphragma sella, visual system involvement indicates suprasellar extension of a pituitary tumor and is a late, not an early, manifestation of chiasmatic mass effect. Acuity, color vision, and pupillary function are not affected unless there is optic nerve involvement.

## Retrochiasmal Lesions

Retrochiasmal lesions produce contralateral homonymous VF defects that respect the vertical meridian. Optic tract and LGB lesions are rare, and characterized by incongruous homonymous hemianopias. In geniculocalcarine pathway (optic radiation) lesions, temporal lobe pathology typically produces contralateral superior quadrantopias, or homonymous hemianopia worse in the upper quadrants; and parietal lobe processes contralateral inferior quadrantopias, or homonymous hemianopia worse in the lower quadrants (Figure 9.4). The more posterior the lesion, the more congruous the defect. Occipital lobe lesions cause contralateral homonymous hemianopias that are highly congruous and tend to spare the macula. Hypotensive watershed infarctions may cause contralateral homonymous paracentral scotomas due to ischemia limited to the macular cortex (Figure 9.4D).

Bilateral occipital lesions may also cause some dramatic defects of cortical function in addition to the visual loss. Anton syndrome is cortical blindness due to bilateral homonymous hemianopias, with extreme visual impairment in which the patient is unaware of, and denies the existence of, the deficit.

# CHAPTER 10

# The Ocular Motor Nerves

T he oculomotor, or third cranial nerve (CN III) arises from the oculomotor nuclear complex in the midbrain and conveys motor fibers to extraocular muscles, plus parasympathetic fibers to the pupil and ciliary body. A single midline structure, the central caudal nucleus, supplies the levator palpebrae muscles on both sides. The periaqueductal gray matter is also involved with eyelid function. The Edinger-Westphal (EW) subnucleus is a single structure that provides parasympathetic innervation to both eyes. The fibers of CN III course anteriorly through the mesencephalon, traversing the medial portion of the red nucleus and the substantia nigra. The nerve exits from the interpeduncular fossa on the anterior surface of the midbrain. It passes between the superior cerebellar and posterior cerebral arteries, then runs forward parallel to the posterior communicating artery. In its course toward the cavernous sinus, it lies on the free edge of the tentorium cerebelli, medial to the temporal lobe. CN III penetrates the dura just lateral and anterior to the posterior clinoid processes and enters the cavernous sinus. In the cavernous sinus, CN III has important relationships with the carotid artery, ascending pericarotid sympathetics, and CNs IV, V, and VI. CN III separates into its superior and inferior divisions in the anterior cavernous sinus, then enters the orbit through the superior orbital fissure.

The trochlear, or fourth cranial, nerve (CN IV) arises from the trochlear nucleus located just anterior to the aqueduct at the level of the inferior colliculus. The nerve filaments curve posteriorly around the aqueduct, decussate in the anterior medullary velum and exit through the tectum. It is the only cranial nerve to exit from the brainstem posteriorly. It penetrates the dura just behind and lateral to the posterior clinoid processes. Leaving the cavernous sinus, it traverses the superior orbital fissure, enters the orbit, and crosses over CN III to terminate on the superior oblique muscle on the side opposite the nucleus of origin.

The nucleus of the abducens, or sixth cranial, nerve (CN VI) lies in the mid to lower pons, encircled by the looping fibers of the facial nerve. The nerve exits anteriorly at the pontomedullary junction, then ascends the clivus in the prepontine cistern. It passes near the Gasserian ganglion, pierces the dura at the dorsum sellae, and enters the cavernous sinus in company with CNs III and IV, where it lies below and medial to CN III and just lateral to the internal carotid artery. CN VI is the only nerve that lies free in the lumen of the sinus; the others are in the wall. It enters the orbit through the superior orbital fissure to innervate the lateral rectus.

Examination of the eyes begins with inspection—looking for any obvious ocular malalignment, abnormal lid position, or abnormalities of the position of the globe within the orbit. Abnormalities of the external eye may occasionally be of diagnostic significance in neurologic patients.

Tortuous ("corkscrew") blood vessels in the conjunctiva occur with carotid cavernous fistula, or there may be jaundice, evidence of iritis, Kayser-Fleischer rings, chemosis, dysmorphic changes (e.g., epicanthal folds), xanthelasma due to hypercholesterolemia, keratoconjunctivitis sicca, premature cataract, or ocular complications of upper facial paralysis. Basal skull fractures often cause bilateral periorbital ecchymosis (raccoon eyes).

## Exophthalmos

The globe may be abnormally positioned within the orbit so that it protrudes (exophthalmos, proptosis) or recedes (enophthalmos). Subtle proptosis can often be better appreciated by looking down at both eyes from above the vertex of the head, or by comparing side views. Exophthalmos is usually bilateral and most commonly due to thyroid eye disease ([TED], Graves ophthalmopathy, Graves orbitopathy); thyroid disease can have a host of neurologic complications. Some of the neurologically significant causes of unilateral proptosis include orbital mass lesion, carotid cavernous fistula, cavernous sinus thrombosis, sphenoid wing meningioma, meningocele, and mucormycosis.

## The Eyelids

Patients may couch the complaint of ptosis in ways other than droopy eyelid (e.g., eye has shrunk). Ptosis may have been present for a very long time before coming to the patient's attention. Looking at old photographs is often helpful. Note the position of the eyelids and the width of the palpebral fissures bilaterally. Note the amount of iris or pupil covered by the lid. The normal upper eyelid in primary position crosses the iris between the limbus (junction of the iris and sclera) and the pupil, usually 1 mm to 2 mm below the limbus; the lower lid touches or crosses slightly above the limbus. Normally there is no sclera showing above the iris. The width of the palpebral fissures should be equal on both sides, although a slight difference occurs in many normal individuals. The palpebral fissures are normally 9 mm to 12 mm from upper to lower lid margin. Measurement can also be made from the lid margin to the corneal light reflex. The upper lid margin is normally 3 mm to 4 mm above the light reflex. Patients may try to compensate for ptosis by contracting the frontalis muscle, causing a telltale wrinkling of the ipsilateral forehead. If the examiner fixes the frontalis muscle with her finger, the patient may be unable to raise the eyelid.

With ptosis, the lid droops down and may cross at the upper margin of the pupil, or cover the pupil partially or totally. With complete ptosis, the eyelid is down and the eye appears closed (Figure 10.1). Ptosis may be unilateral or bilateral, partial or complete, and occurs in many neurologic conditions (Figure 10.2). With eyelid retraction, the upper lid pulls back and frequently exposes a thin crescent of sclera between the upper limbus and the lower lid margin. Lid retraction is a classic sign of thyroid disease, but occurs in neurologic disorders as well. In addition to observing the lid position at rest, notice the relationships of the lid to the globe during eye movement.

Total unilateral ptosis only occurs with complete third nerve palsy. Mild to moderate unilateral ptosis occurs as part of Horner syndrome, or with partial third nerve palsy. Mild to moderate bilateral ptosis occurs in some neuromuscular disorders, such as myasthenia gravis (MG), muscular dystrophy, or ocular myopathy.

The ptosis in MG is frequently asymmetric and may be unilateral, though it will tend to shift from side to side (Figure 10.3). It characteristically fluctuates from moment to moment and is worsened by prolonged upgaze (fatigable ptosis). The Cogan lid twitch sign, characteristic of myasthenia, consists of a brief overshoot twitch of lid retraction following sudden return of the eyes to primary position after a period of downgaze. When the ptosis is asymmetric, manually raising the more ptotic lid may cause increased ptosis on the other side (curtain sign, seesaw ptosis). Compensation for mild ptosis on one side may cause the involved eye to appear normal and the other eye to have lid retraction.

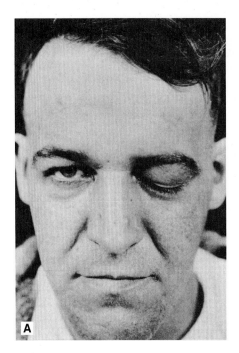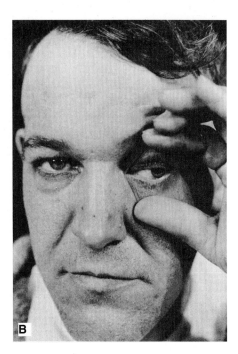

***FIGURE 10.1*** ●    Paralysis of the left oculomotor nerve in a patient with an aneurysm of the left internal carotid artery. **A.** Only ptosis can be seen. **B.** On elevating the eyelid, it is seen that the pupil is dilated and the eyeball is deviated laterally.

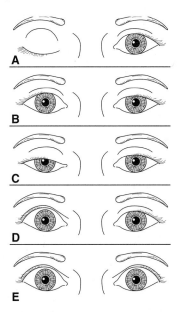

***FIGURE 10.2*** ●    Characteristics of different causes of abnormal lid position. **A.** Right third cranial nerve palsy with complete ptosis. **B.** Left Horner syndrome with drooping of upper lid and slight elevation of lower lid. **C.** Bilateral, asymmetric ptosis in myasthenia gravis. **D.** Right lid retraction in thyroid eye disease. **E.** Bilateral lid retraction with a lesion in the region of the posterior commissure (Collier sign).

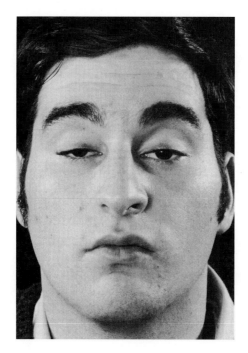

*FIGURE 10.3* ● Bilateral ptosis in a patient with myasthenia gravis.

## Lid Retraction

Lid position is abnormal if there is a rim of sclera showing above the limbus, indicating either lid retraction or lid lag. Thyroid eye disease is a common cause of lid abnormalities, including lid retraction in primary gaze and lid lag in downgaze. Lid retraction in primary gaze also occurs with lesions involving the posterior commissure (Collier sign). Lid retraction with posterior commissure lesions is bilateral, but may be asymmetric. With Collier sign, the levators relax appropriately and the lids usually descend normally on downgaze without lagging behind as they do in TED. In addition, the lid retraction may worsen with attempted upgaze (Figure 10.4). Aberrant regeneration of CN III may cause lid retraction on adduction. Lid retraction may also be mechanical, due to trauma or surgery. Lid retraction may be confused with ipsilateral proptosis or contralateral ptosis.

## The Pupils

The function of the pupil is to control the amount of light entering the eye, ensuring optimal vision for the lighting conditions. The pupils should be equal in size, round, regular, centered in the iris, and should exhibit specific reflex responses.

Pupillary size depends primarily on the balance between sympathetic and parasympathetic innervation and the level of ambient illumination. The most important determinants are the level of illumination and the point at which the eyes are focused. Accurate measurements are important. Measurements should be made with a pupil gauge or a millimeter ruler; estimates are surprisingly inaccurate. The size of the pupils should be determined at distance in ambient and dim light and at near. The normal pupil is 2 mm to 6 mm in diameter. In ordinary ambient light the pupils are usually 3 mm to 4 mm in diameter. The pupils are small and poorly reactive at birth and in early infancy, becoming normal size around ages 7 to 8. They are normally larger in adolescents and young adults, about 4 mm in diameter and perfectly round. In middle age, they are typically 3.5 mm in diameter and regular, and in old age 3 mm or less and often slightly irregular.

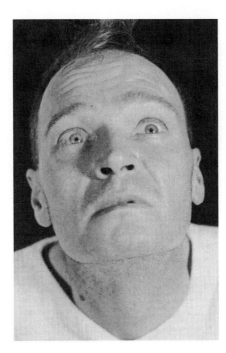

*FIGURE 10.4*    ●    Paresis of upward gaze in a patient with a neoplasm of the posterior third ventricle.

Pupils less than 2 mm in diameter are miotic. Common causes of acquired miosis include old age, hyperopia, alcohol abuse, and drug effects. Neurologically significant causes of miosis include neurosyphilis, diabetes, levodopa therapy, and Horner syndrome. Acute, severe brainstem lesions, such as pontine hematoma, may cause bilaterally tiny, "pinpoint" pupils that still react.

Pupils more than 6 mm in diameter are dilated. Common causes of bilateral mydriasis include anxiety, fear, pain, myopia, and drug effects—especially anticholinergics. Only severe, bilateral lesions of the retina or anterior visual pathways, enough to cause near blindness, will affect the resting pupil size. Neurologically significant bilateral mydriasis occurs in midbrain lesions, in comatose patients following cardiac arrest, in cerebral anoxia, and as a terminal condition.

The normal pupil is round, with a smooth, regular outline. Gross abnormalities in shape are usually the result of ocular disease such as iritis or eye surgery. Synechia, a congenital coloboma (a gap in the iris), prior trauma, or iridectomy may all cause pupil irregularity. A slight change in shape, however, such as an oval pupil, slight irregularity in outline, serration of the border, or slight notching, may be significant in the diagnosis of neurologic disease. The pupils are generally of equal size. A difference of 0.25 mm in pupil size is noticeable, and a difference of 2 mm is considered significant. Physiologic anisocoria, mild degrees of inequality with less than 1 mm of difference between the two sides, occurs in 15% to 20% of normal individuals. With such physiologic anisocoria, the degree of inequality remains about the same in light and dark, and the pupils react normally to all stimuli and to instilled drugs (Figure 10.5). Unequal pupils may be caused by primary eye disorders, such as iritis. Unilateral mydriasis is never due to isolated, unilateral visual loss. The reactivity of the normal eye and the consensual light reflex will ensure pupil size remains equal.

## The Pupillary Reflexes

The principal pupillary reflex responses assessed on examination are the light response and the near response ("accommodation"). The normal pupil constricts promptly in response to light.

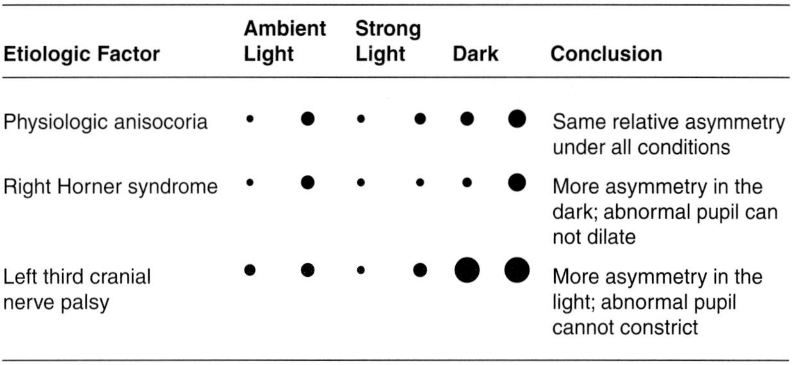

| Etiologic Factor | Ambient Light | Strong Light | Dark | Conclusion |
|---|---|---|---|---|
| Physiologic anisocoria | • ● | • ● | ● ● | Same relative asymmetry under all conditions |
| Right Horner syndrome | • ● | • • | • ● | More asymmetry in the dark; abnormal pupil can not dilate |
| Left third cranial nerve palsy | ● ● | • ● | ● ● | More asymmetry in the light; abnormal pupil cannot constrict |

FIGURE 10.5 ● Behavior of unequal pupils in light and dark conditions.

Pupillary constriction also occurs as part of the near response, along with convergence and rounding up of the lens for efficient near vision. Normally, the light and near responses are of the same magnitude.

## The Light Reflex

The light reflex should be tested in each eye individually. The examining light should be shone into the eye obliquely with the patient fixing at distance to avoid eliciting a confounding near response. A common error in pupil examination is to have the patient fixing at near, as by instructing her to look at the examiner's nose. This technique provides both a light stimulus and a near stimulus simultaneously, and the pupils may well constrict to the near target of the examiner's nose even when the reaction to light is impaired or absent. Using this technique, the examiner would invariably miss light-near dissociation. Always have the patient fix at a distance when checking the pupillary light reaction. The normal pupillary light reflex is brisk constriction followed by slight dilatation back to an intermediate state (pupillary escape). The responses may be noted as prompt, sluggish, or absent, graded from 0 to 4+, or measured and recorded numerically (e.g., 4 mm → 2 mm.) In comatose patients, it is often important, but difficult, to see if the pupillary light reaction is preserved, especially if there is a question of brain death. A useful technique is to use the ophthalmoscope: focus on the pupil with high positive magnification, dim the ophthalmoscope, and then rapidly reilluminate. Even a small residual reaction may be seen.

## The Accommodation Reflex

The accommodation or near reflex is elicited by having the patient relax accommodation by gazing into the distance, then shifting gaze to some near object. The best near object is the patient's own finger or thumb. The response consists of thickening of the lens (accommodation), convergence of the eyes, and miosis. The pupils constrict at near to increase the depth of focus. The midbrain mechanisms for pupillary constriction to near are separate from those for the light reflex; one response may be abnormal while the other is preserved.

## Effects of Drugs on the Pupil

Many systemically acting as well as locally acting drugs may influence pupil size and reactivity. An abnormal pupil may fail to respond appropriately, or respond excessively because of denervation supersensitivity. Sympathomimetics and anticholinergics cause pupillary dilation, and parasympathomimetics or sympathetic blockers cause pupillary constriction. Agents that cause mydriasis include the anticholinergics atropine, homatropine, and scopolamine and the sympathomimetics epinephrine,

## TABLE 10.1

**Summary of Pharmacologic Pupillary Testing for Horner Syndrome**

|  | First Order | Second Order | Third Order |
|---|---|---|---|
| Cocaine | No response | No response | No response |
| Hydroxyamphetamine | Dilates | Dilates | No response |

norepinephrine, phenylephrine, hydroxyamphetamine, and cocaine. Agents that cause miosis include the cholinomimetics pilocarpine, methacholine, muscarine, and opiates, and the cholinesterase inhibitors physostigmine and neostigmine. Pupillary pharmacology can be applied in the neurologic examination, primarily in the evaluation of Horner syndrome and Adie pupil (see Table 10.1).

### Disorders of the Pupil

Pupils can be abnormal for numerous reasons. Common problems include pupils that are too large or too small, unilaterally or bilaterally, or pupils that fail to demonstrate normal reflex responses.

The two conditions most commonly causing a unilaterally large pupil are third cranial nerve palsy and Adie tonic pupil. In CN III palsy, the large pupil has impaired reactions to light and to near; abnormalities of extraocular movement and eyelid position generally betray the origin of the abnormal pupil. With total CN III palsy there is complete ptosis; lifting the eyelid reveals the eye resting in a down and out position (Figure 10.1). Although CN III palsies often affect the pupil more than other functions, some ptosis and ophthalmoparesis is usually present. Since the pupillary parasympathetics occupy a position on the dorsomedial periphery of the nerve as it exits the brainstem, compressive lesions such as aneurysms generally affect the pupil prominently. Ischemic lesions tend to affect the interior of the nerve and spare the pupil, as in diabetic third nerve palsies, because the periphery of the nerve has a better vascular supply. This rule is not absolute. The pupil is usually involved early and prominently with third nerve compression due to uncal herniation (Hutchinson pupil).

The patient presenting with Adie tonic pupil is typically a young woman who suddenly notes a unilaterally enlarged pupil, with no other symptoms. The pupillary reaction to light may appear absent, although prolonged illumination may provoke a slow constriction. The reaction to near, although slow, is better preserved. Once constricted, the tonic pupil redilates very slowly when illumination is removed or the patient looks back at distance, often causing a transient reversal of the anisocoria. Adie syndrome is the association of the pupil abnormality with depressed or absent deep tendon reflexes, particularly in the lower extremities.

The term "tectal pupils" refers to the large pupils with light near dissociation sometimes seen when lesions affect the upper midbrain. Such pupils may accompany the impaired upgaze and convergence/retraction nystagmus of Parinaud syndrome. The variably dilated, fixed pupils reflecting midbrain dysfunction in a comatose patient carry a bleak prognosis. Acute angle closure glaucoma can cause severe frontotemporal headache and a dilated, poorly reactive pupil. Deliberately or accidentally instilled mydriatics will produce a dilated, fixed pupil.

Small pupils occur for many reasons. The pupils in the elderly are normally smaller. Many systemic drugs, such as opiates, may symmetrically shrink the pupils. Important neurologic conditions causing an abnormally small pupil include Horner syndrome and neurosyphilis.

### Horner Syndrome

In Horner syndrome, sympathetic dysfunction produces ptosis, miosis, and anhidrosis. Lack of sympathetic input to the accessory lid retractors results in ptosis and apparent enophthalmos. The ptosis of the upper lid is only 1 mm to 3 mm, never as severe as with a complete CN III palsy, although it may simulate partial third nerve palsy. The ptosis can be subtle and is often missed. The lower lid is frequently elevated 1 mm to 2 mm because of loss of the action of the lower lid accessory retractor that holds the lid down (inverse ptosis). The resulting narrowing of the palpebral fissure causes apparent enophthalmos. Since the fibers mediating facial sweating travel up the external carotid, lesions distal to the carotid bifurcation produce no facial anhidrosis except for perhaps a small area of medial forehead that is innervated by sympathetic fibers traveling with the internal carotid.

The small pupil in Horner syndrome dilates poorly in the dark. Pupillary asymmetry greater in the dark than in the light generally means Horner syndrome. Recall that physiologic anisocoria produces about the same degree of pupillary asymmetry in the light and dark. In contrast, third nerve palsy and Adie pupil cause greater asymmetry in the light because of the involved pupil's inability to constrict. Examining the eyes under light and dark conditions can help greatly in sorting out asymmetric pupils (Figure 10.5 and Figure 10.6). Should the examiner err by having the patient fixate at near during testing, the pupillary constriction in the good eye may lessen the asymmetry and cause the abnormal pupil to be missed. The pupil in Horner syndrome not only dilates less fully, it dilates less rapidly. In the first few seconds after dimming the lights, the slowness of dilation of the affected pupil may cause the anisocoria to be even more pronounced (dilation lag). There is more anisocoria at 4 to 5 seconds after lights out than at 10 to 12 seconds.

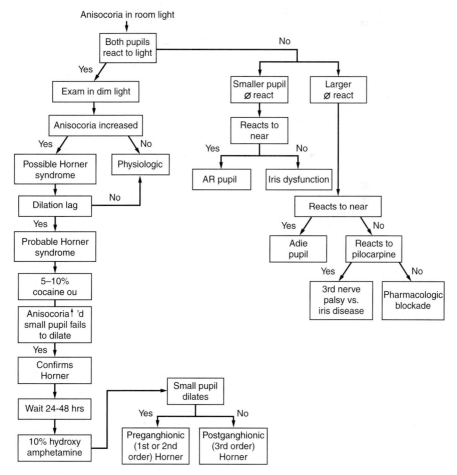

**FIGURE 10.6** ● Flow diagram for the evaluation of anisocoria.

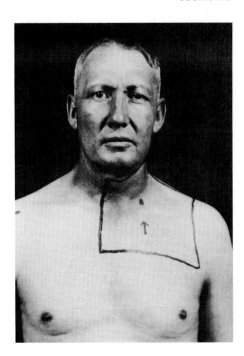

*FIGURE 10.7*  ●  Left Horner syndrome in a patient with a pulmonary sulcus tumor.

The causes of Horner syndrome are legion and include the following: brainstem lesions (especially of the lateral medulla), cluster headache, internal carotid artery thrombosis or dissection, cavernous sinus disease, apical lung tumors, neck trauma, and other conditions (Figure 10.7).

## Argyll Robertson Pupil

Argyll Robertson (AR) pupils are small (1 mm to 2 mm), irregular in outline, and have light near dissociation. They react poorly or not at all to light, but very well to near. Argyll Robertson pupils are the classic eye finding of neurosyphilis. Other conditions may cause an AR-like pupil. With the declining incidence of neurosyphilis, AR-like pupils with light near dissociation are increasingly likely to be of some other etiology.

## Pupils with Abnormal Reactions

Disruption of the afferent or efferent limbs of the pupillary reflex arcs, or disease of the brainstem pupil control centers, may alter pupil reactivity to light or near, as may local disease of the iris sphincter (e.g., old trauma). Disease of the retina does not affect pupil reactivity unless there is involvement of the macula severe enough to cause near blindness. Cataracts and other diseases of the anterior segment do not impair light transmission enough to influence the pupil. Because of the extensive side-to-side crossing of pupillary control axons through the posterior commissure, light constricts not only the pupil stimulated (the direct response) but also its fellow (the consensual response). The eye with a severed optic nerve will show no direct response, but will have a normal consensual response to a light stimulus in the other eye, as well as constriction to attempted convergence (amaurotic pupil). Lesser degrees of optic nerve dysfunction can often be detected by checking for an afferent pupillary defect (see next section). The pupil frozen because of third nerve palsy will have no near response and no direct or consensual light response, but the other eye will exhibit an intact consensual response on stimulation of the abnormal side (Table 10.2).

## TABLE 10.2

**Direct and Consensual Light Reaction**

Comparison of direct and consensual light reflex and pupillary constriction to the near reflex in the presence of a complete lesion of the right optic nerve versus the right oculomotor nerve. In both instances, the right pupil is frozen to direct light stimulation, and the distinction is made by the other reactions

|  | Complete Lesion CN II OD | | Complete Lesion CN III OD | |
|---|---|---|---|---|
|  | Response OD | Response OS | Response OD | Response OS |
| **Light stimulus OD** | No response | No response | No response | Normal |
| **Light stimulus OS** | Normal | Normal | No response | Normal |
| **Near reflex** | Normal | Normal | No response | Normal |

OD, right eye; OS, left eye.

The pupillary reaction to light is normally equal to or greater than the reaction to near. Light near dissociation refers to a disparity between the light and near reactions. The most common form is a poor light response but good constriction with the near response; it is relatively common, and there are a number of causes. The converse, better reaction to light than to near, is rare. In the routine case, if the pupillary light reaction is normal there is little to be gained by examining the near reaction.

The fibers mediating the pupillary light reflex enter the dorsal brainstem, but the near response fibers ascend to the EW nucleus from the ventral aspect. Disorders that affect the dorsal rostral brainstem may affect the light reaction but leave the near reaction intact. This anatomical arrangement likely explains many instances of the phenomenon of light near dissociation of the pupils. Pressure on the pupillary fibers in the region of the pretectum and posterior commissure (e.g., from pinealoma) impairs the light reaction. However, fibers mediating the near response, the EW nucleus, and the efferent pupil fibers are spared, which leaves the near response intact. Causes of light near dissociation include neurosyphilis, other lesions involving the dorsal rostral midbrain, diabetic autonomic neuropathy, Lyme disease, Adie pupil, aberrant regeneration of CN III, sarcoidosis, multiple sclerosis (MS), and severe retinal or optic nerve disease.

### Afferent Pupillary Defect

When testing the light reflex, the amplitude of the initial pupillary constriction and subsequent slight escape depend greatly on the specific circumstances of illumination. Therefore, the status of the light reflex must be judged by comparing the two eyes. With mild to moderate optic nerve disease, it is difficult to detect any change in pupil reactivity to direct light stimulation. Marcus Gunn described pathologic pupillary escape following 10 to 20 seconds of continued exposure, or the adapting pupillary response, due to optic nerve disease. Levitan described looking for the Marcus Gunn pupillary sign by swinging a light back and forth between the two eyes (swinging flashlight test, alternating light test; Levitan P. Pupillary escape in disease of the retina or optic nerve. *Arch Ophthalmol* 1959;62:768–779). He thought moving the light back and forth amplified the asymmetry of the pupillary escape. The swinging flashlight test is a very useful technique that can quickly and accurately compare the initial constriction and subsequent escape of the two pupils. It is a key clinical technique in the evaluation of suspected optic neuropathy, and it can often detect a side-to-side difference even when the lesion is mild and there is no detectable difference in the direct light reflex when testing each eye individually. An APD is an extremely useful and important neurologic sign. Some modify the term with "relative" (RAPD) to emphasize that the finding depends on the difference between the two eyes—the state of the afferent system and activity of the light reflex in one eye relative to the other eye. The shorter form, APD, is currently in more widespread use.

The presence of an APD depends on asymmetry in the afferent signal. A bilateral APD cannot occur, although a severe bilateral afferent defect may cause light near dissociation or abnormal pupillary escape. An APD can occur with bilateral optic neuropathy only if there is significant asymmetry of involvement. Media opacities will not cause an APD. In fact, mature cataract may so scatter the incoming light as to actually increase the light reflex and cause a minor APD in the opposite eye. Only severe retinal or macular disease will cause an APD, and then it will be slight. Maculopathy with 20/200 vision might cause a 1+ APD while optic neuropathy with 20/30 vision would cause a 3+ to 4+ APD. For simulation of an APD see *http://www.richmondeye.com/apd.asp.*

## Ocular Motility

The eyes move in the service of vision, bringing objects of regard into the field of vision and following them if they move. The different eye movement control systems (e.g., saccade, pursuit, vergence) normally function harmoniously to secure and maintain vision. The globe rotates around one or more of three primary axes that intersect at right angles at the center of rotation, 15.4 mm behind the cornea. Movement takes place perpendicular to the axis of rotation. Abduction and adduction are rotation in the horizontal plane about the vertical axis going from superior to inferior. Elevation and depression are up and down movements around the horizontal axis that runs from medial to lateral across the eye. The third axis runs from anterior to posterior; rotation about this axis is referred to as torsion. Intorsion is movement of the upper pole of the eye toward the nose; extorsion is movement away from the nose.

The eyes are said to be in primary position when gaze is straight ahead and the visual axes of the two eyes are parallel. Since the orbits diverge, primary position must be obtained by precisely adjusted contractions of the extraocular muscles, which are controlled by the cerebral cortex. When regarding an object, the extraocular muscles move the eyes so that the visual axes meet at the proper point to ensure that the object's image falls on corresponding points on each macula. The point where the visual axes meet is called the fixation point. Normal eye movements are usually conjugate in order to maintain binocular vision and stereopsis. The medical longitudinal fasciculus (MLF) coordinates the contractions of the yoked muscles and the relaxation of their antagonists so that the two eyes move together.

Monocular eye movements are referred to as ductions. During a duction, the agonist contracts and the antagonist relaxes. Binocular movements are referred to as versions. During version movements, the extraocular muscles work as yoked pairs (e.g., the lateral rectus in one eye contracts with the medial rectus in the other eye) (Figure 10.8). The yoke muscles are paired agonists for the binocular movement, and in each eye their respective antagonists must be reciprocally inhibited. Hering's law, or the law of equal innervation, states that the same amount of innervation goes to an extraocular muscle and to its yoked fellow. The amount of innervation to the yoked pair is always determined by the fixating eye. Hering's law is important in understanding the topic of primary and secondary deviations.

Patients with diplopia become symptomatic because of visual confusion. The confusion results because of discordant retinal images—one real, one not. Historical details are often helpful in deciphering the cause of diplopia. The first step should be to determine whether the diplopia is binocular or monocular. With binocular diplopia, covering one eye eliminates the visual confusion. Monocular diplopia persists when using the affected eye alone. Monocular diplopia is often considered a nonorganic symptom, but there are many organic causes, primarily ophthalmologic conditions such as cataract, corneal astigmatism, lens subluxation, retinal detachment, and macular disease.

Observant patients may be able to state whether the diplopia is horizontal or vertical, worse at near or distance, or worse in a particular direction of gaze; all are pertinent observations.

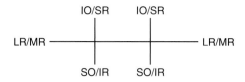

**FIGURE 10.8** ● The yoke muscles control extraocular movement in the six cardinal directions of gaze.

Horizontal diplopia usually results from dysfunction of the medial or lateral rectus muscles. Vertical diplopia tends to result from disorders of the oblique muscles, less often of the vertically acting recti. Patients with sixth nerve palsy have difficulty diverging the eyes and tend to have more diplopia at distance. The lateral recti are not active when the eyes are converging for near vision, and patients have less diplopia at near (reading) as compared to distance (driving). Conversely, patients with medial rectus weakness have difficulty converging with more diplopia at near and less at distance. Diplopia is worse with gaze in the direction of the involved muscle. The patient with either a right sixth nerve palsy or a left third nerve palsy will have more diplopia on right gaze. Patients with fourth nerve palsy often describe an obliquity or tilt to the image. A patient with diplopia may keep one eye closed or may tilt or turn the head to minimize the visual confusion. Associated symptoms may be important. Diplopia accompanied by ptosis may occur with third nerve palsy, as well as with myasthenia gravis and other neuromuscular disorders. Pain in the head or eye in association with diplopia suggests such conditions as diabetic third nerve palsy, posterior communicating aneurysm, ophthalmoplegic migraine, Tolosa-Hunt syndrome (painful ophthalmoplegia), and giant cell arteritis.

## Examination of Eye Movements

Assessment of ocular movements should include an assessment of visual acuity. When acuity is impaired, the patient may not be able to adequately fixate. This influences the results of various maneuvers used to assess motility, particularly the cover test. Note the position of the patient's head. Many patients with ocular malalignment will hold their head in an unusual position. Usually there is a turn or tilt that minimizes the diplopia.

Assuming reasonable visual acuity and normal head position, the motility examination begins with an assessment of fixation. A normal patient can fixate steadily on an object of regard, whether near or distant. Inability to maintain normal steady fixation may occur because of fixation instability, or saccadic intrusions, transient deviations away from fixation with a quick return.

In routine cases where there are no eye complaints and the likelihood of abnormality is low, the ocular motility examination is usually limited to assessing versional pursuit movements in the six cardinal positions of gaze, including full lateral gaze to each side, as well as upgaze and downgaze when looking to either side (Figure 10.8 and Figure 10.9). The target should slowly trace a large letter "H" for the patient to follow. Some add primary gaze plus upgaze and downgaze in the center to make nine cardinal positions. Eye movements should remain smooth and conjugate throughout. The six cardinal positions are designed to search for dysfunction of individual muscles or nerves, as well as supranuclear abnormalities of horizontal gaze. Assessment of upgaze and downgaze in primary position assesses the supranuclear vertical gaze mechanisms. Pursuit versions are done by asking the patient to follow a target held about 0.5 m to 1.0 m away, such as an examining light, a pointer, a pen, or the examiner's finger. A linear target should be held perpendicular to the direction of gaze, vertical for testing horizontal gaze, and horizontal for vertical gaze. Use of an examining light adds the ability to assess the corneal reflection, which gives objective evidence of ocular malalignment. The light reflection should be just medial to the center of the pupil and at corresponding points in each eye. The patient should indicate if she sees more than one target at any point. Pursuit movements are normally smooth. In certain disease states with abnormal pursuit,

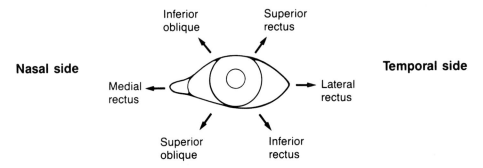

**FIGURE 10.9**  ●  Actions of the extraocular muscles on the left eye. Arrows denote the main directions of action for each muscle, resulting from a combination of movements of the globe in the three dimensions.

the tracking movements become disrupted by superimposed saccades, creating a ratchety or jerky movement termed saccadic pursuit (cogwheel eye movements). The finding is nonspecific and can occur bilaterally with fatigue, inattention, decreased consciousness, basal ganglia disorders, diffuse hemispheric disease, drug effects, or if the target velocity is too fast. Abnormal pursuit in one direction may indicate an ipsilateral deep occipito-parietal lobe lesion involving the pursuit pathways.

Normally the eyes can move through a range of about 45 degrees to either side of primary position. In absolute terms for the normal adult eye, the excursions are about 10 mm for adduction, abduction, and elevation, and about 7 mm for depression. The last 10 degrees of abduction is difficult to maintain and holding there may result in end point nystagmus, a normal physiologic phenomenon. In full lateral gaze, the temporal limbus abuts the lateral canthus; in full medial gaze, about the inner third of the nasal limbus is buried. A small rim of sclera showing on extreme abduction is not abnormal. Normally, the amount of scleral show on abduction is symmetric in the two eyes. Greater scleral show on full abduction in one eye than the other may be a subtle sign of abduction impairment.

The vergence system comes into play when an object moves toward or away from the observer. Dysconjugate eye movements, convergence or divergence, are required. The central mechanisms subserving adduction of the eyes for convergence are different from the mechanisms for adduction during conjugate gaze. Testing convergence is helpful in some circumstances, such as when the pupillary light reflex is not crisply normal (in order to look for light near dissociation of the pupils), or when there is anything to suggest an internuclear ophthalmoplegia (INO).

The saccadic system can be tested by having the patient rapidly refixate between two targets. The patient is instructed to switch gaze between one target, such as the examiner's nose, and an eccentric target, such as the examiner's finger held to one side. The examiner assesses the velocity, magnitude, and accuracy of the saccades, and compares adduction and abduction saccades in each eye and saccades in the two eyes. Saccadic velocity may be decreased globally in some conditions, such as MG, or selectively, such as slow adduction saccades in the involved eye in a unilateral INO. Saccades may be hypometric, falling short of target and requiring additional, smaller saccades to attain fixation, or hypermetric, overshooting the target and requiring saccades back in the opposite direction. In some conditions, reflex eye movements may be present when other movements are impaired. Vestibulo-ocular reflex movements can be examined by having the patient fix on a target, then passively moving the head from side to side, or up and down.

## Evaluation of Ocular Malalignment

Testing for diplopia and ocular malalignment may be subjective or objective. The subjective tests depend on the patient's observation of images, the objective tests on the examiner's observation of eye movements during certain maneuvers. Common subjective bedside evaluations include the red lens and Maddox rod tests; common bedside objective tests are the corneal light reflex tests and the cover tests (cover–uncover and alternate cover). The objective tests only require the patient to fixate; they do not require any subjective responses or interpretation of the color or separation of images.

## Subjective Tests

When a patient has diplopia due to extraocular muscle weakness, she sees two images. The real image falls on the macula of the normal eye. The false image falls on the retina beside the macula of the paretic eye. The brain is accustomed to images falling off the macula coming from peripheral vision, so it projects the false image peripherally. The farther away from the macula that the image falls, the farther peripherally the misinterpretation of its origin. As the eye moves in the direction of the paretic muscle, the separation of images increases, and the false image appears to be more and more peripheral. The false image is also usually fainter than the true image because extramacular vision is not as acute. The clarity, however, depends on the visual acuity in the two eyes. These considerations lead to three "diplopia rules" to identify the false object: (a) the separation of images is greatest in the direction of action of the weak muscle, (b) the false image is the more peripheral, and (c) the false image comes from the paretic eye.

The false image may be identified in different ways. The simplest is to move the patient's eyes into the position with the greatest separation of images. Then cover one eye. If the more peripheral image disappears, the covered eye is the paretic eye. The red lens (red glass) and Maddox rod tests are attempts to be more precise (see Toolkit). They may be especially useful when the diplopia is mild and the weak muscle or muscles not apparent from examination of ocular versions. The theory of the red lens test is sound, but often the results of testing in clinical practice are less than clear. One reason is that the red lens breaks fusion just enough to bring out unrelated phorias, which muddy the findings. The results of the red lens test may be drawn to aid interpretation. There should be a notation as to whether the diplopia fields are drawn as seen by the patient or as seen by the examiner (Figure 10.10).

## Objective Tests

The corneal light reflex test depends on observing the reflection of an examining light on the cornea, and estimating the amount of ocular deviation depending on the amount of displacement of the reflection from the center of the pupil. The test can only be done at near because distant reflections are too dim, so the confounding effects of the near reflex must be reckoned with. Each millimeter of light displacement from the center indicates 18 degrees of eye deviation.

## Cover Tests

The cover tests are predicated on forcing one eye or the other to fixate by occluding its fellow, and determining the drift of the nonfixing eye while it is under cover. Varieties of cover testing include

FIGURE 10.10 ● Red lens diplopia fields, drawn as seen by the examiner. The red lens is placed over the right eye, and the eyes move through the six cardinal positions of gaze with the patient looking at an examining light. White circles depict images coming from the left eye (white light); dark circles, images from the right eye (red light); and intermediate circles, images from both eyes (pink light).

the cover–uncover test and the alternate cover test. The cover–uncover test is used primarily by ophthalmologists to evaluate patients with congenital strabismus where there is an obvious squint. When neurologic patients have an obvious malalignment, its nature is usually apparent. The alternate cover test is used to evaluate more subtle deviations. For simulation of cover tests see http://www.richmondeye.com/eyemotil.asp.

## Optokinetic (Opticokinetic, Optomotor) Nystagmus

Optokinetic nystagmus (OKN) is a normal, physiologic phenomenon sometimes affected by disease. It is sometimes useful in evaluating disturbed ocular motility. Optokinetic nystagmus is conjugate nystagmus induced by a succession of moving visual stimuli. Optokinetic nystagmus occurs whenever the eyes must follow a series of rapidly passing objects, such as telephone poles zipping by a car or train window. Clinical testing entails moving a striped target, a rotating drum, or a cloth tape bearing stripes or squares in front of the patient and requesting that she "count" the stripes on the drum or the stripes or squares on the tape (Figure 10.11). A typical OKN tape would consist of a series of 2-in-square red patches placed 2 in apart on a white tape 1 yard long, which is drawn across the patient's field of vision. The toolkit contains a rudimentary OKN tape. Although OKN is more complex, it can be viewed for clinical purposes as testing pursuit ipsilateral to the direction of target movement, and contralateral saccades. The ipsilateral parieto-temporo–occipital junction mediates pursuit of the acquired stripe via connections that run in the internal sagittal stratum, deep in the parietal lobe medial to the geniculocalcarine radiations and adjacent to the atrium of the lateral ventricle. When ready to break off, it communicates with the ipsilateral frontal lobe, which then generates a saccadic movement in the opposite direction to acquire the next target. In normal, alert individuals, an OKN stimulus induces brisk nystagmus with the fast phase in the direction opposite tape movement. The response is intensified if the subject looks in the direction of the quick phase. Responses in one direction are compared with responses in the other direction. A vertically moving stimulus can evaluate upgaze and downgaze.

Patients with hemianopsias due to occipital lobe disease have a normal OKN response, despite their inability to see into the hemifield from which the tape originates. Because of interruption of the OKN pathways, patients with hemianopsias due to disease of the optic radiations in the deep parietal lobe have abnormally blunted or absent OKN responses. The patient is unable to pursue normally toward the side of the lesion and is unable to generate contraversive saccades into the blind hemifield.

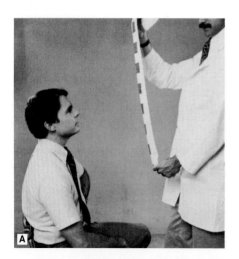 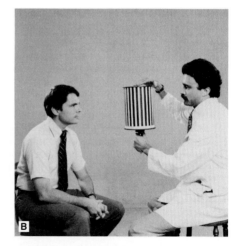

*FIGURE 10.11*  ●  Testing for optokinetic nystagmus. **A.** Using optokinetic tape. **B.** Using the rotating drum.

The significance of OKN asymmetry lies in the vascular anatomy and the differing pathologies that affect the parietal and occipital lobes. The primary clinical utility of OKN testing is investigation of patients with parieto-occipital lesions, but the OKN tape has other uses. It may be used to crudely check visual acuity, especially in infants, and for estimating visual function in patients with depressed consciousness. It may provide a clue to the presence of psychogenic visual loss. Optokinetic nystagmus testing can demonstrate the slowed adducting saccades of a subtle INO, and sometimes accentuate the nystagmus in the abducting eye. Optokinetic nystagmus forced upward saccades may induce convergence retraction nystagmus in patients with Parinaud syndrome.

## Disordered Ocular Motility

Abnormal eye movements can occur for many reasons. Disorders can be broadly divided into peripheral (infranuclear and nuclear) and central (internuclear and supranuclear). Peripheral disorders involve the extraocular muscles (e.g., MG or ocular myopathy) or the cranial nerves (e.g., fourth nerve compression). Peripheral disorders include things that affect the cranial nerve nuclei, fascicles, or peripheral trunks. Although the nuclei and fascicles are "central" in that they lie within the parenchyma of the CNS, the clinical characteristics of conditions involving these structures is much more akin to other infranuclear conditions than to supranuclear disorders. Central disorders can be divided into supranuclear, involving the optomotor control centers, and internuclear, involving the pathways connecting and coordinating the activity of the ocular motor nuclei, primarily the MLF. For simulation of disordered ocular motility see http://cim.ucdavis.edu/eyes/version1/eyesim.htm.

## Peripheral Disorders of Ocular Motility

Disturbances of ocular motility may result from processes involving the orbit causing mechanical limitation of eye movement, or from ocular myopathies, neuromuscular transmission disorders, or a palsy of an individual ocular motor nerve.

### Orbital Disease

Masses within the orbit may mechanically inhibit movement of the globe, often causing telltale proptosis as well. Following trauma to the orbit, individual extraocular muscles may become caught in fracture fragments. The muscles may also be injured directly. Mechanically limited eye excursions exist for passive as well as active movements. Forced ductions involve pushing or pulling on the anesthetized globe in order to passively move it through the impaired range. An eye affected by ocular muscle weakness, MG, or an ocular motor nerve palsy moves freely and easily through a full range. An eye affected by restrictive myopathy or an entrapped muscle cannot be moved passively any better than actively.

### Muscle Disease

Primary ocular muscle disease may cause impaired motility because of weakness or because of restriction of movement. A number of myopathies and muscular dystrophies may affect eye muscles. Muscle disorders may be divided into myopathies and restrictive orbitopathies. The most common restrictive orbitopathy is TED. Muscle involvement by restrictive myopathy is easily confused with weakness of the antagonist (e.g., restrictive myopathy of the medial rectus simulating weakness of the lateral rectus). Forced ductions are often done to clarify matters. The possibility of TED must be constantly borne in mind when dealing with ocular motility disturbances.

Primary muscle disorders cause weakness of the extraocular muscles, usually accompanied by ptosis. Associated weakness of eye closure due to myopathic involvement of the facial muscles is often present. Weakness of eye closure is strongly suggestive of ocular myopathy or neuromuscular transmission disorder as the cause of eye muscle weakness. Few other conditions affect both eye muscles and facial muscles. The common conditions causing ocular myopathy are chronic progressive external ophthalmoplegia and oculopharyngeal muscular dystrophy.

## Neuromuscular Transmission Disorders

Myasthenia gravis, the most common neuromuscular transmission disorder, frequently involves the extraocular muscles, affecting any muscle or combination of muscles. Ocular involvement occurs early in 50% to 70% of patients, and it eventually develops in 90%. Patients typically present with ptosis or diplopia, or both. The hallmark of MG is fatigable weakness. The weakness gets worse with repetitive contraction of the muscle. The ptosis in MG is "fatigable"; it gets progressively worse with prolonged upgaze. The eyelid signs of MG are discussed above. Fluctuating ptosis and diplopia, and worsening symptoms toward the end of the day are characteristic. The ptosis and ophthalmoparesis of MG are usually asymmetric and may vary from minute to minute. These features, along with accompanying weakness of eye closure, are virtually diagnostic. Myasthenia gravis should be considered in the differential diagnosis of virtually any patient with external ophthalmoplegia, but involvement of the pupil excludes MG.

## Individual Nerve Palsies

The same basic processes cause third, fourth, and sixth nerve palsies, but with different frequencies. As many as 25% of cases are idiopathic, and of these 50% recover spontaneously. Some processes may affect more than one ocular motor nerve. Trauma is the most common cause of fourth nerve palsy and the second most common cause of third and sixth nerve palsy. Microangiopathic vascular disease due to diabetes or hypertension is the most common etiology of nontraumatic third and sixth nerve palsies. Aneurysms are an important etiology of third nerve disease. Increased intracranial pressure may cause third nerve palsies because of uncal herniation and sixth nerve palsies as a nonspecific and nonlocalizing effect. Neoplasms may affect any of these nerves. Basilar meningitis, migraine, viral infection, immunizations, cavernous sinus disease, sarcoid, vasculitis, and Guillain-Barré syndrome are occasional etiologies; the list of rare etiologies is long.

## The Oculomotor Nerve

CN III palsy produces varying degrees and combinations of extraocular muscle weakness, ptosis, and pupil involvement. Internal ophthalmoplegia means involvement limited to the pupillary sphincter and ciliary muscle; external ophthalmoplegia means involvement of only the extraocular muscles; complete ophthalmoplegia is both. The most common identifiable etiologies are ischemia, aneurysm, tumor, and trauma; some 20% remain unexplained. Uncal herniation from mass effect of any sort may result in compression as the temporal tip crowds through the tentorial hiatus and traps CN III against the sharp edge of the tentorium. Posterior communicating or distal internal carotid aneurysms commonly cause third nerve palsy (Figure 10.12). With third nerve palsy, processes affecting the nucleus or fascicles within the brainstem generally produce accompanying neighborhood signs permitting localization (e.g., Weber or Benedikt syndrome). In its long course along the base of the brain, CN III may be affected in isolation. In the cavernous sinus (Figure 10.13) or orbit, accompanying deficits related to involvement of other structures usually permit localization.

Complete paralysis of the third nerve causes severe ptosis of the upper lid, impairment of medial, upward, and downward gaze and loss of accommodation, with a dilated pupil that does not react to light, directly or consensually, or to near (Figure 10.1). The eye rests in a down and out position due to preservation of the lateral rectus and superior oblique functions. Incomplete CN III lesions, causing paresis rather than paralysis and affecting certain functions more than others, are more common than complete ones.

## Localization of Oculomotor Nerve Lesions

Cranial nerve III palsy can occur because of lesions anywhere along its course from the oculomotor nucleus in the midbrain to the orbit. Midbrain lesions are usually accompanied by neighborhood signs that permit localization. Processes involving the third nerve nucleus may cause characteristic

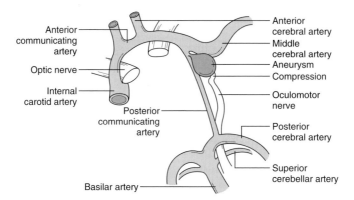

**FIGURE 10.12** ● Anatomy of the oculomotor nerve in relation to the major arteries at the base of the brain. An aneurysm arising from the posterior communicating artery is compressing and distorting the nerve.

patterns of weakness not seen with lesions at other locations. Processes involving the subarachnoid course of the nerve usually produce isolated unilateral CN III palsy with few associated findings to assist in localization. The most pressing diagnostic consideration in an isolated third nerve palsy is posterior communicating artery or basilar artery aneurysm. Ischemic third nerve palsies most often occur because of microvasculopathy related to diabetes and hypertension. Traumatic CN III palsy usually occurs only with major head injuries, severe enough to cause loss of consciousness or skull fracture. Increased intracranial pressure with uncal herniation most often compresses the ipsilateral nerve; the earliest sign is usually an abnormal pupil. Compression of the contralateral cerebral peduncle causing a false localizing hemiparesis ipsilateral to the lesion is not uncommon (Kernohan's notch syndrome). Cavernous sinus disease usually affects other structures in addition to CN III.

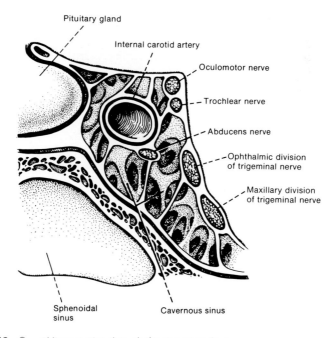

**FIGURE 10.13** ● Oblique section through the cavernous sinus.

## The Trochlear Nerve

Cranial nerve IV is slender and has a long intracranial course; these two factors increase its vulnerability to injury. The most common etiology of fourth nerve palsy is head trauma; bilateral involvement is not uncommon. Nontraumatic cases are usually microvascular, idiopathic, or congenital. A patient with a congenital fourth nerve palsy may decompensate as an adult and present as an apparently new onset condition. Patients with fourth nerve palsies may not complain of diplopia, but rather blurry vision or some vague problem when looking down—as when reading a book or descending stairs. The diplopia is vertical or diagonal and maximal in downgaze. Patients may tilt the head to the opposite side to eliminate diplopia, tucking the chin so the affected eye may ride up and into extorsion, out of the field of action of the weak superior oblique. Some fourth nerve palsies, particularly in children, present with head tilt rather than diplopia.

On examination there is extorsion and impairment of depression of the adducted eye. The involved eye has incomitant hypertropia or hyperphoria; with the patient looking down and in, alternate cover testing shows corrective downward refixations indicating upward drift of the affected eye under cover. The Bielschowsky head tilt test consists of tilting the head to each side, localizing the fourth nerve palsy by the changes in diplopia that result. Forcing the involved eye to intort worsens the diplopia. If diplopia improves with head tilt to the left and worsens with tilt to the right, the patient has a right fourth nerve palsy.

## The Abducens Nerve

Sixth nerve palsies are common, and many resolve with no explanation. With a complete CN VI palsy, the eye cannot be abducted and often rests in a position of adduction (Figure 10.14). Incomplete palsies are common. Patients present with horizontal diplopia worse at distance. There may be esotropia in primary position. Examination shows paralytic (noncomitant) strabismus, worse in the direction of action of the involved muscle. Mild weakness may show only esophoria on alternate

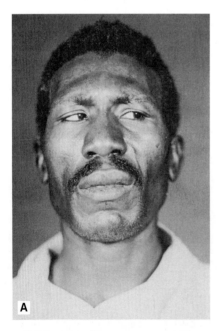 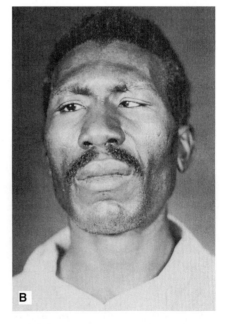

**A** **B**

*FIGURE 10.14* ● Paralysis of the right abducens nerve in a patient with a posterior fossa neoplasm. **A.** Patient looking to left. **B.** Patient attempting to look in the direction of action of the paralyzed muscle.

cover testing when the patient looks toward the side of the involved muscle. Neoplasms, trauma, and microvascular neuropathy are the most common identifiable etiologies. As many as 25% of cases remain unexplained. Neighborhood signs usually permit localization when the nerve is involved in the brainstem, cavernous sinus, or orbit. Sixth nerve palsies occur with increased intracranial pressure, after head injury, with structural disease in the middle or posterior fossa, with nasopharyngeal tumors, and for numerous other reasons. Cranial nerve VI palsies are the most common and classic of all false localizing signs: they are nonspecific and bear no necessary anatomical relationship to the central nervous system (CNS) pathology producing them. Bilateral sixth nerve palsies are not uncommon. Not all abduction failure is due to CN VI palsy. Some of the other causes include entrapment of the medial rectus by a medial orbital fracture, TED, MG, convergence spasm, divergence insufficiency, Duane syndrome, orbital pseudotumor, and Möbius syndrome.

## CENTRAL DISORDERS OF OCULAR MOTILITY

Central disorders can be divided into supranuclear and internuclear. Supranuclear disorders include those that affect the supranuclear gaze centers in the hemispheres and brainstem, as well as other areas that influence eye movements, such as the basal ganglia and cerebellum. Internuclear disorders affect the connections between the ocular motor nerve nuclei in the brainstem.

### Internuclear Ophthalmoplegia

Lesions of the MLF cause an INO. The contralateral medial rectus receives no signal to contract when the pontine paramedian reticular formation (PPRF) and sixth nerve nucleus act to initiate lateral gaze. As a result, gaze to one side results in abduction of the ipsilateral eye, but no adduction of its fellow. Typically the abducting eye has nystagmus as well, which may be sustained or only a few beats. Failure of the medial rectus to adduct is an isolated abnormality in the affected eye; normality of the lid and pupil distinguish an INO from a third nerve palsy. By convention, the INO is labeled by the side of the adduction failure; a right INO produces adduction failure of the right eye. Many brainstem lesions can cause an INO, but the common conditions are MS and brainstem stroke. Internuclear ophthalmoplegias due to MS are usually bilateral and seen in young patients, whereas those due to brainstem vascular disease are more often unilateral and seen in older patients.

### Gaze Palsies and Gaze Deviations

The frontal eye fields move the eyes into contralateral conjugate horizontal gaze. The eyes normally remain straight ahead because of a balance of input from the frontal eye fields in each hemisphere. Seizure activity in one frontal lobe drives the eyes contralaterally. In an adversive seizure, the eyes and then the head deviate to one side, after which the seizure may generalize. With destructive frontal lobe lesions, most often ischemic stroke, the patient is unable to move the eyes contralaterally—a gaze palsy, or, if less severe, a gaze paresis. The intact, normal hemisphere maintains its tonic input, the imbalance causing the eyes to move contralaterally, toward the diseased side—a gaze deviation. Patients may have gaze palsy without gaze deviation. The presence of gaze deviation usually means gaze palsy to the opposite side, but it may occasionally signal seizure activity.

Similar considerations apply to disease of the pons. The PPRF governs ipsilateral, conjugate horizontal gaze. The PPRF draws the eyes ipsilaterally, in contrast to the frontal eye fields, which force the eyes contralaterally. Destructive lesions of the PPRF impair the ability to gaze ipsilaterally, resulting in a gaze deviation toward the intact side as the normal PPRF pulls the eyes over. Pontine gaze palsies affect all functions, voluntary and reflex; even ice water calorics will not move the eyes.

When faced with a patient whose eyes rest eccentrically to one side, the possibilities are (a) frontal lobe seizure activity, (b) frontal lobe destructive lesion, and (c) pontine destructive lesion. Patients with destructive frontal lesions gaze away from the side of the hemiparesis; patients with pontine strokes gaze toward the hemiparesis. Epileptogenic gaze deviations are usually betrayed by a component of jerky eye movement and subtle twitches elsewhere.

## Vertical Gaze Abnormalities

Two common disorders affecting vertical gaze are Parinaud syndrome and progressive supranuclear palsy.

### Parinaud Syndrome

The core feature of Parinaud syndrome is impaired upgaze (Figure 10.4). Patients are unable to look up, and when they attempt it the eyes may spasmodically converge and retract backward into the orbits (convergence–retraction nystagmus). The convergence–retraction movements readily appear during forced upward saccades in response to a down-moving OKN tape. The retraction movement is best seen from the side. Parinaud syndrome usually results from a mass lesion involving the region of the posterior third ventricle and upper dorsal midbrain, such as a pinealoma. Other frequent signs include eyelid retraction and abnormal pupils. The pupils in Parinaud syndrome have a poor, rarely absent, light response and much better near response (tectal pupils).

### Progressive Supranuclear Palsy

In progressive supranuclear palsy, degenerative changes in the rostral brainstem and thalamus result in impairment first of downgaze, then of upgaze, and eventually in global gaze paresis. Reflex eye movements are preserved until late in the disease. The gaze abnormalities are accompanied by parkinsonian signs and a pronounced tendency to extensor axial rigidity.

### Nystagmus and Other Ocular Oscillations

Nystagmus is a complex topic. When faced with a patient with nystagmus or similar appearing movements, the usual clinical exercises include the following two steps: (a) deciding if the nystagmus indicates neurologic pathology and (b) if so, whether the pathology is central or peripheral. There are normal, physiologic forms of nystagmus. A few beats of nystagmus at the extremes of lateral gaze (end-point nystagmus) occur commonly in normals and have no pathologic significance. A whole host of conditions can cause nystagmus, including ocular disease, drug effects, peripheral vestibular disease, and CNS disease. Nystagmus may also be congenital. Schemes have classified nystagmus in many different ways. This discussion focuses on the types of nystagmus commonly encountered in neurologic practice and on the differentiation between nystagmus that likely signifies neurologic disease (neuropathologic) and the kind that does not (nonneuropathologic).

Nystagmus is classified in multiple ways: pendular (both phases of equal amplitude and velocity) versus jerk (a fast phase and a slow phase); central versus peripheral; induced versus spontaneous; and physiologic versus pathologic. Further characterizations include rapid/slow, coarse/fine, manifest/latent, sensory/motor, and horizontal/vertical. Pendular nystagmus is classified by its plane of movement, usually horizontal. Pendular nystagmus only rarely signifies neurologic disease, and this discussion is focused primarily on jerk nystagmus. Jerk nystagmus is classified by the direction of the fast phase. Alexander's law states that jerk nystagmus increases with gaze in the direction of the fast phase. First-degree nystagmus is present only with eccentric gaze (e.g., right-beating nystagmus on right gaze). Second-degree nystagmus is present in primary gaze and increases in intensity with gaze in the direction of the fast component (e.g., right-beating nystagmus in primary gaze increasing with gaze to the right). With third-degree nystagmus, the fast component continues to beat even with gaze in the direction of the slow component (e.g., right-beating nystagmus persisting even with gaze to the left). Dissociated nystagmus is different in the two eyes (e.g., the nystagmus in the abducting eye in INO).

### Nonneuropathologic Nystagmus

Nystagmus that does not signify neurologic disease may be physiologic, or due to ocular disease (e.g., poor vision), or other conditions.

## Physiological Nystagmus

Types of physiologic nystagmus include end-point, OKN, and induced vestibular. Although these types of nystagmus are normal, they may be altered when disease is present in such a way as to assist in localization. End-point nystagmus is fine, variably sustained nystagmus at the extremes of lateral gaze, especially with gaze eccentric enough to eliminate fixation by the adducting eye. Symmetry on right and left gaze, abolition by moving the eyes a few degrees toward primary position, and the absence of other neurologic abnormalities generally serve to distinguish end-point from pathologic nystagmus. End-point nystagmus is the most common form of nystagmus seen in routine clinical practice. Although OKN is a normal response, its characteristics may be altered in disease. Changes in OKN occur primarily with deep parietal lobe lesions. Vestibular nystagmus can be induced by rotation (e.g., Barany chair) or by irrigation of the ear with hot or cold water.

## Other Forms of Nonneuropathologic Nystagmus

Types of nystagmus that are not physiologic, but do not result from neurologic disease include voluntary nystagmus, drug induced nystagmus, congenital nystagmus, and nystagmus due to ocular disease.

## Neuropathologic Nystagmus

Nystagmus is a frequent manifestation of disease of the nervous system. Common types include vestibular, positional, gaze evoked, and gaze paretic nystagmus. Symmetric, equal activity of the vestibular systems on each side normally maintains the eyes in straight-ahead, primary position. Vestibular imbalance causes the eyes to deviate toward the less active side as the normal side overcomes the weakened tonic activity from the hypoactive side. In an alert patient, the frontal eye fields generate a saccade to bring the eyes back toward primary position, creating the fast phase of vestibular nystagmus. When the cortex does not generate a correcting saccade, as in coma, only the tonic deviation develops; the eyes deviate toward the ice-water-irrigated ear.

Degenerative changes in the otoliths frequently produce the syndrome of positional vertigo and nystagmus. Nystagmus occurs after a latency of up to 30 seconds, beats with the fast phase toward the down ear, quickly fatigues despite holding the position, and adapts with repeated attempts to elicit it. Positional nystagmus is a very common condition. While generally peripheral it may occur with central disease (tumor, stroke, MS, degenerative disease).

Any nystagmus not present in primary gaze but appearing with gaze in any direction with the fast phase in the direction of gaze is referred to as gaze-evoked nystagmus. Normal physiologic end-point nystagmus is gaze evoked, but only present horizontally and at extremes of gaze. Abnormal gaze-evoked nystagmus occurs short of extreme gaze and is more sustained than end point. Drug-induced nystagmus is gaze evoked, usually horizontally and in upgaze. Nystagmus with the same appearance in the absence of drug effects is nonspecific but usually indicates disease of the cerebellum or cerebellar connections. Gaze paretic nystagmus is a form of gaze-evoked nystagmus seen in patients with incomplete gaze palsies. Rather than having an absolute inability to gaze in a particular direction, the patient achieves full lateral gaze transiently but is not able to maintain it. The eyes drift back toward neutral and then spasmodically jerk back in the desired gaze direction.

## Other Disorders of Ocular Motility

Other types of abnormal eye movements include ocular bobbing, ocular flutter, and opsoclonus. Ocular flutter and opsoclonus are types of saccadic intrusions, spontaneous saccades away from fixation; they may be confused with nystagmus. Ocular dysmetria is an over- or under-shooting of the eyes on rapid refixation of gaze toward either side or on returning to the primary position that requires corrective saccades.

# CHAPTER 11

# The Trigeminal Nerve

The trigeminal, or fifth cranial, nerve (CN V) has a large sensory part that innervates the face, teeth, oral and nasal cavities, the scalp back to the vertex, and the intracranial dura; and a much smaller motor part that innervates the muscles of mastication. The sensory component has 3 divisions: the first, or ophthalmic division (CN $V_1$), the second or maxillary division (CN $V_2$), and the third or mandibular division (CN $V_3$). The motor and principal sensory nuclei are located in the midpons. The spinal tract and nucleus, which subserve pain and temperature, extend from the pons down into the upper cervical spinal cord. The mesencephalic root receives proprioceptive fibers.

## Examination of the Motor Functions

Assessment of trigeminal motor function is accomplished by examining the muscles of mastication. Bulk and power of the masseters and pterygoids can be gauged by palpating these muscles as the patient clenches the jaw. An effective technique is to place the examining fingers along the anterior, not lateral, border of the masseters bilaterally. When the jaw is clenched the fingers will move forward; this movement should be symmetric on the two sides. Unilateral trigeminal motor weakness causes deviation of the jaw toward the weak side on opening (Figure 11.1). Subtle deviation on jaw opening is often the earliest clue to the presence of an abnormality. It is occasionally difficult to be certain whether the jaw is deviating or not. Note the relationship of the midline notch between the upper and lower incisor teeth; it is a more reliable indicator than lip movement. The tip of the nose and the interincisural notches should line up. A straightedge against the lips can help detect deviation. Another useful technique is to draw a vertical line across the midline upper and lower lips. Failure of the two vertical marks to match when the jaw is opened indicates deviation. If there is any suggestion of a problem, have the patient move the jaw from side to side. With unilateral weakness the patient is unable to move the jaw contralaterally. With facial weakness there may be apparent deviation of the jaw, and of the tongue, because of the facial asymmetry. Holding up the weak side manually will sometimes eliminate the pseudodeviation.

Other techniques for examining trigeminal motor function include having the patient protrude and retract the jaw, noting any tendency toward deviation; and having the patient bite on tongue depressors with the molar teeth, comparing the impressions on the two sides and comparing the difficulty of extracting a tongue depressor held in the molar teeth on each side.

Unilateral weakness of CN V innervated muscles generally signifies a lesion involving the brainstem, Gasserian ganglion, or the motor root of CN V at the base of the skull. Severe bilateral weakness of the muscles of mastication with inability to close the mouth (dangling jaw) suggests

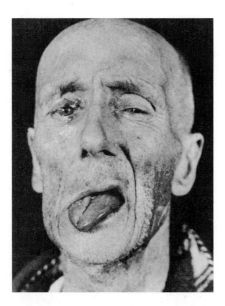

**FIGURE 11.1** ● Infranuclear paralysis of the right trigeminal, facial, and hypoglossal nerves in a patient with metastatic carcinoma, showing deviation of the tongue and mandible to the right.

motor neuron disease, a neuromuscular transmission disorder, or a myopathy. With significant atrophy of one masseter, a flattening of the jowl on the involved side may be apparent (Figure 11.2). With temporalis atrophy there may be a hollowing of the temple. Rarely, fasciculations or other abnormal

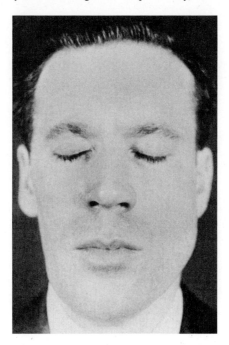

**FIGURE 11.2** ● Infranuclear paralysis of the right trigeminal nerve with atrophy of the muscles of mastication.

involuntary movements occur. There is no reliable or realistic method for examination of the other muscles supplied by CN V. Because of bilateral innervation, unilateral upper motor neuron lesions rarely cause significant impairment of trigeminal motor function. There may be mild, transitory unilateral weakness. The amount of involvement depends on the extent of decussation. In bilateral supranuclear lesions there may be marked paresis.

## Examination of the Sensory Functions

In testing facial sensation, touch, pain, and occasionally temperature are examined in the same manner as elsewhere on the body, searching for areas of altered sensation. It is better to ask the patient if the stimuli feel the same on the two sides, rather than suggesting they might feel different. Sometimes it is useful to examine the nostrils, gums, tongue, and insides of the cheeks. Proprioception cannot be adequately tested, but one can test for extinction and the ability to identify figures written on the skin.

There are three common exercises in evaluating facial sensation: (a) determining whether sensory loss is organic or nonorganic, (b) determining which modalities are involved, and (c) defining the distribution. Complaints of facial numbness are common, and not all are organic. However, real facial sensory loss can be a serious finding, occasionally signifying underlying malignancy. The various methods and tricks for detecting nonorganic sensory loss are not entirely reliable, and this diagnosis should be made with caution. Patients with nonorganic sensory loss may have a demarcation of the abnormal area at the hairline rather than the scalp vertex. On the lower face functional sensory loss tends to follow the jaw line and involve the notch over the masseter muscle, which is not trigeminal innervated (Figure 11.3). On the trunk, organic sensory loss typically stops short of midline because of the overlap from the opposite side, and splitting of the midline suggests

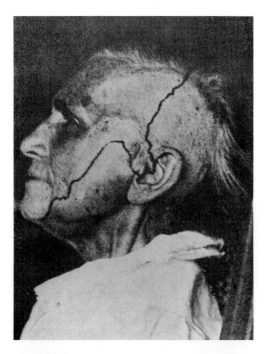

**FIGURE 11.3** ● The distribution of sensory loss following complete section of the trigeminal root. Note the large area at the angle of the jaw that is innervated by C2 through the greater auricular nerve, and the inclusion of the tragus of the ear in the trigeminal distribution.

nonorganicity. This finding is not reliable on the face because there is less midline overlap on the face, so organic facial sensory loss may extend to the midline. The corneal and sternutatory reflexes should be normal in nonorganic sensory loss. Splitting of vibration along the midline is reputedly a nonorganic sign. Because the frontal bone and mandible are single bones, there should be no difference in vibratory sensibility on either side of midline. Patients who report a difference in vibratory sensibility on testing just to either side of midline may have nonorganic sensory loss. The reliability of this sign has not been validated; it can be misleading. Other signs suggestive of nonorganicity include dissociation between pinprick and temperature, variability from trial to trial, history of hypochondriasis, secondary gain, la belle indifference, nonanatomical sensory loss, and changing boundaries of hypalgesia.

## Examination of the Reflexes

The corneal, sternutatory, and jaw reflexes are the reflexes most often assessed in evaluating the trigeminal nerve. Many other reflexes have been described, but they are of limited value and are seldom used. The afferent limbs of these reflexes are trigeminal mediated. In some the efferent limb is also trigeminal (e.g., the jaw jerk); in others the efferent limb is executed through connections with CN III, CN VII, or other pathways.

## The Jaw, Masseter, or Mandibular Reflex

To elicit the jaw (or jaw muscle) reflex, the examiner places an index finger or thumb over the middle of the patient's chin, holding the mouth open about midway with the jaw relaxed, then taps the finger with the reflex hammer. The response is an upward jerk of the mandible. Other methods to elicit the reflex include tapping the chin directly and placing a tongue blade over the tongue or the lower incisor teeth and tapping the protruding end. All of these cause a bilateral response. A unilateral response may sometimes be elicited by tapping the angle of the jaw or by placing a tongue blade over the lower molar teeth along one side and tapping the protruding end.

The afferent impulses of this reflex are carried through the sensory portion of the trigeminal nerve, possibly through the mesencephalic root, and the efferent impulses through its motor portion; the reflex center is in the pons. In normal individuals, the jaw jerk is minimally active or absent. Its greatest use is in distinguishing limb hyper-reflexia due to a cervical spine lesion (where the jaw jerk is normal) from a state of generalized hyper-reflexia (where the jaw jerk is increased along with all of the other reflexes). The jaw reflex is exaggerated with lesions affecting the corticobulbar pathways above the motor nucleus, especially if bilateral, as in pseudobulbar palsy or amyotrophic lateral sclerosis (ALS). It is sometimes possible to elicit extra beats or jaw clonus.

## The Corneal Reflex

The corneal reflex is elicited by lightly touching the cornea with a wisp of cotton or tissue. It is used to assess CN $V_1$ function. The stimuli should ideally be delivered to the upper cornea, because the lower cornea may be CN $V_2$ innervated in some individuals. The stimulus should be brought in from below or from the side so the patient cannot see it (Figure 11.4). The stimulus must be delivered to the cornea, not the sclera. If there is any evidence of eye infection, different pieces of cotton or tissue should be used for the two eyes. Crude stimuli, such as a large blunt object or fingertip should never be used, even in comatose patients.

In response to the corneal stimulus, there should be blinking of the ipsilateral (direct reflex) and contralateral (consensual reflex) eyes. The afferent limb of the reflex is mediated by CN $V_1$, the efferent limb by CN VII.

With a unilateral trigeminal lesion both the direct and consensual responses may be absent; neither eye blinks. Stimulation of the opposite eye produces normal direct and consensual responses. With a unilateral CN VII lesion the direct response may be impaired, but the consensual reflex should

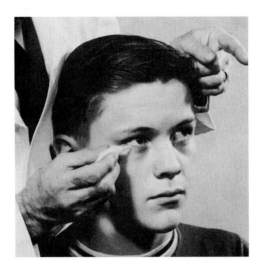

**FIGURE 11.4** ● Eliciting the corneal reflex. The stimulating object should be brought in outside the patient's vision. The patient should look upward as the object is brought in from below, or laterally as the object is brought in from the other side. The stimulus must be applied to the cornea, not the sclera.

be normal. Stimulation of the opposite side produces a normal direct response but an impaired consensual response. These patterns are summarized in Table 11.1. Lesions involving the brainstem polysynaptic trigeminofacial connections may produce impairment of both direct and consensual responses. The corneal reflex may be depressed with lesions of the contralateral hemisphere, especially if there is thalamic involvement. Because of the descent of the spinal tract and nucleus of CN V into the upper cervical cord, lesions there sometimes affect the corneal reflex. Corneal sensation may be impaired in contact lens wearers, even when the lenses are out.

## The Sternutatory (Nasal, Sneeze) Reflex

Stimulation of the nasal mucous membrane with cotton, a spear of tissue, or similar object causes wrinkling of the nose, eye closure, and often a forceful exhalation resembling a feeble sneeze, as

## TABLE 11.1

**Patterns of Direct and Consensual Corneal Reflex Abnormality with Trigeminal and Facial Nerve Lesions**

|  |  | Direct Corneal Reflex | Consensual Corneal Reflex |
|---|---|---|---|
| Complete Trigeminal Nerve Lesion |  |  |  |
|  | Stimulate involved eye | Absent | Absent |
|  | Stimulate opposite eye | Normal | Normal |
| Complete Facial Nerve Lesion |  |  |  |
|  | Stimulate involved eye | Absent | Normal |
|  | Stimulate opposite eye | Normal | Absent |

the nose tries to rid itself of the foreign object. The ophthalmic, not the maxillary, division of the trigeminal innervates the nasal septum and the anterior nasal passages. The afferent limb of the reflex arc is carried over CN $V_1$, the efferent limb over CNs V, VII, IX, X, and the motor nerves of the cervical and thoracic spinal cord. The reflex center is in the brainstem and upper spinal cord. The primary clinical use of the sternutatory reflex is as a cross-check on the corneal reflex.

## DISORDERS OF FUNCTION

Trigeminal nerve lesions may cause weakness, abnormal involuntary movements, sensory loss or other sensory abnormalities, facial pain, trophic abnormalities, autonomic dysfunction, or abnormalities of the reflexes mediated by the trigeminal nerve. The conditions most commonly seen are facial pain, particularly trigeminal neuralgia, and facial numbness.

### Motor Dysfunction

Because of the bilateral hemispheric innervation, weakness in the trigeminal distribution does not often occur with upper motor neuron lesions, although slight weakness of the contralateral muscles with an exaggerated jaw reflex can occur. Bilateral supranuclear lesions, as in pseudobulbar palsy or ALS, can cause marked weakness, often with a grossly exaggerated jaw reflex. In supranuclear lesions no atrophy or fasciculations occur.

Significant weakness in the trigeminal motor distribution is most often the result of a neuromuscular transmission disorder or ALS. Patients with myasthenia gravis may have chewing difficulties with masticatory fatigue, especially when eating difficult-to-chew things such as tough meat. Patients with severe polymyositis, rarely with other myopathies, may also have difficulty with jaw power. Patients with giant cell arteritis commonly have jaw claudication with focal pain in the masseter when chewing, which can be confused with weakness. Amyotrophic lateral sclerosis commonly causes a jaw drop, often with dysphagia and difficulty swallowing saliva, requiring the patients to constantly keep absorbent materials at their mouth. Lesions anywhere along the course of the lower motor neuron can cause weakness accompanied by atrophy, sometimes marked; fasciculations; and a decreased jaw jerk (Figure 11.1).

Abnormal involuntary movements commonly affect the jaw. Oromandibular dystonia produces a variety of abnormal movements: jaw opening, jaw closing, lateral movements, bruxism, and combinations of these. Jaw dystonia may occur as part of an extrapyramidal syndrome due to psychoactive drugs, and abnormal jaw movements are a common manifestation of tardive dyskinesias. Meige syndrome is oromandibular dystonia and blepharospasm. Chewing movements and grinding of the teeth are sometimes present in psychoses, and chewing or tasting movements in complex partial seizures. Trismus is marked spasm of the muscles of mastication. The teeth are tightly clenched, the muscles hard and firm, and the patient is unable to open the jaw. It is a classical manifestation of tetanus. Some myopathies, especially polymyositis, may result in fibrosis of the masseters, which causes painless trismus.

### Sensory Dysfunction

Supranuclear lesions, particularly of the parietal lobe or sensory radiations, may raise the sensory threshold of the contralateral face; a thalamic lesion may cause facial hypesthesia with hyperpathia or allodynia. Lesions of the principal sensory nucleus in the pons may cause diminished tactile sensation involving both skin and mucous membranes on the involved side, and loss of reflexes in which the afferent arc is mediated by the trigeminal nerve. Lesions of the spinal tract or nucleus cause a disturbance of the pain and temperature modalities, and, possibly to a lesser extent, of tactile sense.

Dissociation of sensation, with different degrees of involvement of light touch as compared to pain and temperature suggests a lesion in the substance of the brainstem (intramedullary), where the different sensory pathways are running in widely separate locations. Extramedullary lesions are characterized by loss or diminution of all types of exteroceptive sensation, dysesthesias or paresthesias, or spontaneous pain. A lesion central to or at the Gasserian ganglion will affect all three divisions; a lesion peripheral to the ganglion will involve only isolated divisions or branches. There may also be reflex changes, such as absence of the corneal or sternutatory.

The most common disorder to involve trigeminal sensory function is trigeminal neuralgia (TN), or tic douloureux. Trigeminal neuralgia causes paroxysms of fleeting but excruciating unilateral facial pain. It usually involves the second or third division, rarely the first. The lancinating pain lasts only seconds, but it may occur many times per day. Stimulation of some specific area, a trigger zone, in the involved nerve distribution will often provoke a paroxysm of pain. Pain may be brought on by activities such as talking, chewing, brushing teeth, exposure to cold, or by wind on the face. Male patients may present with the trigger zone unshaven. The patient may be reluctant to allow neurologic examination of the involved area for fear of triggering a paroxysm of pain. Patients with idiopathic TN have no clinical motor or sensory deficit in the distribution of the involved nerve.

The most common cause of TN is compression of the sensory root by an ectatic arterial loop of the basilar artery, most commonly the anterior inferior cerebellar or superior cerebellar. Rarely, structural lesions may cause facial pain resembling TN. These may cause sensory loss in the involved distribution, motor dysfunction, or involve neighboring structures. Examples include multiple sclerosis (MS), tumors involving the Gasserian ganglion or its branches, and other tumors in the cerebellopontine angle. MRI in idiopathic trigeminal neuralgia is rarely abnormal except for vascular loops. The presence of a complaint of numbness, impaired sensation on examination, other neurologic abnormalities, history of symptom progression, and duration of symptoms of less than 1 year greatly increase the likelihood of an abnormal imaging study.

Trigeminal neuralgia occurs in MS patients much more commonly than in the general population; it is usually caused by a demyelinating lesion involving the trigeminal root entry zone in the pons.

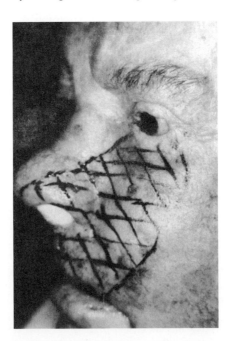

*FIGURE 11.5* ●  Patient with infraorbital neuropathy from carcinomatous infiltration. Note that the maxillary division innervates only the side of the nose distally. This patient had numbness of only the anterior teeth and gums, which proved the lesion was at the infraorbital foramen and not intracranially. (From Campbell WW. The numb cheek syndrome: a sign of infraorbital neuropathy. *Neurology* 1986;36:421–3.)

## TABLE 11.2

### Some Causes of Trigeminal Sensory Neuropathy

Idiopathic
Connective tissue disorder
   Sjögren syndrome
   Scleroderma
   Mixed connective tissue disorder
   Other
Sarcoidosis
Wegener granulomatosis
Giant cell arteritis
Multiple sclerosis
Tumor
Diabetes
Syringobulbia
Toxins
   Trichlorethylene
   Stilbamidine
   Mefloquine

Bilateral tic douloureux is especially suggestive of MS. Most TN patients are in the fifth decade or beyond; the onset in a young person should prompt consideration of demyelinating disease. The term atypical facial pain is used to refer to a syndrome of facial pain that does not have the characteristics of TN. The pain in atypical facial pain is typically chronic, not restricted to a single trigeminal division,

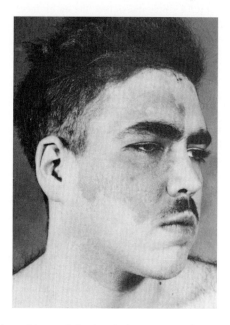

*FIGURE 11.6* ● A patient with encephalotrigeminal angiomatosis (Sturge-Weber syndrome).

not lancinating, and not associated with any trigger zone. No identifiable etiology is usually apparent, and the pain is often attributed to depression or other emotional factors.

Acute herpes zoster (HZ) of the trigeminal nerve is extremely painful. It is usually seen in elderly or immunocompromised patients. HZ most often affects CN $V_1$, causing pain and vesicles over the forehead, eyelid, and cornea (herpes ophthalmicus), but may affect any of the trigeminal divisions, and there may be motor involvement. Ophthalmic involvement may lead to keratitis, corneal ulcerations, residual corneal scarring, and sometimes results in blindness.

## Postherpetic Neuralgia

In some patients with trigeminal HZ, particularly the elderly, the pain of the acute phase evolves into a dreadful, persistent neuralgic pain syndrome called postherpetic neuralgia. Pain persisting for more than one month after the acute eruption is appropriately labeled as postherpetic neuralgia. The pain is probably related to deafferentation and mediated centrally. It is typically dysesthetic with a burning component, constant but with superimposed paroxysms of lancinating pain that may be provoked by touching certain spots within the affected area. There may be hypesthesia or hyperesthesia in the affected area.

## Facial Numbness

Isolated facial numbness is a common problem. A number of processes, some ominous, may be responsible. The numb chin syndrome refers to hypesthesia and sometimes paresthesias involving the lower lip and chin, approximately in the distribution of the mental nerve. The numb chin syndrome is often due to a neoplastic process, with metastasis either to the mental foramen of the mandible or to the intracranial meninges or skull base, often from carcinoma of the breast or lung. The numb cheek syndrome is similar but usually due to a lesion involving the infraorbital nerve (Figure 11.5). The numb chin or cheek syndrome can be the presenting manifestation of cancer. Unusual causes of trigeminal sensory dysfunction include pontine hemorrhage, Wegener granulomatosis, localized hypertrophic mononeuropathy, and a midbrain lesion affecting the crossed trigeminothalamic fibers.

Trigeminal sensory neuropathy refers to a syndrome of isolated facial numbness, usually gradual in onset, which may involve a single division or the entire face; it is occasionally bilateral. Some cases are idiopathic, but many underlying diseases, particularly connective tissue disorders, can cause trigeminal sensory neuropathy (Table 11.2).

## Other Trigeminal Nerve Disorders

Pathology involving the trigeminal nerve and its connections may result in misdirection of nerve fibers, producing unusual and interesting effects. Congenital ocular aberrant innervation syndromes are a complex group of disorders involving abnormal miswiring of the extraocular muscles. The Marcus Gunn phenomenon, or jaw-winking, occurs in patients with congenital ptosis; opening the mouth, chewing, or lateral jaw movements cause an exaggerated reflex elevation of the ptotic lid. The phenomenon may be the result of proprioceptive impulses from the pterygoid muscles being misdirected to the oculomotor nucleus. Involuntary closure of one eye on mouth opening (reversed Gunn phenomenon, inverse jaw winking, or Marin Amat sign) is a synkinesia due to aberrant regeneration of the facial nerve; it occurs most often following Bell palsy. The auriculotemporal (Frey) syndrome produces flushing, warmness, and excessive perspiration over the cheek and pinna on one side following ingestion of spicy food. This syndrome is due to misdirection of the secretory fibers to the parotid gland to the sweat glands and vasodilator endings in the auriculotemporal nerve distribution; it usually follows trauma or infection of the parotid gland or local nerve injury. In encephalotrigeminal angiomatosis (Sturge-Weber syndrome, or Weber-Dimitri disease), there are congenital nevi or angiomas over one side of the face in the trigeminal distribution with associated ipsilateral leptomeningeal angiomas and intracortical calcifications with attendant neurologic complications (Figure 11.6).

# CHAPTER 12

# The Facial Nerve

T he facial, or seventh, cranial nerve (CN VII) has two components: the motor root, which makes up about 70% of the fibers, and the sensory root, which accounts for 30%. The motor portion innervates the muscles of facial expression and the muscles of the scalp and ear. The sensory root (nervus intermedius of Wrisberg) contains both sensory and autonomic fibers. It carries parasympathetic secretory fibers to the submandibular and sublingual salivary glands and to the lacrimal gland. Its most important sensory function is to mediate taste from the anterior two-thirds of the tongue. Anatomically the motor division of the nerve is separate from the sensory and parasympathetic portions.

The supranuclear innervation to the muscles of facial expression arises from the lower third of the contralateral precentral gyrus in the facial area of the motor homunculus and descends in the corticobulbar tract into the pons, then decussates to converge on the facial nuclei. The portion of the nucleus that innervates the lower half to two-thirds of the face has predominantly contralateral supranuclear control; the portion that innervates the upper third to half has bilateral control.

## Examination of the Motor Functions

Examination of facial nerve motor functions centers on assessment of the actions of the muscles of facial expression. A great deal can be learned from simple inspection. At rest the face is generally symmetric, at least in young individuals. With aging, the development of character lines may cause asymmetry that does not indicate disease. Note the tone of the muscles of facial expression, and look for atrophy and fasciculations. Note the resting position of the face and whether there are any abnormal muscle contractions. Note the pattern of spontaneous blinking for frequency and symmetry. A patient with parkinsonism may have infrequent blinking and an immobile, expressionless, "masked" face. Facial dystonia causes an abnormal fixed contraction of a part of the face, often imparting a curious facial expression. Progressive supranuclear palsy may cause a characteristic facial dystonia with knitting of the brows and widening of the palpebral fissures (omega sign). Synkinesias are abnormal contractions of the face, often subtle, synchronous with blinking or mouth movements; they suggest remote facial nerve palsy with aberrant regeneration. Spontaneous contraction of the face may be due to hemifacial spasm (HFS). Other types of abnormal involuntary movements that may affect the facial muscles include tremors, tics, myoclonic jerks, chorea, and athetosis.

Observe the nasolabial folds for depth and symmetry and note whether there is any asymmetry in forehead wrinkling or in the width of the palpebral fissures with the face at rest. A flattened nasolabial fold with symmetric forehead wrinkles suggests a central (upper motor neuron) facial

119

palsy; a flattened nasolabial fold with smoothing of the forehead wrinkles on the same side suggests a peripheral (lower motor neuron) facial nerve palsy. Eyelid position and the width of the palpebral fissures often provide subtle but important clinical clues. A unilaterally widened palpebral fissure suggests a facial nerve lesion causing loss of tone in the orbicularis oculi muscle, the eye closing sphincter; this is sometimes confused with ptosis of the opposite eye. It is a common misconception that facial nerve palsy causes ptosis.

Observe the movements during spontaneous facial expression as the patient talks, smiles, or frowns. Have the patient grin, vigorously drawing back the angles of the mouth and baring the teeth. Note the symmetry of the expression, how many teeth are seen on each side and the relative amplitude and velocity of the lower facial contraction. Have the patient close her eyes tightly and note the symmetry of the upper facial contraction. How completely the patient buries the eyelashes on the two sides is a sensitive indicator of comparative orbicularis oculi strength.

Other useful movements include having the patient raise the eyebrows, singly or in unison, and noting the excursion of the brow and the degree of forehead wrinkling; close each eye in turn; corrugate the brow; puff out the cheeks; frown; pucker; whistle; alternately smile and pucker; contract the chin muscles; and pull the corners of the mouth down in an exaggerated frown to activate the platysma. The platysma can also be activated by having the patient open the mouth against resistance or clinch the teeth. The patient may smile spontaneously after attempting to whistle, or the examiner may make an amusing comment to assess emotional facial movement. Because of their paucity of facial expression, patients with Parkinson disease may fail to smile after being asked to whistle: the whistle-smile (Hanes) sign.

Trying to gently push down the uplifted eyebrow may detect mild weakness. It is difficult to pry open the tightly shut orbicularis oculi in the absence of weakness. Vigorously pulling with the thumbs may sometimes crack open a normal eye. If the examiner can force the eye open with her small fingers, then the orbicularis oculi is definitely weak. Likewise, it is difficult to force open the tightly pursed lips in a normal individual. When the orbicularis oris sphincter is impaired, the examiner may be able to force air out of the puffed cheek through the weakened lips. With stapedius weakness, the patient may complain of hyperacusis, especially for low tones.

## Examination of the Sensory Functions

Testing of CN VII sensory functions is limited to taste. The peripheral receptors are the taste buds embedded in the tongue epithelium, and to a lesser extent in the soft palate and epiglottis. Taste is also carried through CN IX and probably CN X. There are four primary tastes, in order of decreasing sensitivity in humans: bitter, sour, sweet, and salty. A fifth modality, umami (delicious or savory), may exist in response to compounds of some amino acids. The many flavors encountered in life are a combination of the four primary tastes plus olfaction and oral sensory information ("mouth feel"). Sweet and salty substances are most commonly employed for clinical bedside testing due to their ready availability. Cranial nerve VII only subserves taste on the anterior two-thirds of the tongue. When the tongue is retracted into the mouth, there is rapid dispersion of the test substance outside the area of interest. The tongue must therefore remain protruded throughout testing of an individual substance, and the mouth must be rinsed between tests.

Since the patient will be unable to speak with the tongue protruded, instructions must be clear in advance. A damp applicator stick may be dipped into a packet of sugar, artificial sweetener or salt and coated with the test substance, then placed on one side of the patient's tongue and rubbed around. The patient signals whether she can identify the substance. Most patients will identify the test substance in less than 10 seconds. Taste sensation is less on the tip of the tongue, and the substance is best applied to the dorsal surface at about the junction of the anterior and middle third of the tongue. The sweetness of artificial sweeteners such as saccharine and aspartame is more intense, and they may make better test substances than ordinary sugar.

## TABLE 12.1

**Possible Causes of Disturbed Taste**

Oral and perioral infections (e.g., candidiasis, gingivitis, periodontitis)
Bell palsy
Medications
Dental procedures
Dentures and other dental devices
Age
Nutritional compromise (e.g., vitamin $B_{12}$ deficiency, zinc deficiency,
   malnutrition, chronic disease)
Lesions involving neural taste pathways
Head trauma
Toxic chemical exposure
Radiation treatment of head and neck
Psychiatric conditions (e.g., depression, anorexia nervosa, bulimia)
Epilepsy (gustatory aura)
Migraine headache (gustatory aura)
Sjögren syndrome
Multiple sclerosis
Endocrine disorders (e.g., diabetes mellitus, hypothyroidism)

Modified from Bromley, SM. Smell and taste disorders: a primary care approach. *Am Fam Physician* 2000;61:427–36,438.

The most common situation calling for assessment of taste is the evaluation of facial nerve palsy. If a patient with a peripheral pattern of facial weakness has impaired taste, the lesion is proximal to the junction with the chorda tympani. A lesion at or distal to the stylomastoid foramen (e.g., in the parotid gland) does not affect taste.

Ageusia is the complete inability to taste. With hypogeusia, taste perception is blunted or delayed. Perversions or abnormal perceptions of taste are parageusias. Some causes of disturbed taste are listed in Table 12.1.

## DISORDERS OF FUNCTION

Motor abnormalities, either weakness or abnormal movements, account for the preponderance of clinical abnormalities of facial nerve function. Changes in sensation, primarily taste, and in secretory function sometimes occur as a sidebar, but are rarely if ever the major manifestation of disease of CN VII. Changes in these functions can help to localize the lesion along the course of the nerve. The major branches in sequence are the greater superficial petrosal, nerve to the stapedius, and chorda tympani, after which the nerve continues to the facial muscles. The mnemonic tear-hear-taste-face may help recall the sequence.

### Facial Weakness

There are two types of neurogenic facial nerve weakness: peripheral, or lower motor neuron; and central, or upper motor neuron. Peripheral facial palsy (PFP) may result from a lesion anywhere from the CN VII nucleus in the pons to the terminal branches in the face. Central facial palsy (CFP) is due to a lesion involving the supranuclear pathways before they synapse on the facial nucleus. PFP results from an ipsilateral lesion, whereas CFP, with rare exception, results from a contralateral lesion.

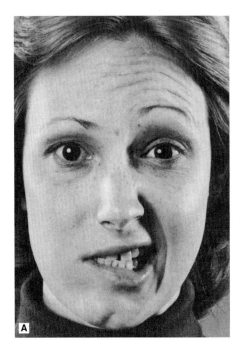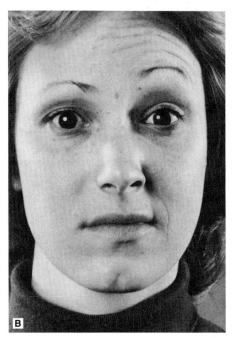

**FIGURE 12.1** ● A patient with a peripheral facial nerve palsy on the right. **A.** Patient is attempting to retract both angles of the mouth. **B.** Patient is attempting to elevate both eyebrows.

### Peripheral Facial Palsy

With PFP, there is flaccid weakness of all the muscles of facial expression on the involved side, both upper and lower face, and the paralysis is usually complete. The affected side of the face is smooth; there are no wrinkles on the forehead; the eye is open; the inferior lid sags; the nasolabial fold is flattened; and the angle of the mouth droops (Figure 12.1). The patient cannot raise the eyebrow, wrinkle the forehead, frown, close the eye, laugh, smile, bare the teeth, blow out the cheeks, whistle, pucker, retract the angle of the mouth, or contract the chin muscles or platysma on the involved side. She talks and smiles with one side of the mouth, and the mouth is drawn to the sound side on attempted movement. The cheek is flaccid and food accumulates between the teeth and the paralyzed cheek; the patient may bite the cheek or lip when chewing. Food, liquids, and saliva may spill from the corner of the mouth. The cheek may puff out on expiration because of buccinator weakness. The facial asymmetry may cause an apparent deviation of the tongue. A patient with an incomplete PFP may be able to close the eye, but not with full power against resistance. Inability to wink with the involved eye is common. The palpebral fissure is open wider than normal, and there may be inability to close the eye (lagophthalmos). During spontaneous blinking, the involved eyelid tends to lag behind, sometimes conspicuously. Attempting to close the involved eye causes a reflex upturning of the eyeball (Bell phenomenon). The iris may completely disappear upwardly.

A sensitive sign of upper facial weakness is loss of the fine vibrations palpable with the thumbs or fingertips resting lightly on the lids as the patient tries to close the eyes as tightly as possible. Labials and vowels are produced by pursing the lips; patients with peripheral facial weakness have a great deal of difficulty in articulating these sounds. Because of weakness of the lower lid sphincter, tears may run over and down the cheek, especially if there is corneal irritation because of inadequate eye protection. A lack of tearing may signal very proximal involvement, above the origin of the greater superficial petrosal nerve. With severe weakness, the eye never closes, even in sleep.

The facial weakness in PFP is obvious on both voluntary and spontaneous contraction. There is no dissociation. With a severe lesion, the passage of time may lead to atrophy of the involved muscles. With PFP the motor limb of the direct corneal reflex is impaired but the consensual is intact; in the opposite eye the direct response is intact and the consensual impaired (Table 12.1); in other words, the involved eye does not blink no matter which side is stimulated, and the normal eye does blink no matter which side is stimulated. In comatose or otherwise uncooperative patients, facial movements can be elicited by painful pressure over the supraorbital nerves, or by other painful stimuli applied to the face to elicit an avoidance response.

## Localization of Peripheral Facial Nerve Palsy

The weakness of the muscles of facial expression is the same with lesions anywhere along the course of the nerve proximal to the pes anserinus. Diagnostic localization depends on the associated findings, such as hyperacusis, decreased tearing, impaired taste, and involvement of neural structures beyond CN VII. The most common cause of PFP by far is Bell palsy.

## Bell Palsy

Idiopathic facial paralysis (Bell palsy) frequently follows a viral infection or an immunization. Symptoms often begin with pain behind the ear, followed within a day or two by facial weakness. There is peripheral facial weakness involving both upper and lower face. The paralysis is complete in approximately 70% of patients. About 25% of patients report some degree of facial numbness that is often dismissed as an odd sensation related to the immobility. Depending on the relationship of the lesion to the geniculate ganglion, to the takeoff of the chorda tympani, and to the takeoff of the branch to the stapedius, patients may note loss of taste sensation on the ipsilateral anterior two-thirds of the tongue, dryness of the eye, or hyperacusis for low tones.

Aberrant regeneration is common after Bell palsy and after traumatic nerve injury. Axons destined for one muscle regrow to innervate another, so that there is abnormal twitching of the face outside the area of intended movement. On blinking or winking, the corner of the mouth may twitch. On smiling the eye may close (Marin Amat sign, Figure 12.2). These synkinesias can be

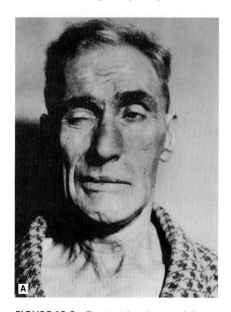
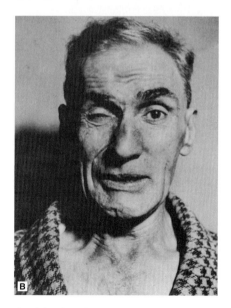

*FIGURE 12.2* ● Facial synkinesias following right peripheral facial paralysis. **A.** Patient attempting to close the eye. **B.** Patient attempting to retract the angle of the mouth.

prominent in some patients; more often they are subtle, such as a slight twitch of the orbicularis oris synchronous with blinking of the eye. Aberrant regeneration may also involve autonomic and taste fibers. The syndrome of crocodile tears is a gustatory-lacrimal reflex, characterized by tearing when eating, especially highly flavored foods. It is due to misdirection of salivary axons to the lacrimal gland. Frey auriculotemporal syndrome is similar, but with sweating and flushing over the cheek rather than lacrimation.

## Other Causes of Peripheral Facial Weakness

There are numerous other causes of PFP. Common processes involving the motor neurons of the CN VII nucleus in the pons include motor neuron disease and Möbius syndrome. In spinobulbar muscular atrophy (Kennedy syndrome), facial fasciculations and facial weakness are often prominent. Facial nerve paralysis, unilateral or bilateral, may be congenital. Möbius syndrome (congenital oculofacial paralysis) is the association of congenital facial nerve palsy with paralysis of the extraocular muscles, especially the lateral rectus, due to hypoplasia or aplasia of the cranial nerve nuclei.

Lesions involving the facial nerve fibers in the pons may cause PFP. There are usually associated findings to indicate the lesion is intramedullary. Many disorders may affect the intrapontine fibers of CN VII. Ischemic lesions are common. Because of the proximity of the nucleus and fibers of CN VII to the nucleus and fibers of CN VI, pontine lesions frequently cause both an ipsilateral facial paralysis and an ipsilateral lateral rectus paralysis.

Mass lesions in the cerebellopontine angle, such as acoustic neuroma and meningioma, commonly extend to involve CN VII, the nervus intermedius, CN VIII, CN V, the cerebellar peduncles, and the cerebellum. There is usually hearing loss, facial sensory changes, ipsilateral ataxia, and nystagmus. In Ramsay Hunt syndrome (herpes zoster oticus) the PFP is due to a reactivation of varicella zoster virus involving the geniculate ganglion. There may be vesicles on the tympanic membrane, in the external auditory canal, on the lateral surface of the pinna and in the cleft between the ear and mastoid process.

Patients with diabetes mellitus have a four- to fivefold increased risk of developing acute PFP. Slowly progressive facial weakness can occur with neoplasms involving either the pons or the facial nerve peripherally. Both HIV infection and Lyme disease can occasionally present with facial neuropathy. PFP due to Lyme disease is particularly prone to be bilateral. Fractures of the petrous bone due to closed head injury may injure the facial nerve. Melkersson syndrome (Melkersson-Rosenthal syndrome) is characterized by recurrent attacks of facial palsy, nonpitting facial and lip edema, and a congenitally furrowed and fissured tongue (lingua plicata, scrotal tongue); it is sometimes familial and usually begins in childhood. Its cause is unknown.

Bilateral facial palsy (facial diplegia) refers to bilateral PFP; it is much less common but much more ominous than unilateral PFP. Bilateral facial weakness can also occur because of neuromuscular disorders, including myasthenia gravis, bulbospinal neuronopathy, and muscle disease. Myopathic facies are particularly typical of facioscapulohumeral muscular dystrophy.

When bilateral facial weakness is due to disease of CN VII, the differential diagnosis includes bilateral Bell palsy, sarcoidosis, Lyme disease, diabetes, head trauma, HIV infection, Guillain-Barré syndrome, Miller Fisher syndrome, carcinomatous or lymphomatous meningitis, tuberculous or fungal meningitis, pontine tumor, Melkersson-Rosenthal syndrome, pseudotumor cerebri, Möbius syndrome, and a long list of other conditions.

## Facial Weakness of Central Origin

In a supranuclear, upper motor neuron or central facial palsy (CFP), there is weakness of the lower face, with relative sparing of the upper face. The upper face has both contralateral and ipsilateral supranuclear innervation, and cortical innervation of the facial nucleus may be more extensive for the lower face than the upper. The paresis is rarely complete.

A lesion involving the corticobulbar fibers anywhere prior to their synapse on the facial nerve nucleus will cause a CFP. Lesions are most often in the cortex or internal capsule. There is considerable individual variation in facial innervation, and the extent of weakness in a CFP may vary from the lower half to two-thirds of the face. The upper face is not necessarily completely spared, but it is always involved to a lesser degree than the lower face.

Even if there is some degree of upper facial involvement in a CFP, the patient is always able to close the eye, Bell phenomenon is absent, the corneal reflex is present, and the orbicularis oculi reflex may be exaggerated. In CFP the lower face is weak, the nasolabial fold is shallow, and facial mobility is decreased. However, the lower face weakness is never as severe as with a PFP, which suggests that there may be some direct cortical innervation to the lower face as well as the upper. Separating CFP and PFP is rarely difficult.

There are two variations of CFP: (a) volitional, or voluntary; and (b) emotional, or mimetic. In most instances of CFP, the facial asymmetry is present both when the patient is asked to smile or show the teeth, and during spontaneous facial movements such as smiling and laughing. However, spontaneous movements and deliberate, willful movements may show different degrees of weakness. When asymmetry is more apparent with one than the other, the facial weakness is said to be dissociated. Facial asymmetry more apparent with spontaneous expression, as when laughing, is called a mimetic, emotive, or emotional facial palsy; weakness more marked on voluntary contraction, when the patient is asked to smile or bare her teeth, is called a volitional facial palsy. Volitional facial palsy may result from a lesion in the cortex or in the subcortical corticobulbar pathways as they go through the internal capsule, the cerebral peduncle, or the pons above the facial nucleus. Facial weakness seen only with emotional movements most commonly results from thalamic or striatocapsular lesions, usually infarction, rarely with brainstem lesions.

## Abnormal Facial Movements

Some conditions involving the face produce abnormal movements rather than weakness. Common disorders causing abnormal facial movements include aberrant regeneration due to facial nerve palsy, blepharospasm, hemifacial spasm, and facial myokymia. Hemifacial spasm (HFS) usually arises de novo, due to intermittent compression by an ectatic arterial loop in the posterior circulation, most often a redundant loop of the anterior inferior cerebellar artery. The compression is usually near the anterior aspect of the root exit zone; arterial pulsations are thought to cause demyelination and focal nerve damage leading to ephaptic transmission and ectopic excitation. Hemifacial spasm usually develops in older patients. Twitching usually begins in the orbicularis oculi, and initially may be subtle and difficult to distinguish from facial synkinesias. Fully developed HFS causes repetitive, paroxysmal, involuntary, spasmodic, tonic, and clonic contractions of the muscles innervated by the facial nerve on the involved side of the face. The mouth twists to the affected side, the nasolabial fold deepens, the eye closes, and there is contraction of the frontalis muscle (Figure 12.2). Synkinesias due to aberrant regeneration following PFP may cause movements resembling HFS. The essential difference is that synkinesias are provoked by a voluntary movement, whereas HFS is a spontaneous, involuntary contraction. Blepharospasm causes involuntary twitching that primarily involves the orbicularis oculi and frontalis muscles. Blepharospasm is most often idiopathic or "essential" and is a form of focal dystonia. It is most often bilateral. Tic, or habit spasm, can cause a movement resembling HFS or blepharospasm. Bizarre grimacing movements of the face are usually habit spasms.

Facial myokymia is a continuous, involuntary muscular quivering that has a rippling, worm-like, appearance. It is usually unilateral. Facial myokymia has been reported with numerous conditions, most intrinsic to the brainstem. It is a classic feature of multiple sclerosis, but may also occur with pontine tumor, Guillain-Barré syndrome, and other conditions. Disease of the basal ganglia or extrapyramidal system may involve the facial muscles causing hypokinesia or hyperkinesia. Parkinson disease causes hypokinesia. Forms of facial hyperkinesias include dyskinesias, choreiform, athetoid, dystonic, grimacing, and myoclonic movements and tremors. Oral-facial dyskinesias are common, most often as a tardive manifestation of psychoactive drug use.

## Other Abnormalities

Except for disturbances of taste, sensory abnormalities are not a common part of facial nerve lesions. Taste may be affected with lesions of the facial nerve proximal to the takeoff of the chorda tympani. Geniculate neuralgia causes paroxysmal pain deep in the ear, sometimes radiating to the face. Cranial nerve VII is involved in lacrimation and salivation; lesions of the nerve at or proximal to the geniculate ganglion can cause abnormalities of these functions.

# CHAPTER 13

# The Acoustic (Vestibulocochlear) Nerve

The vestibulocochlear, acoustic, or eighth cranial nerve (CN VIII) has two components, the vestibular and the cochlear, blended into a single trunk. The cochlear portion subserves hearing; the vestibular nerve subserves equilibration, coordination, and orientation in space.

## THE COCHLEAR NERVE

### Clinical Examination

Some information about hearing may be obtained simply by observation and gauging the patient's ability to understand soft and loud tones and low and high pitches; note signs of deafness, such as a tendency to turn the head when listening, lip reading, or speaking with a loud voice. Any history of hearing difficulty, such as trouble using the telephone or hearing conversation in noisy environments, or complaints from family members, should prompt a careful evaluation. Before testing hearing, otoscopic examination should be done to ensure the tympanic membrane is intact, and to exclude the presence of wax, pus, blood, foreign bodies, and exudate. The mastoid region should be examined for swelling and tenderness.

Conductive hearing loss is that due to impaired conduction of sound to the cochlea and may be due to occlusion of the external auditory canal, middle ear disease (e.g., otitis), or abnormality of the ossicular chain (e.g., otosclerosis). Sensorineural hearing loss is that due to disease of the cochlea (e.g., Ménière disease) or eighth cranial nerve (e.g., acoustic neuroma). Central hearing loss is that due to disease of the central pathways. Central hearing loss is very rare because of the bilaterality and redundancy of the auditory system; unilateral lesions of the central auditory pathways typically do not cause any deficit detectable by routine clinical testing.

There are many ways to assess hearing at the bedside. All are crude compared to the information that can be obtained with a formal audiogram. Bedside clinical testing of hearing may theoretically use any available instrument that is capable of making a sound. Because the ability to hear and understand speech is the most important functional aspect of audition, whispered voice is useful; clinically significant hearing loss is usually detectable using this simple modality. In certain types of deafness, loss of speech discrimination is of clinical significance, even though pure tone and even speech thresholds are normal. One key to the effective use of whisper is unpredictability of the stimulus, for example, the numbers, "1, 2, 3" in one ear and "7, 8, 9" in the other. Monosyllables are preferable to common stock questions such as "How are you?" in which hearing a small part may enable the patient to "hear" the rest in context. Alternating words and numbers is a challenging test of hearing. Other useful sounds for bedside testing include finger rub and pure tones created by a tuning fork.

Detailed testing of hearing is done monaurally, ideally while occluding the opposite ear, as by pressing the tragus over the canal, and the patient is asked to compare the sound intensity between the two ears. The examiner may also compare the distance from each ear at which a sound of the same intensity can be heard.

Tuning forks—typically 128, 256, or 512 Hz—are sometimes used to give more specific information and to assess air conduction (AC) and bone conduction (BC). The patient may be asked to compare the loudness of the vibrating fork in the two ears, or the examiner may compare the distance on each side at which the fork begins or ceases to be heard. The examiner with good hearing may compare the patient's air and bone conduction with his own. In evaluating BC, be certain the patient hears rather than feels the tuning fork.

The Rinne test compares the patient's AC and BC; it can be done in at least two ways. An activated fork may be placed first on the mastoid process, then immediately beside the ear (or vice versa), and the patient asked which is louder; it should always be louder by the ear. The more time-consuming, traditional method is to place the tuning fork on the mastoid and when no longer heard then move it beside the ear, where it should still be audible. The fork should be heard twice as long by AC as by BC. The Rinne test is normal or positive when AC is better than BC. In conductive hearing loss, AC is impaired but BC is preserved; sound is not conducted normally through the canal or from the tympanic membrane through the ossicular chain to the cochlea, but the sensorineural mechanisms are intact. In sensorineural hearing loss (SNHL), both AC and BC are impaired while retaining their normal relationship of AC better than BC

In the Weber test, a vibrating tuning fork is placed in the midline on the vertex of the skull. It may be placed anywhere in the midline, over the nasal bridge, forehead, or maxilla, but works best over the vertex. Normally, the sound is heard equally in both ears or seems to resonate somewhere in the center of the head; it is "not lateralized." In conductive hearing loss, the sound is heard better on ("lateralized to") the involved side. In sensorineural deafness, the sound is heard best in the normal ear.

In summary, with unilateral conductive hearing loss (CHL) there is primarily loss of AC; BC is preserved or even exaggerated and the Weber lateralizes to the involved side (Table 13.1). With unilateral SNHL, AC and BC are both diminished, but AC remains better than BC, and the Weber lateralizes to the normal ear. With CHL, low tones are lost, as are some of the broad or flat consonants and vowels such as m, n, l, r, o, and u. Impairment of speech discrimination parallels the loss for pure tones. There is no recruitment, and tone decay is normal. Patients with CHL tend to hear speech better in a noisy background than in a quiet setting. In SNHL, the hearing loss is worse for higher frequencies, and there is greater difficulty with sibilants, sharp consonants, and short vowels (e.g., in the words sister, fish, twenty, water, and date). Auditory reflex responses that

## TABLE 13.1

### Rinne and Weber Tests

Normally the auditory acuity is equal in both ears, air conduction is greater than bone conduction (Rinne test normal or positive) bilaterally, and the Weber test is nonlateralizing (midline). The table depicts the pattern on the involved side with *unilateral* conductive or sensorineural hearing loss

|  | Auditory Acuity | Rinne Test | Weber Test |
|---|---|---|---|
| Conductive hearing loss | Decreased | BC > AC (Rinne negative or abnormal) | Lateralizes to abnormal side |
| Sensorineural hearing loss | Decreased | AC > BC (Rinne positive or normal) | Lateralizes to normal side |

produce a blink or reflex eye closure in response to a loud, sudden noise are occasionally useful in evaluating hearing in children, patients with altered mental status, and in hysteria or malingering. Mixed hearing loss, with elements of both CHL and SNHL, is not uncommon.

## Disorders of Function

Dysfunction of the cochlear nerve and its connections usually causes either diminution or loss of hearing (hypacusis or anacusis), with or without tinnitus. Conductive hearing loss is due to interference with the transmission of sound to the cochlea. Sensorineural hearing loss is due to disease of the cochlea or its central connections. In essence, CHL is due to disease external to the oval window, and SNHL is due to disease central to the oval window. Some causes of hearing loss are listed in Table 13.2.

Sensorineural hearing loss may be due to disease of the cochlea (end-organ deafness), such as in Ménière disease, or to disease of CN VIII or more central structures (retrocochlear), as in acoustic neuroma. Audiographic findings typical of cochlear disease are loss of acuity for pure tones with a parallel impairment of speech discrimination, recruitment, and tone decay. Recruitment is an abnormal loudness of sounds due to cochlear dysfunction, which can cause a paradoxical increase in the perception of louder sounds, sometimes accompanied by sound distortion. Retrocochlear lesions tend to cause a loss of speech discrimination out of proportion to the loss for pure tones, no recruitment, and abnormal auditory adaptation by tone decay.

The cochlear and vestibular nerves run together in a common sheath from the brainstem to their respective end organs, and disorders of the eighth nerve between the cochlea and brainstem may cause hearing loss. Some disease processes affect both divisions peripherally (e.g., labyrinthitis) or centrally (e.g., brainstem neoplasm). In its course across the cerebellopontine angle (CPA), the most important disorder to affect both divisions is a neoplasm. Acoustic neuroma (acoustic

## TABLE 13.2

### Causes of Hearing Loss

Conductive hearing loss
    External auditory canal obstruction (e.g., cerumen, foreign bodies, water, blood)
    Perforation of the tympanic membrane
    Disease of the middle ear
    Disease of the nasopharynx with obstruction of the eustachian tube
Sensorineural hearing loss
    Disease of the cochlea
        Acoustic trauma
        Ménière disease
        Infections
        Congenital conditions (e.g., congenital rubella)
        Presbycusis
    Disease of the cochlear nerve or nuclei
        Tumors (e.g., acoustic neuroma)
        Trauma (e.g., skull fracture)
        Infection (meningitis, syphilis)
        Toxins or drugs
        Presbycusis
        Nuclear lesions (e.g., vascular, inflammatory, or neoplastic)
Lesions of the central auditory pathways

neurinoma, acoustic schwannoma) is the most common, but neurofibroma, meningioma, facial nerve schwannoma, cholesteatoma, epidermoid cyst, and other tumors may arise in the CPA as well. Other conditions that may cause both hearing loss and vertigo include Ménière disease, labyrinthitis, viral infection (especially herpes), trauma, meningitis, vascular occlusion (internal auditory or anterior inferior cerebellar), Susac syndrome, Cogan syndrome, Fabry disease, perilymphatic fistula, toxins, and drugs.

Nonorganic hearing loss refers to hearing loss in the absence of any organic disease, or hearing loss that is exaggerated. It is more common for real hearing loss to be exaggerated in severity than for it to be feigned with entirely normal hearing. In most instances nonorganic hearing loss is a transient symptom related to acute emotional stress. It may be partial or total, unilateral or bilateral. It is often bilateral and total, and the patient makes no attempt to hear what is said or to read the speaker's lips. The mainstay of diagnosis is inconsistency in the performance on hearing tests and the absence of verifiable abnormalities on objective tests. Psychogenic hearing loss may be associated with other nonorganic symptoms, such as mutism and blindness. Patients simulating bilateral deafness do not behave as a deaf person does. Deaf individuals usually raise their voices during conversation and keep their eyes fixed on the speaker's face and lips, watching for any gesture that may help understanding. A deaf man eager to hear will automatically turn his best ear toward the speaker. Experienced lip readers have difficulty with sound-alike words; the dissembler may do better than expected because the words are actually heard.

Many tests have been devised for detection of unilateral nonorganic deafness. The diagnosis is best made audiometrically; discrepancies and inconsistencies on repeated audiometric examinations are typical. With some trickery, a stethoscope—with one earpiece occluded—can be put with the occluded earpiece in the good ear and the open earpiece into the bad ear, to demonstrate that the "deaf" ear can hear. In the yes-no test, the examiner whispers into the patient's deaf ear after instructions to "say yes if you hear it and no if you don't."

Tinnitus is spontaneous noise in the ears originating inside the head. There are many types, and the causes are protean. In many cases no precise etiology can be established. The most common identifiable cause is noise exposure. Objective tinnitus refers to noise audible to both the patient and the examiner, as occurs in carotid stenosis. Most tinnitus is subjective tinnitus. It may vary in pitch and intensity, and may be continuous or intermittent. It may be described in many ways, such as ringing, buzzing, blowing, whistling, swishing, or roaring. Tinnitus is commonly associated with deafness. It is common in presbycusis and in other types of SNHL, and is a fairly constant feature of otosclerosis. Most cases are due to disease of the cochlea or eighth nerve; some are due to CNS disease. Tinnitus is often more noticeable at night when environmental noises are diminished, and it may interfere with sleep. To the patient, tinnitus may be more distressing than the accompanying deafness, and it may cause depression in elderly individuals.

Pulsatile tinnitus is synchronous with the pulse; it is in reality a bruit. Causes include carotid stenosis, arteriovenous malformations, particularly of the dura, glomus tumors, venous hums, and hypertension. Pulsatile tinnitus is fairly common in pseudotumor cerebri, and it occurs occasionally in increased intracranial pressure of other origins. The perilymphatic duct connects the perilymph-filled spaces of the cochlea and an extension of the subarachnoid space in the region of the jugular foramen. Through this channel, pulsations in the subarachnoid space are transmitted to the cochlea. Vascular tinnitus may occasionally be affected by carotid artery compression. Rhythmic tinnitus not synchronous with the pulse may occur with palatal myoclonus (palatal microtremor).

Other causes of tinnitus include cerumen impaction, medications (particularly ototoxic drugs), Ménière disease, acoustic neuroma, and Arnold-Chiari malformation. Muscle spasm, contraction of the tensor tympani, nasopharyngeal sounds, and temporomandibular joint clicking may also simulate tinnitus. Tinnitus may be psychogenic. Bizarre types of tinnitus may occur with pontine and cerebral lesions. Auditory hallucinations may occur in lesions of the temporal lobe; these are frequently epileptic auras. More bizarre hallucinations occur in psychotic and drug-induced states.

## THE VESTIBULAR NERVE

### Clinical Examination

The conditions that may present as dizziness range from trivial to life threatening, and are often difficult to evaluate and manage. The nebulousness of the patient's description of dizziness often produces frustration on the part of the clinician, yet in few other conditions are the historical details so pivotal in correct diagnosis. Fortunately, the truly serious conditions that present as dizziness are rare. The first step in understanding the symptom is to have the patient describe what he means by "dizziness." Patients use the word dizzy to describe vertigo, as well as a number of other sensations, such as lightheadedness or giddiness, sometimes referred to as pseudovertigo. Concomitant dysfunction in several systems may cause dizziness. Conflicting sensory information may certainly cause dizziness; the sensory mismatch from watching a motion picture with dramatic movement in the visual panorama while sitting in a stationary seat illustrates the effect.

In a classic study of 100 dizzy patients in an ambulatory setting, the causes were as follows: vestibulopathy (54), psychiatric disorders (16), multifactorial (13), unknown (8), presyncope (6), dysequilibrium (2), and hyperventilation (1) (Drachman DA, Hart CW. An approach to the dizzy patient. *Neurology* 1972;22:323–334). The most common treatable conditions were benign positional, or benign paroxysmal positional, vertigo (BPV or BPPV), and psychiatric disorders. Other studies have shown a similar distribution. Some of the causes of dizziness are listed in Table 13.3. Table 13.4 lists causes of dizziness due to labyrinthine or vestibular pathway dysfunction. Before discussing vestibular disease, some discussion of nonspecific dizziness is warranted, since patients with such complaints make up a large proportion of the dizzy population.

## TABLE 13.3

### Some Causes of "Dizziness"

| Symptom Description | Characteristics | Possible Etiologies |
|---|---|---|
| Vertigo (spinning, whirling, tilting, falling) | Illusion of motion of self or environment | Dysfunction of the vestibular system, peripheral or central |
| Disequilibrium (poor balance but not "dizzy") | Impaired balance, unsteady gait | Bilateral vestibular dysfunction, deafferentation (peripheral neuropathy, posterior column disease), brainstem lesion, cerebellar lesion, extra-pyramidal disorder, drug effects |
| Presyncope (lightheaded, drunk, woozy, faint) | Lightheadedness; often with systemic symptoms (e.g., diaphoresis, nausea, graying of vision) inciting event | Global cerebral hypoperfusion (numerous causes) |
| Multiple sensory deficits | Elderly patient, vague complaints, difficulty walking | Multiple concurrent problems |
| Ill defined | Histrionic but vague description and nonspecific complaints | Psychogenic |

## TABLE 13.4

### Some Common Causes of Vertigo

Otologic disorders
   Benign paroxysmal positional vertigo
   Ménière disease
   Vestibular neuronitis
Neurologic disorders
   Migraine-associated vertigo
   Vertebrobasilar ischemia

Cerebral hypoperfusion produces a sensation of lightheadedness, drunkenness, or impending syncope without spinning, whirling, or any illusion of environmental motion. Such hypoperfusion may occur under a variety of circumstances, all of which may lead the patient to seek medial attention because of "dizziness." In hyperventilation syndrome (HVS), hypocapnia induced cerebral arterial constriction and the resultant hypoperfusion induces lightheadedness along with other symptoms, such as chest pain, headache; numbness and tingling of the hands, feet, and circumoral region; and occasionally outright syncope. Frequently, patients are unaware of their overbreathing, but the high minute volume of respiration produces dryness of the mouth, which the patient may describe spontaneously or respond to on specific questioning. Induced hyperventilation may reproduce the symptom complex. Orthostatic hypotension due to drugs, prolonged standing, dehydration, increased vagal tone, or dysautonomia likewise may present as lightheadedness or faintness. Accompanying symptoms are few, and only a careful history eliciting the relationship of the dizziness to posture will make the diagnosis. Global cerebral hypoperfusion may also result from decreased cardiac output via any number of mechanisms; arrhythmia is the primary concern.

Elderly patients "deafferented" because of separate disease processes affecting different sensory systems may present with complaints of vague dizziness, unsteadiness, and difficulty with balance, particularly when turning (multiple sensory defect vertigo). Patients can apparently tolerate problems with any one afferent system, but when multiple systems are involved imbalance and dizziness result. The term presbylibrium has been applied to poor balance due to aging.

Numerous terms have been employed to describe the clinical phenomenology of vestibular disease; not all are helpful. Vertigo is the sensation of environmental motion (spinning, whirling, lateropulsion, tilt). The term "true vertigo" is sometimes used to describe this symptom. When true vertigo is present, the problem is usually an acute peripheral vestibular disturbance. Objective vertigo creates the sensation that the environment is spinning, whereas subjective vertigo creates the sensation that the patient is spinning. The absence of true vertigo does not exclude peripheral vestibular disease, especially if bilateral pathology exists, such as in ototoxicity due to drugs. Central vertigo is due to CNS disease; peripheral vertigo is due to disease of the peripheral vestibular apparatus or its connections. Patients with CNS lesions may not have true vertigo. Acoustic neuroma causes a gradual unilateral loss of vestibular function and is more prone to cause imbalance than true vertigo. Some other serious conditions may present as dizziness without true vertigo, such as cardiac dysrhythmias and dysautonomic orthostasis. Physicians should not make too much of the presence or absence of true vertigo in judging how seriously to take a patient's complaint of dizziness.

Dizziness may be present constantly or intermittently. If intermittent, as in BPPV, one of the most common causes of dizziness, the episodes may occur so frequently that the initial description may lend the impression the symptoms are constant. If the episodes are intermittent, the duration of the attacks is important. Attack duration is one of the most important features in distinguishing between central and peripheral vertigo. In vertigo due to BPPV, the attacks last 10 to 30 seconds; in other peripheral vestibulopathies, such as Ménière disease, the attacks last hours; and in vertebrobasilar insufficiency, the episodes last for minutes. Exploring the precipitating factors is very helpful. Dizziness may be provoked by head or body movement, standing, lying down or occur spontaneously. The presence of associated symptoms, such as nausea, vomiting, staggering, deviation of the eyes, disturbances of balance, prostration, tinnitus, hearing loss, or loss of consciousness, is important. Table 2.8 reviews some of the pertinent history to explore in a dizzy patient.

Useful bedside testing of vestibular function includes assessment of vestibulospinal reflexes (past pointing, Romberg, Fukuda stepping test), tests of vestibulo-ocular reflexes (oculocephalic reflex, head thrust test, dynamic visual acuity, and caloric responses), and searching for nystagmus (spontaneous, positional, or after head shaking). In recalling the expected pattern of responses to some of these, remember that the vestibular system tends to push (eyes, limbs, body) to the opposite side; when the system is in balance the eyes are midline and the limbs and body can accurately find a target. When disease is present the involved labyrinth is usually hypoactive and the uninvolved labyrinth pushes toward the abnormal side. The bedside tests of vestibular function are listed in Table 13.5.

## Vestibulospinal Reflexes

Past pointing is a deviation of the extremities caused by either cerebellar or vestibular disease. It is a poor term because it implies the patient points beyond the target, when in fact it simply means the patients misses the target, most often to one side or the other. Testing is usually done with the upper extremities. A quick and effective technique is simply to have the patient close his eyes while doing traditional cerebellar finger-to-nose testing. If past pointing is present, the limb will deviate to the side of the target because of the absence of visual correction. This method will usually bring out past pointing if it is present. The traditional method is to have the patient extend the arm and place his extended index finger on the examiner's index finger; then with eyes closed raise the arm directly overhead; then bring it back down precisely onto the examiner's finger.

## TABLE 13.5

### Useful Bedside Tests and Signs to Elicit in the Evaluation of Vestibular Function

Note: Frenzel lenses and/or hyperventilation may bring out some of these signs.
Observation for spontaneous nystagmus
Evaluation of eye movements
Head thrust test
Dynamic visual acuity
Subjective visual vertical
Vibration induced nystagmus
Head-shaking nystagmus
Head-tapping test
Past pointing
Dix-Hallpike maneuver
Evaluation of gait, especially tandem
Romberg test
Walking straight line, eyes closed
Star walking test
Fukuda stepping test
Calorics

Cerebellar and vestibular past pointing have different patterns. With acute vestibular imbalance, the normal labyrinth will push the limb toward the abnormal side, and the patient will miss the target to one side. The past pointing will always be to the same side of the target and will occur with either limb. With a cerebellar hemispheric lesion, the ipsilateral limbs have ataxia and incoordination; past pointing occurs only with the involved arm and may be to the side of the lesion or erratically to either side of the target. In vestibulopathy, the past pointing is with both limbs, and to the same side of the target, in cerebellar disease, it occurs only with one upper extremity, and to either side of the target with no consistent pattern. The lower limbs would behave similarly but are more difficult to test. In vestibulopathy, after a period of compensation the past pointing disappears and may even begin to occur in the opposite direction.

Romberg's test is described in more detail in Chapter 33. In brief, the Romberg compares balance as the patient stands with eyes open and eyes closed. The feet should be brought as close together as will allow the patient to maintain eyes open balance. A normal individual can stand feet together and eyes open without difficulty, but not all patients can. The critical observation is eyes open v. eyes closed. Inability to maintain balance with eyes open and feet together is not a positive Romberg. In unilateral vestibulopathy, if balance is lost with eyes closed the patient will tend to fall toward the side of the lesion, as the normal vestibular system pushes him over. If the patient has spontaneous nystagmus due to a vestibular lesion, the fall will be in the direction of the slow phase. In peripheral vestibular disease the direction of the fall can be affected by changing head position; the patient will fall toward the abnormal ear. With a right vestibulopathy and facing straight ahead, eye closure will cause the patient to fall to the right; looking over his right shoulder, he will fall backward; and looking over his left shoulder, he will fall forward. The sharpened Romberg (tandem Romberg), which is done by having the patient stand tandem with eyes closed, may be useful in some circumstances.

The patient with an acute vestibulopathy may have difficulty with tandem gait with a tendency to fall to the side of the lesion, but normal straightaway walking may appear unimpaired because visual cues compensate for the vestibular abnormality. But straightaway walking with eyes closed may be informative. A normal individual can walk without visual clues well enough to point his index finger at the palm of the examiner's hand, close his eyes, walk along a path of 20 ft or so, and then touch the finger to the examiner's palm. The patient with acute vestibulopathy may drift toward the side of the lesion and end up well off the target, the gait equivalent of past pointing.

The Fukuda stepping test is analogous. The patient, eyes closed, marches in place for one minute. A normal individual will continue to face in the same direction, but a patient with acute vestibulopathy will slowly pivot toward the side of the less active labyrinth. In the star walking test, the patient, eyes closed, takes several steps forward then several steps backward, over and over. A normal individual will begin and end oriented approximately along the same line. A patient with acute vestibulopathy will drift toward the less active side walking forward, and continue to drift during the backward phase. The resulting path traces out a multipointed star pattern. As with past pointing, the direction of gait drift, pivoting on the stepping test, and similar findings do not reliably indicate the side of the lesion in patients with chronic vestibulopathy after compensation has occurred.

## Vestibulo-Ocular Reflexes

The vestibulo-ocular reflex (VOR) serves to move the eyes at an equal velocity but in the direction opposite the head movement; this keeps the eyes still in space and maintains visual fixation while the head is in motion. There are several ways to examine the VOR, including the doll's eye test, head thrust test, dynamic visual acuity, and calorics.

## Oculocephalic Reflex (Doll's Eye Test)

The oculocephalic response is primarily useful in the evaluation of comatose patients. Turning the head in one direction causes the eyes to turn in the opposite direction. This response indicates that the pathways connecting the vestibular nuclei in the medulla to the extraocular nuclei in the pons and midbrain are functioning and that the brainstem is intact. In an alert patient, visuomotor and ocular fixation mechanisms come into play, limiting the drawing of any conclusions about vestibular function.

## Head Thrust

The doll's eye test utilizes side-to-side head movements in a comatose patient; the head thrust test is done in an awake patient. Abrupt, rapid movements are made in each direction while the patient attempts to maintain fixation straight ahead, as on the examiner's nose. The ocular smooth pursuit mechanism cannot compensate for head movements done at such high velocity, but normally the VOR will maintain fixation and the eyes will hold on target. When the VOR is impaired, the compensatory eye movement velocity is less than the head movement velocity; the eyes lag behind the head movement and a corrective "catch-up" saccade must be made to resume fixation in the eccentric position.

## Dynamic Visual Acuity

The ability of the VOR to maintain ocular fixation means that a patient can read even while shaking the head to and fro. The dynamic visual acuity test is performed by obtaining a baseline acuity, and then determining the acuity during rapid head shaking. Degradation by more than three lines on the Snellen chart suggests impaired vestibular function.

## Caloric Tests

Caloric responses are frequently used to check for brainstem integrity in comatose patients. Ice water instilled into one ear canal will abruptly decrease the tonic activity from the labyrinth on the irrigated side. Cold calorics in a comatose patient with an intact brainstem cause tonic deviation of the eyes toward the side of irrigation as the normally active labyrinth pushes the eyes toward the hypoactive, irrigated labyrinth. In an awake patient, cold calorics cause nystagmus with the fast component away from the irrigated side because the cerebral cortex produces a compensatory saccade that jerks in the direction opposite the tonic deviation. The familiar mnemonic "COWS" (cold opposite, warm, same), refers to the fast phase of the nystagmus, not to the tonic gaze deviation. Nystagmus is seen only when the cortex is functioning normally. Warm water irrigation has opposite effects. Bilateral simultaneous cold calorics induce tonic downgaze, warm calorics upgaze.

In comatose patients, large volumes of ice water, 30 cc to 50 cc, are commonly used since it is imperative to elicit the response if it is present. Calorics can also be done to assess vestibular function in dizzy patients, either using much smaller volumes, 2 cc to 10 cc of an ice and water slush (minicalorics), or larger volumes of water less cold. The latency to onset and the duration of the nystagmus elicited is compared on the two sides. A difference of more than 20% in nystagmus duration suggests a lesion on the side of the decreased response.

Whether in comatose or awake patients, the head is positioned so as to bring the horizontal canal into a position to elicit a maximal response. In comatose patients lying supine this is with the head flexed 30 degrees to bring the horizontal canal vertical. For awake patients, the same position may be used, or the head may be extended with the seated patient looking at the ceiling.

## Nystagmus

Nystagmus is discussed in greater detail in Chapter 10. The characteristics of vestibular nystagmus will be briefly reviewed. Nystagmus due to vestibular disease may occur spontaneously or be produced by various maneuvers.

## Spontaneous Nystagmus

The slow phase of spontaneous vestibular nystagmus is usually in the direction of the lesion, with the fast phase away, because an acute vestibular lesion typically causes hypoactivity of the labyrinth. The findings are similar to those produced by ice water irrigation of the ear, and are due to the normal labyrinth pushing the eyes toward the diseased side with the cortex generating a corrective saccade away from the abnormal side. Because of the influence of the three different semicircular canals, vestibular nystagmus may beat in more than one direction, the summation of which creates an admixed rotatory component rarely seen with other conditions. Vestibular nystagmus typically is fine, often present but easily overlooked in primary position. Third degree nystagmus (fast component opposite to the direction of gaze) rarely occurs with any other nystagmus type. Vertigo, deafness, and tinnitus also help mark nystagmus as vestibular. When evaluating nystagmus, the presence of a torsional component suggests a peripheral origin. The amplitude increases with gaze in the direction of the fast phase. Peripheral vestibular nystagmus (i.e., that due to disease of the labyrinth or eighth nerve) is markedly inhibited by visual fixation. Inhibiting fixation with Frenzel lenses (strongly convex spectacles that block visual fixation) will often make the nystagmus more obvious by both blocking fixation and magnifying the eyes. When Frenzel lenses are used, torsional nystagmus is often more prominent because vertical and horizontal nystagmus are more easily suppressed by visual fixation. Another technique is to have the patient close the eyelids gently, then partially lift one lid and look for abnormal movements of the scleral vessels. The fundoscopic examination may bring out subtle vestibular nystagmus. The dim lighting lessens visual fixation, and the disc is magnified. A rhythmic jerking of the disc to the patient's right indicates left beating nystagmus. Formal eye movement studies are done in darkness with recording of the eye movements by electrodes in order to remove the effects of visual fixation. Failure of visual fixation to suppress nystagmus suggests the nystagmus may be of central origin, usually a cerebellar or brainstem lesion. The spontaneous nystagmus due to a central lesion may be purely horizontal or purely vertical.

Nystagmus can sometimes be induced by having the patient rapidly turn the head back and forth with the eyes closed for about 30 seconds, then opening the eyes (head-shaking nystagmus). No nystagmus occurs in normal individuals, but patients with vestibular imbalance may have brief spontaneous nystagmus beating away from the abnormal side. Alternately, the patient may wear Frenzel lenses while shaking the head. Spontaneous nystagmus can occasionally be produced by tapping on the head or by low frequency vibration applied to the mastoid. Hyperventilation may also help bring out vestibular nystagmus.

## Positional Nystagmus

When not present spontaneously, nystagmus can sometimes be elicited by placing the patient's head into a particular position. To perform the Dix-Hallpike (Hallpike or Nylen-Bárány) maneuver, the patient is moved from a seated position to a supine position with the head extended 45 degrees and turned 45 degrees to one side so that one ear is dependent. In BPPV, nystagmus begins after a latency of about 3 to 10 seconds, occasionally as long as 40 seconds; persists for 20 to 30 seconds, rarely as long as a minute; and then gradually abates even though the head remains in the provoking position. The nystagmus is commonly torsional with the fast component toward the dependent ear. The response is usually much more dramatic in one particular head position. Typically, the patient will experience whirling, occasionally nausea, and rarely vomiting. The response is fatigable, and repeating the maneuver several times consecutively provokes less of a response each time until eventually the nystagmus and vertigo are nil. This type of positional nystagmus is most often due to peripheral vestibular disease. Although rare, positional vertigo can occur with a central lesion, especially one near the fourth ventricle, but the characteristics of the nystagmus are different. With a central lesion, there may be no latency, and the nystagmus often begins as soon as the head is placed in the provoking position. Central positional nystagmus is typically vertical (either up- or downbeating), without the rotatory component seen with peripheral lesions. In addition, the nystagmus and associated symptoms may persist for a prolonged period, longer than 30 to 40 seconds, sometimes continuing as long as the head position is maintained. With central lesions there may be a mismatch in the severity of the nystagmus, vertigo, and nausea, in contrast to peripheral lesions where nystagmus, vertigo, and nausea are generally of comparable intensity.

Positional nystagmus can be divided into a paroxysmal type that is fleeting, fatigable, often difficult to reproduce, and associated with prominent vertigo, and a static type that does not fatigue, persisting as long as the head is maintained in the provoking position, often with little associated vertigo. The static type can occur with either central or peripheral vestibular lesions, but a lack of visual suppression increases the likelihood of a central lesion.

The characteristics of peripheral versus central positional nystagmus and related findings are summarized in Table 13.6.

## Disorders of Function

The primary manifestation of disorders of the vestibular nerve is vertigo and related symptoms such as imbalance. Vertigo will be used in this discussion as a surrogate for all similar symptoms. One of the primary concerns when dealing with a vertiginous patient is to separate central vertigo, due to CNS disease, from peripheral vertigo, due to peripheral vestibular disease. Disease of the

## TABLE 13.6

### The Characteristics of Central Versus Peripheral Positional Nystagmus on Dix-Hallpike Maneuver

| Finding | Peripheral | Central |
|---|---|---|
| Latency | Yes, typically 3–10 sec, rarely as long as 40 sec | No |
| Fatigability* (habituation) | Yes, individual episode typically lasts 10–30 sec, rarely as long as 1 min | No |
| Adaptability* (fatigability) | Yes, maneuver done several times consecutively provokes less of a response each time | No |
| Nystagmus direction | Direction fixed, typically mixed rotational upbeating with small horizontal component; quick phase of intorsion movement toward the dependent ear, upbeat toward forehead | Direction changing, variable, often purely vertical (either upbeating or downbeating) or purely horizontal |
| Suppression of nystagmus by visual fixation | Yes | No |
| Severity | Severe, marked vertigo, intense nystagmus, nausea | Mild vertigo, less obvious nystagmus, inconspicuous nausea |
| Consistency (reproducibility) | Less consistent | More consistent |
| Past pointing | In direction of nystagmus slow phase | May be in direction of fast phase |

*Adaptability and fatigability are not used consistently in the literature.

peripheral vestibular apparatus or eighth cranial nerve produces peripheral vertigo. Disease of the central vestibular connections produces central vertigo. The vestibular nuclei lie within the CNS in the dorsolateral medulla; disease there may act like either peripheral or central forms. Central vertigo is much less common than peripheral. Certain features are helpful in making the distinction. Central vertigo is typically less severe, and other neurologic signs and symptoms are usually present. Peripheral vestibular disorders cause more nausea, vomiting, and autonomic symptoms than do central disorders. Imbalance tends to be more severe with central lesions, and the patients are often unable to stand or walk. Associated symptoms are helpful if present. Aural symptoms (hearing loss, tinnitus, pain or fullness in the ear) suggest a peripheral cause. Facial weakness or numbness occurs with lesions involving the eighth nerve in the cerebellopontine angle. Processes in the brainstem typically cause prominent neighborhood signs; isolated vertigo is rare. Occasionally, vertigo can be a manifestation of disease of the more rostral vestibular pathways, including the temporal lobe.

Distinguishing central from peripheral nystagmus is a common clinical exercise. The most helpful features are of course the presence of aural symptoms and signs in peripheral nystagmus and the presence of CNS symptoms and signs with central nystagmus. Peripheral vestibular nystagmus does not change direction, although it may vary in amplitude depending on the direction of gaze, and is strongly suppressed by visual fixation. Central nystagmus typically changes direction and may not be affected by visual fixation.

Because of the effects of fixation and other compensatory mechanisms, peripheral nystagmus is seldom prominent after the first 12 to 24 hours, but central nystagmus may persist for weeks or months. The vestibular apparatus pushes not only the eyes, but also the limbs and the body to the opposite side. With acute peripheral vestibulopathy, the patient will past point, fall on Romberg, turn on the stepping test, and drift walking eyes closed in the direction of the nystagmus slow phase. Failure to follow these rules (e.g., past pointing in the direction of the fast phase) suggests a central lesion, but can occur with a compensated peripheral lesion. Peripheral nystagmus is often positional, and the vertigo and vegetative symptoms are in proportion to the nystagmus. With positional nystagmus, latency to onset, fatigability, and adaptability all support a peripheral process. Minimal vertigo with prominent nystagmus, or lack of latency, fatigability, and adaptability suggests a central process. Peripheral nystagmus often has a rotary component, and the horizontal nystagmus beats in the same direction in all fields of gaze (may even be third degree). Central nystagmus tends to change directions. Visual fixation inhibits peripheral nystagmus but has no effect on central nystagmus.

Involvement of the vestibular nuclei may cause vertigo that has central features. Common processes that involve the brainstem and that are likely to cause vertigo include ischemia, demyelinating disease, and neoplasms. Less common brainstem lesions causing central vestibular dysfunction include arteriovenous malformation, syringobulbia, hematoma, and spinocerebellar degeneration. Lesions in the cerebellopontine angle affect both the auditory and vestibular portions of CN VIII.

Vertebrobasilar transient ischemic attacks, or "vertebrobasilar insufficiency," commonly causes vertigo, most often along with other signs and symptoms. Rare patients may have transient vertigo without accompanying symptoms. A syndrome of acute vertigo mimicking labyrinthitis may occur with acute cerebellar infarction or hemorrhage. The most common misdiagnosis in one series of patients with cerebellar hematoma was labyrinthitis. In acute cerebellar lesions, the patient will tend to fall toward the side of the lesion on Romberg testing; the nystagmus may also be maximal with gaze toward the lesion. As a result, the patient may fall in the direction of the fast phase, opposite the pattern seen in acute peripheral vestibulopathy.

Dizziness, vertigo, and dysequilibrium occur commonly in patients with multiple sclerosis (MS). In one instance, an MS lesion in the medulla caused clinical symptoms mimicking vestibular neuronitis. However, MS patients are not immune from developing the common syndrome of BPPV, and peripheral vestibulopathy may be a more common cause of vertigo in such patients than MS exacerbation.

There is a relationship between migraine and episodic vertigo. Motion sensitivity is common in migraineurs, and episodic vertigo occurs in as many as 25%. Isolated attacks of vertigo have been labeled as a migraine equivalent. Occasionally, migraine patients may also develop cochlear symptoms, perhaps due to spasm of the labyrinthine microvasculature. Migraine can mimic Ménière disease. In some patients there may be a channelopathy involved.

Disorders of the peripheral vestibular apparatus are the most common cause of vertigo and related symptoms. Table 13.4 lists some of the causes of peripheral vertigo. In BPPV, the most common peripheral vestibulopathy, vertigo is induced by assumption of a particular head position or by rapid head movement. Classically, such patients experience vertigo when first lying down or when rolling over in bed at night, bending over, or looking up. Benign paroxysmal positional vertigo attacks are brief, generally 10 to 30 seconds, and frequent. BPPV probably results from otoliths that have become detached from the macula of the utricle and formed free floating debris that settles into the posterior canal, the most dependent portion of the vestibular labyrinth. Movement of the debris causes the attacks of vertigo. The Dix-Hallpike maneuver causes the debris to move and reproduces the symptoms. The disorder predominantly affects the posterior semicircular canal; about 5% involve the horizontal canal and about 1% the anterior canal. Common identifiable antecedents are head trauma and viral neurolabyrinthitis. Rarely, patients with posterior fossa tumors have a clinical picture nearly identical to BPPV.

In vestibular neuronitis or labyrinthitis, more severe attacks prostrate the patient for several days. Although often used interchangeably, technically labyrinthitis is accompanied by cochlear dysfunction, whereas vestibular neuronitis is purely vestibular. Mild, brief attacks of vertigo similar to BPPV may plague the patient for months to years after seeming recovery. Some instances of apparent labyrinthitis are likely due to internal auditory artery ischemia. In Ménière disease, the attacks of vertigo typically last several hours and patients describe other symptoms, either along with the vertigo or independently, including hearing loss (classically fluctuating), tinnitus, and a sensation of vague pain or fullness in the ear. Inner ear disease can occasionally cause drop attacks.

# CHAPTER 14

# The Glossopharyngeal and Vagus Nerves

The glossopharyngeal (CN IX) and vagus (CN X) nerves are intimately related and similar in function. Both have motor and autonomic branches with nuclei of origin in the medulla. Both conduct general somatic afferents as well as general visceral afferents fibers to related or identical fiber tracts and nuclei in the brainstem and both have a parasympathetic, or general visceral efferent and a branchiomotor, or special visceral efferent component. The two nerves leave the skull together, remain close in their course through the neck, and supply some of the same structures. They are often involved in the same disease processes, and involvement of one may be difficult to differentiate from involvement of the other. For these reasons the two nerves are discussed together.

## THE GLOSSOPHARYNGEAL NERVE

Cranial nerve IX is difficult to examine because most or all of its functions are shared by other nerves and because many of the structures it supplies are inaccessible. It is possible to examine pain and touch sensation of the pharynx, tonsilar region, and soft palate, and the gag reflex. The only muscle to receive its motor innervation purely from CN IX is the stylopharyngeus. The only deficit that might be detectable is a slight lowering of the palatal arch at rest on the involved side. Other palatal motor functions are subserved either by CN X, or the two nerves working together.

The gag reflex is elicited by touching the lateral oropharynx in the region of the anterior faucial pillar, or by touching one side of the soft palate or uvula, with a tongue blade, applicator stick, or similar object. The afferent limb of the reflex is mediated by CN IX and the efferent limb through CNs IX and X. The reflex center is in the medulla. The motor response is constriction and elevation of the oropharynx. This causes the midline raphe of the palate and the uvula to elevate, and the pharyngeal constrictors to contract. The activity on the two sides is compared. The gag reflex is protective; it is designed to prevent noxious substances or foreign objects from going beyond the oral cavity. There are three motor components: elevation of the soft palate to seal off the nasopharynx, closure of the glottis to protect the airway, and constriction of the pharynx to prevent entry of the substance.

When unilateral pharyngeal weakness is present, the midline raphe will deviate away from the weak side and toward the normal side. This movement is usually dramatic. Minor movements of the uvula and trivial deviations of the raphe are not of clinical significance. There is variation in the intensity of the stimulus required. The gag reflex may be bilaterally absent in some normal individuals. Unilateral absence signifies a lower motor neuron lesion. Like most bulbar muscles the pharynx receives bilateral supranuclear innervation, and a unilateral cerebral lesion does not cause detectable weakness.

The gag reflex is often used to predict whether or not a patient will be able to swallow or guard the airway. A decreased gag reflex may portend inadequate guarding of the airway and increased aspiration risk, but the status of the gag reflex is not a completely reliable indicator. Patients with an apparently intact gag reflex may still aspirate, and a patient with a depressed gag reflex may not. The clinical assessment of swallowing, a major component of which is the status of the gag reflex, underestimates the probability of aspiration in patients who are at risk, and overestimates it in patients who are not. The gag reflex may be hyperactive in some normal individuals, even to the point of causing retching and vomiting. A hyperactive gag reflex may occur with bilateral cerebral lesions, as in pseudobulbar palsy and amyotrophic lateral sclerosis (ALS).

## Disorders of Function

Isolated lesions of CN IX are extremely rare if they ever occur. In all instances, the nerve is involved along with other cranial nerves, especially CN X. In glossopharyngeal neuralgia or "tic douloureux of the ninth nerve," the patient experiences attacks of severe lancinating pain originating in one side of the throat or tonsilar region and radiating along the course of the eustachian tube to the tympanic membrane, external auditory canal, behind the angle of the jaw and adjacent portion of the ear. There may be trigger zones, usually in the pharyngeal wall, fauces, tonsilar regions, or base of the tongue. The pain may be brought on by talking, eating, swallowing, or coughing. It can lead to syncope, convulsions, and rarely to cardiac arrest because of stimulation of the carotid sinus reflex. Glossopharyngeal neuralgia must be differentiated from other craniofacial neuralgias, and from pain due to a structural lesion of the nerve.

## THE VAGUS NERVE

Despite its size and importance, CN X is difficult to evaluate at the bedside. Formal autonomic function assessment can sometimes provide useful information.

### Examination of the Motor Functions

The motor branches of CN X supply the soft palate, pharynx, and larynx in the same distribution as for CN IX, and are examined in the same manner. The gag reflex is discussed in the section on CN IX.

The character of the voice and the ability to swallow provide information about the branchiomotor functions of the vagus. With acute unilateral lesions the speech may have a nasal quality and dysphagia is often present; this is more marked for liquids than solids with a tendency to nasal regurgitation. Examination of the soft palate includes observation of the position of the palate and uvula at rest, and during quiet breathing and phonation. The median raphe of the palate rises in the midline on phonation. With a unilateral lesion of the vagus there is weakness of the levator veli palatini and musculus uvulae, which causes a droop of the palate and flattening of the palatal arch. Preserved function of the tensor veli palatini (innervated by CN V) may prevent marked drooping of the palate. On phonation, the medial raphe deviates toward the normal side. The gag reflex may be lost on the involved side because of interruption of the motor rather than sensory path.

With bilateral vagus involvement the palate cannot elevate on phonation; it may or may not droop depending on the function of the tensor veli palatini. The gag reflex is absent bilaterally. The tendency toward nasal speech and nasal regurgitation of liquids is pronounced. The speech is similar to that of a patient with cleft palate.

Weakness of the pharynx may also produce abnormalities of speech and swallowing. With pharyngeal weakness, dysarthria is usually minimal unless there is also weakness of the soft palate or larynx. Spontaneous coughing and the cough reflex may be impaired. Dysphagia may occur but without the tendency to greater difficulty with liquids and to nasal regurgitation that occurs with palatal weakness. Dysphagia is marked only in acute unilateral or in bilateral lesions. Examination of the pharynx includes observation of the contraction of the pharyngeal muscles on phonation, notation of the elevation of the larynx on swallowing, and testing the gag reflex. Unilateral weakness of the superior pharyngeal constrictor may cause a "curtain movement," with motion of the pharyngeal wall toward the nonparalyzed side on testing the gag reflex or at the beginning of phonation. The normal elevation of the larynx may be absent on one side in unilateral lesions, and on both sides in bilateral lesions.

Cranial nerve X innervates the vocal cords. Normal movement of the vocal cords is necessary for three vital functions: breathing, coughing, and talking. During inspiration and expiration, the cords abduct to allow for free air flow; when speaking the cords adduct and vibrate to accomplish phonation. The cords are also adducted when coughing. Movements of the myriad small muscles that control the larynx are complex and have different effects on laryngeal function. A unilateral lesion of the vagus may cause cord weakness or paralysis. Vocal cord dysfunction alters the character and quality of the voice, and may produce abnormalities of articulation, difficulty with respiration, and impairment of coughing.

Spasmodic dysphonia is a common focal dystonia that involves the vocal cords and causes characteristic voice changes. Spasmodic dysphonia most often causes abnormal adduction spasms of both vocal cords, and the voice is strained and high-pitched. Abductor dysphonia is due to spasmodic contraction of the posterior cricoarytenoid, which causes a failure of normal adduction on phonation; the voice is breathy and hoarse. This type of spasmodic dysphonia is most likely to be confused with a lesion of CN X.

The most common cause of vocal cord paralysis is a lesion of one recurrent laryngeal nerve. The paralysis may evolve from mild abduction impairment due to isolated involvement of the posterior cricoarytenoid to complete paralysis with the cord in the cadaveric position. With slight weakness of the vocal cords or pharynx, hoarseness and dysphagia may be apparent only when the head is turned to either side. Occasionally, even severe weakness of a vocal cord causes little appreciable effect on the voice because of preserved movement of the normal cord.

## Disorders of Function

Nuclear and infranuclear processes that may affect CN IX and X include intramedullary and extramedullary neoplasms and other mass lesions (e.g., glomus jugulare tumor), trauma (e.g., basilar skull fracture or surgical dissection), motor neuron disease, syringobulbia, retropharyngeal abscess, demyelinating disease, birth injury, and brainstem ischemia. Extramedullary, intracranial involvement can occur in processes involving the meninges, extramedullary tumors, aneurysms, and skull fractures. Lesions at the jugular foramen or in the retroparotid space usually involve some combination of IX, X, XI, XII, and the cervical sympathetics. Isolated or multiple lower cranial nerve palsies can be a manifestation of dissecting aneurysm of the cervical internal carotid artery or occur as a complication of carotid endarterectomy. Surgical section or other trauma to the carotid branch of CN IX may cause transient or sustained hypertension. Involvement of CN IX may be related to the cardiovascular dysautonomia that sometimes accompanies Guillain-Barré syndrome.

A unilateral vagal lesion causes weakness of the soft palate, pharynx, and larynx. Acute lesions may produce difficulty swallowing both liquids and solids and hoarseness or a nasal quality to the voice. The only definite sensory change is anesthesia of the larynx due to involvement of the superior laryngeal nerve. It is seldom possible to demonstrate loss of sensation behind the pinna and in the external auditory canal. The gag reflex is absent on the involved side. Autonomic reflexes (vomiting, coughing, sneezing) are not usually affected. Tachycardia and loss of the oculocardiac reflex on the involved side may occur, but usually there are no cardiac symptoms. Gastrointestinal disturbances are inconspicuous. Bilateral complete vagal paralysis is incompatible with life. It causes complete paralysis of the palate, pharynx, and larynx, with marked dysphagia and dysarthria;

tachycardia; slow, irregular, respiration; vomiting; and gastrointestinal atonia. Lesions of individual vagal branches are rare except for involvement of the recurrent laryngeal nerve.

The primary effect of increased vagal activity is bradycardia. The term vasovagal refers to the effects of the vagus nerve on the blood vessels. Vasovagal attacks (fainting, syncope) are characterized by bradycardia, hypotension, peripheral vasoconstriction, and faintness, sometimes with loss of consciousness. Vasovagal attacks are typically induced by strong emotion or pain. The bradycardia and projectile vomiting that occur with increased intracranial pressure may be vagally mediated. Cheyne-Stokes, Biot, and Kussmaul breathing, respiratory tics, forced yawning, and other abnormalities of breathing may be vagally mediated as well.

Rhythmic movements of the palate (palatal myoclonus, palatal microtremor, or palatal nystagmus) can occur with a lesion of the brainstem, usually vascular. The movements are mediated by CN X. Bilateral supranuclear lesions, as from pseudobulbar palsy, cause dysphagia and dysarthria. Extrapyramidal disorders may produce difficulty with swallowing and talking. Laryngeal spasm with stridor may occur in Parkinson disease and other extrapyramidal disorders. Nuclear lesions of the nucleus ambiguus can occur with any intrinsic brainstem disease. A slowly progressive nuclear lesion, such as in bulbar ALS, syringomyelia, and some neoplasms, may cause fasciculations in the palatal, pharyngeal, and laryngeal muscles.

Individual vagal branches may be involved by disease processes in the neck, upper mediastinum, thorax, and abdomen. The recurrent laryngeal nerve is the most frequently affected. This may be damaged by tumors in the neck, aortic aneurysms, mediastinal and apical tumors, stab wounds in the neck, or accidental trauma during a thyroidectomy or other surgical procedure. The superior laryngeal and pharyngeal branches may be involved in trauma, or in neoplasms or abscesses in the neck.

# CHAPTER 15

# The Spinal Accessory Nerve

The spinal accessory (SA) nerve, cranial nerve XI (CN XI), is actually two nerves that run together in a common bundle for a short distance. The smaller cranial portion is a special visceral efferent accessory to the vagus. The cranial root exits through the jugular foramen separately from the spinal portion then blends with the vagus. It is distributed principally with the recurrent laryngeal nerve. The major part of CN XI is the spinal portion. The fibers of the spinal root arise from motor cells in the SA nuclei in the ventral horn from C2 to C5, or even C6. Its axons emerge as a series of rootlets laterally between the anterior and posterior roots. These unite into a single trunk which ascends between the denticulate ligaments and the posterior roots. The nerve enters the skull through the foramen magnum, ascends the clivus for a short distance, then curves laterally. The spinal root joins the cranial root for a short distance, probably receiving one or two filaments from it. It exits through the jugular foramen in company with CNs IX and X.

The supranuclear innervation of CN XI arises from the lower portion of the precentral gyrus. Fibers from the lateral corticospinal tract in the cervical spinal cord communicate with the SA nucleus. There is some controversy, but the bulk of current evidence indicates that both the sternocleidomastoid (SCM) and trapezius receive bilateral supranuclear innervation, but the input to the SCM motor neuron pool is predominantly ipsilateral and that to the trapezius motor neuron pool is predominantly contralateral. The SCM turns the head to the opposite side, and its supranuclear innervation is ipsilateral; therefore the right cerebral hemisphere turns the head to the left.

## Examination of the Spinal Accessory Nerve

The functions of the cranial portion of CN XI cannot be distinguished from those of CN X, and examination is limited to evaluation of the functions of the spinal portion. One SCM acts to turn the head to the opposite side or to tilt it to the same side. Acting together, the SCMs thrust the head forward and flex the neck. The muscles should be inspected and palpated to determine their tone and volume. The contours are distinct even at rest. With a nuclear or infranuclear lesion there may be atrophy or fasciculations.

To assess SCM power, have the patient turn the head fully to one side and hold it there, then try to turn the head back to midline, avoiding any tilting or leaning motion. The muscle usually stands out well, and its contraction can be seen and felt (Figure 15.1). Unilateral SCM paresis causes little change in the resting position of the head. Even with complete paralysis, other cervical muscles can perform some degree of rotation and flexion; only occasionally is there a noticeable head turn.

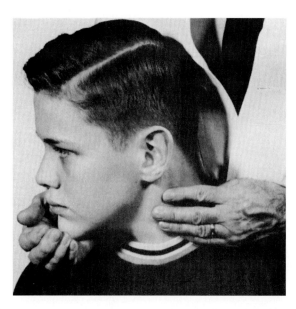

**FIGURE 15.1** ● Examination of the sternocleidomastoid muscle. When the patient turns his head to the right against resistance, the contracting muscle can be seen and palpated.

With bilateral paralysis of CN XI innervated muscles there is diminished but not absent neck rotation, and the head may droop or even fall backward or forward, depending upon whether the SCMs or the trapezei are more involved. The two SCM muscles can be examined simultaneously by having the patient flex his neck while the examiner exerts pressure on the forehead, or by having the patient turn the head from side to side. Flexion of the head against resistance may cause deviation of the head toward the paralyzed side. With unilateral paralysis, the involved muscle is flat and does not contract or become tense when attempting to turn the head contralaterally or to flex the neck against resistance. Weakness of both SCMs causes difficulty in anteroflexion of the neck, and the head may assume an extended position.

With trapezius atrophy the outline of the neck changes, with depression or drooping of the shoulder contour and flattening of the trapezius ridge (Figure 15.2). Severe trapezius weakness causes sagging of the shoulder, and the resting position of the scapula shifts downward. The upper portion of the scapula tends to fall laterally, while the inferior angle moves inward. This scapular rotation and displacement are more obvious with arm abduction.

The strength of the trapezius is traditionally tested by having the patient shrug the shoulders against resistance (Figure 15.3). However, much of shoulder shrugging is due to the action of the levator scapulae. A better test of the upper trapezius is resisting the patient's attempt to approximate the occiput to the acromion. The movement may be observed and the contraction seen and palpated. To examine the middle and lower trapezius, place the patient's abducted arm horizontally, palm up, and attempt to push the elbow forward. Muscle power should be compared on the two sides. In unilateral weakness of the trapezius these movements are impaired.

The trapezius is one of several muscles that act to stabilize the scapula and create a platform for movements of the humerus. The serratus anterior protracts the scapula, moving it forward as in a boxing jab. The trapezius is a synergist to the main mover, the rhomboids, in retracting the scapula. The trapezius and serratus anterior act in concert to rotate the scapula when the arm is abducting. The trapezius brings the glenoid fossa progressively more cephalad so that the abduction motion is unrestricted. In addition, contraction of the upper trapezius adds the final few degrees

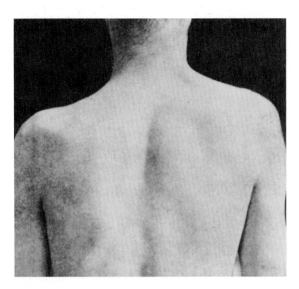

**FIGURE 15.2** ●    Paralysis of the left trapezius muscle. There is a depression in the shoulder contour with downward and lateral displacement of the scapula.

of abduction, after the glenohumeral and acromioclavicular ranges of motion are exhausted, so that the arm can be brought directly overhead.

Weakness of the trapezius disrupts the normal scapulohumeral rhythm and impairs arm abduction. Impairment of upper trapezius function causes weakness of abduction beyond 90 degrees. Weakness of the middle trapezius muscle causes winging of the scapula. The winging due to trapezius weakness is more apparent on lateral abduction in contrast to the winging seen with serratus anterior weakness, which is greatest with the arm held in front. In fact, with winging due to trapezius weakness, the jutting of the inferior angle lessens when the arm is raised anteriorly; in winging due to serratus anterior weakness, it worsens. Scapular winging is discussed further in

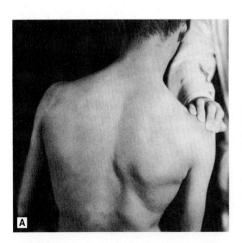
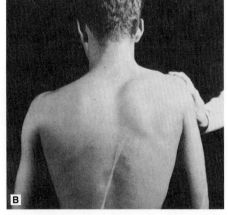

**FIGURE 15.3** ●    Examination of the trapezius muscle. **A.** Examiner pressing shoulder down against patient's resistance. **B.** Patient attempting to elevate shoulder against examiner's resistance.

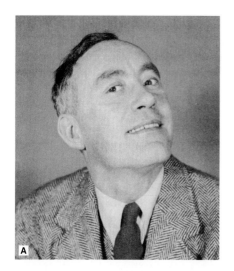
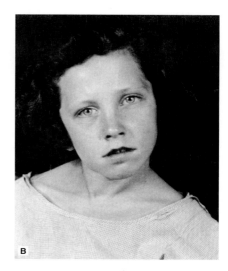

*FIGURE 15.4* ● Two examples (A and B) of cervical dystonia (spasmodic torticollis).

Chapter 18. When the trapezius is weak, the arm hangs lower on the affected side, and the finger-tips touch the thigh at a lower level than on the normal side. Placing the palms together with the arms extended anteriorly and slightly below horizontal shows the fingers on the affected side extending beyond those of the normal side. The two trapezius muscles can be examined simultaneously by having the patient extend his neck against resistance. Bilateral paralysis causes weakness of neck extension. The patient cannot raise his chin, and the head may tend to fall forward (dropped head syndrome).

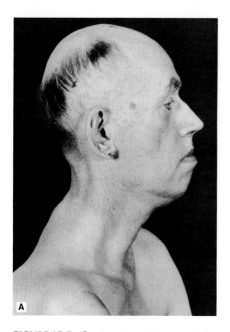
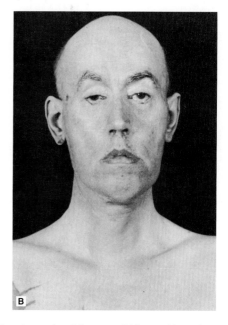

*FIGURE 15.5* ● A patient with myotonic dystrophy. There is atrophy of the sternocleidomastoid muscles.

## DISORDERS OF FUNCTION

Weakness of the muscles supplied by CN XI may be caused by supranuclear, nuclear, or infranuclear lesions. Supranuclear involvement usually causes at worst moderate loss of function since innervation is partially bilateral. In hemiplegia there is usually no head deviation, but testing may reveal slight, rarely marked, weakness of the SCM, with difficulty turning the face toward the involved limbs. There may be depression of the shoulder resulting from trapezius weakness on the affected side. Abnormal involuntary movements of the head and neck are seen in certain movement disorders. The SCM and trapezius are frequently involved in cervical dystonia, a common focal dystonia causing torticollis, anterocollis, or retrocollis (Figure 15.4). With nuclear lesions of CN XI, such as in motor neuron disease, the weakness is frequently accompanied by atrophy and fasciculations.

Infranuclear or peripheral lesions—either extra-medullary but within the skull, in the jugular foramen, or in the neck—are the most common causes of impairment of function of the SA nerve. Basal skull fractures, meningitis, extramedullary neoplasms within the skull, or processes at or just distal to the foramen give rise to a number of syndromes reflecting involvement of the lower cranial nerves. Such conditions affect both the SCM and the trapezius.

In the posterior triangle of the neck, the SA nerve is very vulnerable, since it lies superficially, covered only by skin and subcutaneous tissue. The nerve may be affected by severe cervical adenopathy, neoplasms, trauma, or abscesses. These lesions are generally distal to the SCM and affect only trapezius function. The most common cause of SA neuropathy in the posterior triangle is trauma, often iatrogenic. Surgical trauma may be unavoidable, as in radical neck dissection, or inadvertent, as in lymph node biopsy. Traction injury may occur when the shoulder is pulled down and the head turned in the opposite direction. Carrying heavy loads on the shoulder may cause SA injury due to local trauma or stretch.

Spontaneous, idiopathic cases of isolated SA palsy, often benign and self-limited, are likely comparable to similar focal neuropathies, such as Bell palsy or long thoracic nerve palsy, or may represent a restricted type of neuralgic amyotrophy. In these cases, the onset is typically sudden with pain in the posterior triangle, which resolves and is followed by SA palsy.

Neuromuscular disorders that affect the SCM and trapezius muscles include anterior horn cell disease, myasthenia gravis, polymyositis, dermatomyositis, and facioscapulohumeral dystrophy. Atrophy and weakness of both sternocleidomastoid muscles is a prominent feature of myotonic dystrophy (Figure 15.5). The "dropped head syndrome," characterized by severe neck extensor weakness and an inability to hold the head up, occurs in a variety of neuromuscular disorders, especially polymyositis and myasthenia gravis.

# CHAPTER 16

# The Hypoglossal Nerve

The hypoglossal nerve (CN XII) is a purely motor nerve, supplying the tongue. Its cells of origin are in the hypoglossal nuclei. The paired nuclei extend almost the entire length of the medulla just beneath the floor of the fourth ventricle, close to the midline, under the medial aspect of the hypoglossal trigone. The nerve emerges from the medulla in the sulcus between the pyramid and inferior olive as a series of 10 to 15 rootlets on each side, anterior to the rootlets of CNs IX, X, and XI.

The nerve passes through the hypoglossal canal, descends the neck to the level of the angle of the mandible, then passes forward under the tongue to supply its extrinsic and intrinsic muscles. In the upper portion of its course, the nerve lies beneath the internal carotid artery and internal jugular vein, and near the vagus nerve. It passes between the artery and vein, runs forward above the hyoid bone, and breaks up into a number of fibers to supply the various tongue muscles. At the base of the tongue it lies near the lingual branch of the mandibular nerve.

The cerebral center regulating tongue movements lies in the lower portion of the precentral gyrus near and within the sylvian fissure. The supranuclear fibers run in the corticobulbar tract through the genu of the internal capsule and through the cerebral peduncle. Supranuclear control to the genioglossus muscle is primarily crossed; supply to the other muscles is bilateral but predominantly crossed.

## Examination of the Hypoglossal Nerve

The clinical examination of hypoglossal nerve function consists of evaluating the strength, bulk, and dexterity of the tongue—looking especially for weakness, atrophy, abnormal movements (particularly fasciculations), and impairment of rapid movements. After noting the position and appearance of the tongue at rest in the mouth, the patient is asked to protrude it, move it in and out, from side to side, and upward and downward, both slowly and rapidly. Motor power can be tested by having the patient press the tip against each cheek as the examiner tries to dislodge it with finger pressure. The normal tongue is powerful and cannot be moved. For more precise testing, press firmly with a tongue blade against the side of the protruded tongue, comparing the strength on the two sides.

When unilateral weakness is present, the tongue deviates toward the weak side on protrusion because of the action of the normal genioglossus, which protrudes the tip of the tongue by drawing the root forward (Figure 16.1). Because the tip of the tongue is pushed out of the mouth it deviates toward the weak side. There is impairment of the ability to deviate the protruded tongue toward the nonparetic side and of the ability to push the tongue against the cheek on the normal side, but the patient is able to push it against the cheek on the weak side. Lateral movements of the tip of the nonprotruded tongue, controlled by the intrinsic tongue muscles, may be preserved.

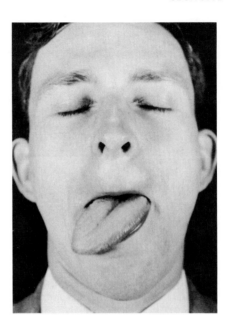

***FIGURE 16.1*** ● Infranuclear paralysis of muscles supplied by the hypoglossal nerve: Unilateral atrophy and deviation of the tongue following a lesion of the right hypoglossal nerve.

Because of the extensive interlacing of muscle fibers from side to side, the functional deficit with unilateral tongue weakness may be minimal. There may be difficulty manipulating food in the mouth, and an inability to remove food from between the teeth and the cheeks on either side. With either weakness or incoordination, rapid tongue movements may be impaired. In bilateral paralysis, the patient may be able to protrude the tongue only slightly, or not at all.

Facial muscle weakness or jaw deviation makes it difficult to evaluate deviation of the tongue. Patients with significant lower facial weakness often have distortion of the normal facial appearance that can produce the appearance of tongue deviation when none is present (Figure 11.1). Protruding the tongue may cause an appearance of deviation toward the side of the facial weakness. Because of the lack of facial mobility the corner of the mouth does not move out of the way and the protruded tongue lies tight against it, making it look as though the tongue has deviated. Manually pulling up the weak side of the face eliminates the "deviation." It may also be helpful to gauge tongue position in relation to the tip of the nose or the notch between the upper incisors.

When tongue atrophy occurs, the loss of bulk is first apparent along the borders or at the tip (Figure 16.2). With advanced atrophy, the tongue is wrinkled, furrowed, and obviously smaller. The epithelium and mucous membrane on the affected side are thrown into folds. As the paralyzed side becomes wasted, the protruded tongue may curve strikingly toward the atrophic side, assuming a sickle shape.

In progressive bulbar palsy and advanced amyotrophic lateral sclerosis, the atrophy may be so severe that the tongue cannot be protruded; it lies inert on the floor of the mouth (glossoplegia). Atrophy may be accompanied by fasciculations, especially in motor neuron disease. In some patients, the tongue is tremulous and it may be difficult to distinguish these fine, rapid tremors from fasciculations, especially when the tongue is protruded. Tremors will usually disappear when the tongue is lying at rest in the mouth, whereas fasciculations persist.

In addition to fasciculations, other abnormal movements of the tongue sometimes occur. Tremors are usually accentuated by protrusion of the tongue or by talking. Coarse tremors of the

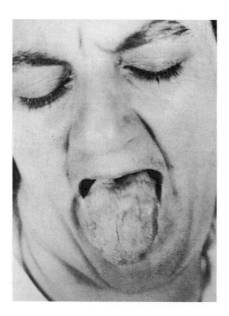

**FIGURE 16.2** ● Nuclear paralysis of muscles supplied by the hypoglossal nerve. Atrophy and fasciculations of the tongue in a patient with amyotrophic lateral sclerosis.

tongue can occur in parkinsonism; a fine tremor can occur in thyrotoxicosis. Chorea may cause irregular, jerky movements of the tongue, and often the patient is unable to keep the tongue protruded (snake tongue, trombone tongue). Abnormal involuntary movements may involve the tongue. It is often prominently involved in orofacial or buccolingual dyskinesias, which usually occur as a type of tardive dyskinesia following the use of psychotropic drugs. Similar dyskinesias may also occur in patients with Parkinson disease related to the use of levodopa and dopamine agonists, and in Meige syndrome. Seizures may involve the tongue, either as part of a Jacksonian seizure or rarely in isolation.

Morphologic changes in the tongue may be of diagnostic significance in many medical conditions. Macroglossia occurs in hypothyroidism, Down syndrome, amyloidosis, acromegaly, and rarely in some myopathies. The term atrophic glossitis refers to atrophy of the epithelium and papillae, causing a smooth, glistening, often reddened tongue. There may be punctate, erythematous lesions from atrophic, hyperemic papillae. Atrophic glossitis occurs in certain deficiency states, especially vitamin $B_{12}$, folate, other B vitamins, and iron. In pernicious anemia, the tongue is smooth, slick, and translucent. In some stages the tongue is pale; in others, it is red. In pellagra and niacin deficiency, the tongue is smooth and atrophic; acutely it is scarlet red and swollen and may have ulcerations. In riboflavin deficiency, the tongue may be a purplish or magenta hue, with prominent, edematous fungiform and filiform papillae that resemble cobblestones. Fusion and atrophy of the papillae and fissuring may cause a geographic, or scrotal, tongue. Burning tongue (glossodynia, glossalgia) with no visible lesions may occur from early glossitis, tobacco abuse, heavy metal intoxication, as a menopausal symptom, and in pellagra. Xerostomia and local irradiation may cause the tongue to be dry and sore. Melkersson-Rosenthal syndrome causes facial nerve palsy and scrotal tongue. Longitudinal lingual fissuring occurs in syphilitic glossitis. Ulcerations of the tongue may be seen in primary syphilis (lingual chancre) and in Behçet disease. Three parallel longitudinal fissures of the tongue is characteristic of myasthenia gravis (trident or triple furrowed tongue). The tongue is often bitten during generalized tonic clonic seizures.

## DISORDERS OF FUNCTION

Lesions of CN XII or its central connections may cause weakness of the tongue. There are no sensory changes. Unilateral weakness may cause few symptoms; speech and swallowing are little affected. With severe bilateral weakness the tongue cannot be protruded or moved laterally; the first stage of swallowing is impaired, and there is difficulty with articulation, especially in pronouncing linguals. Rarely, the tongue tending to slip back into the throat may cause respiratory difficulty.

Tongue weakness may be due to a supranuclear, nuclear, or infranuclear lesion. Supranuclear lesions cause weakness but no atrophy, and the weakness is rarely severe. Since the genioglossus—the principal protractor of the tongue—has mainly crossed supranuclear innervation, the tongue protrudes toward the weak side, but to the side opposite the supranuclear lesion. Supranuclear tongue weakness may occur with a destructive lesion of the cerebral cortex or the corticobulbar tract in the internal capsule, cerebral peduncle, or pons. Pontine lesions may cause supranuclear tongue weakness depending on the relationship to the decussating corticolingual fibers. Supranuclear lesions may cause dysarthria due to tongue weakness and incoordination. Pseudobulbar palsy due to bilateral upper motor neuron disease may cause bilateral tongue weakness. Patients with hemispheric lesions may have apraxia of tongue movements, and are often unable to protrude it on command. Extrapyramidal disorders may cause slowing of tongue movements, with thickness of speech and difficulty in protrusion.

In addition to weakness, nuclear and infranuclear lesions cause atrophy of the involved side. The tongue protrudes toward the weak side, which is also the side of the lesion. Progressive nuclear lesions, such as motor neuron disease, often cause fasciculations in addition to weakness. Common disorders that may involve the hypoglossal nucleus include neoplasms, vascular lesions, and motor neuron disease. Nuclear lesions may be accompanied by involvement of contiguous structures, such as the ascending sensory or descending motor pathways.

Infranuclear lesions may involve the intramedullary fibers between the nucleus and the point of exit. Except for motor neuron disease and similar conditions, causes are generally the same as for nuclear lesions. Processes involving the extramedullary, intracranial course of the nerve include disorders involving the meninges, such as infectious and neoplastic meningitis, subarachnoid hemorrhage, neoplasms and other mass lesions (e.g., schwannoma), inflammation, and trauma. Processes involving the skull base—such as basal skull fractures, basilar impression, and platybasia— may affect the nerve before it leaves the skull. Lesions along the clivus may cause bilateral hypoglossal palsies. Processes involving the extracranial course of the nerve include trauma of various types, especially penetrating wounds (including surgery on the neck, mouth, or tongue), carotid aneurysms (especially dissections), tumors or infections in the retroparotid or retropharyngeal spaces, deep cervical adenopathy, cranial irradiation, and tumors involving the neck, tongue base, or salivary glands. Hypoglossal nerve palsy can also occur as an idiopathic, benign syndrome that resolves spontaneously. Mechanical lesions may result in aberrant regeneration, which causes progressive difficulty with coordinated tongue movements. Rarely, primary neural tumors involve CN XII extracranially. CN XII may be involved with other lower cranial nerves and the cervical sympathetics in lesions in the retroparotid space. Cranial nerve XII may be involved unilaterally or bilaterally in Guillain-Barré syndrome and related polyneuropathies.

Except for myasthenia gravis, neuromuscular junction disorders and myopathies rarely involve the tongue to any clinically significant degree. Tongue weakness and fatigability may occur in myasthenia gravis but generally only with severe involvement.

The tongue may be involved in myotonic disorders, although it rarely causes any symptoms. One way to test for myotonia is to place the edge of a tongue blade across the tongue, then percuss it sharply. Myotonia may cause a temporary focal contraction along the line of percussion, causing the tongue to narrow sharply at that point. The appearance of the resulting constriction has been referred to as the napkin ring sign.

# The Motor Examination

# CHAPTER 17

# Overview of the Motor Examination

**E**xamination of motor functions includes the determination of muscle power, evaluation of muscle tone and bulk, and observation for abnormal movements. Examination of coordination and gait are closely related to the motor examination. Coordination is often viewed as a cerebellar function, but integrity of the entire motor system is essential for normal coordination and control of fine motor movements. Station (standing) and gait (walking) are complex, and involve much more than motor function; they are usually assessed separately from the motor examination.

Both the peripheral and central nervous systems participate in motor activity, and various functional components have to be evaluated individually. The lowest echelon of motor activity is the motor unit, which consists of an alpha motor neuron in the spinal cord or brainstem, its axon, and all of the muscle fibers it innervates. The segmental or spinal cord level mediates simple segmental reflexes, such as the withdrawal reflex, and includes the activity of many motor units and elements of both excitation and inhibition involving agonists, synergists, and antagonists. Various descending suprasegmental motor systems modulate the activity that occurs at the segmental level. The pyramidal (corticospinal) system arises from the primary motor cortex in the precentral gyrus. The corticospinal system is the primary, overarching suprasegmental motor control mechanism. The function of the corticospinal system is modulated and adjusted by the activity of the extrapyramidal and cerebellar systems. The extrapyramidal system arises primarily in the basal ganglia. Centers in the brainstem that give rise to the vestibulospinal, rubrospinal, and related pathways are of importance in postural mechanisms and standing and righting reflexes. The psychomotor, or cortical associative, level of motor control has to do with memory, initiative, and conscious and unconscious control of motor activity that arises primarily from the motor association cortex anterior to the motor strip.

# OVERVIEW OF CLINICAL MANIFESTATIONS OF DISEASE OF THE MOTOR SYSTEM

The most common manifestation of motor system disease is weakness. Other abnormalities include alterations in muscle tone, changes in muscle size and shape, abnormal involuntary movements, and defective coordination.

## Weakness

Weakness is a common abnormality and can follow many patterns. Terminology may become problematic. For instance, weakness may be generalized or localized, symmetric or asymmetric, proximal or distal, or upper motor neuron or lower motor neuron. The term focal is often used to imply asymmetry; a patient with a hemiparesis is said to have a focal examination. The term generalized is often used to imply symmetry, even though the weakness may not truly be generalized. A disease may cause weakness in a particular distribution that is bilaterally symmetric (e.g., the scapuloperoneal syndromes), but these are not generally regarded as focal even though the involvement is very localized. A patient with bilateral carpal tunnel syndrome or bilateral peroneal nerve palsies would most properly be described as having a multifocal pattern of weakness, even though the weakness is bilateral and symmetric. The term nonfocal is often used to describe a patient's neurologic examination, particularly by non-neurologists. The implication is usually that the examination is normal, or at least that there is no asymmetry. It is a poor and not very helpful term. A patient with Guillain-Barré syndrome causing generalized weakness and impending respiratory failure would have a nonfocal examination, yet be critically ill.

## Other Motor System Abnormalities

Muscle tone may be increased (hypertonia) or decreased (hypotonia). Hypertonia comes in two common variants: rigidity and spasticity. When the increased tone occurs to more or less the same degree throughout the range of passive motion of a limb, and is independent of the speed of the movement, it is referred to as rigidity. When the hypertonia is most marked near the middle of the range of motion and is more apparent with fast than with slow passive movement, it is referred to as spasticity. One of the key characteristics of spasticity is that the hypertonus is velocity dependent, most evident with rapid movements. In lead pipe (plastic) rigidity, there is smooth resistance throughout the range independent of the rate of movement. Gegenhalten (paratonia) is an increase in tone in a limb more or less proportional to the examiner's attempt to move it. In cogwheel rigidity there is ratchety, jerky, tremulous variation in the hypertonia, due primarily to superimposed tremor. Spastic hypertonia is typically associated with increased deep tendon reflexes, loss of superficial reflexes, and Babinski signs. Cogwheel rigidity occurs in Parkinson disease and related conditions. Gegenhalten is usually associated with other abnormal neurologic signs depending on the etiology. The term dystonia refers to transient or sustained hypertonic conditions that do not fit into the other categories. Hypotonia occurs in two primary settings in the adult: myopathies and cerebellar disease. Infantile hypotonia (floppy baby) is a common clinical problem. The differential diagnosis of infantile hypotonia is extensive, and the workup of a floppy baby is a frequent exercise in pediatric neurology.

## Muscle Volume and Contour

Muscle mass or volume may be decreased (atrophy) or increased (hypertrophy). Neurogenic atrophy results from a lesion involving the anterior horn cells, nerve root, or peripheral nerve innervating a muscle; it may be severe. Muscle diseases usually cause only mild to moderate atrophy of the involved muscles. Disuse atrophy occurs after immobilization, as when a limb is in a cast, and is usually mild to moderate in severity and recovers quickly with resumption of use.

True muscle hypertrophy results from an increase in the size of the muscle. It is most often physiologic hypertrophy from heavy use, but it can occur in certain neuromuscular disorders. Pseudohypertrophy refers to apparent muscle enlargement due to replacement of diseased muscle by fat and fibrous tissue. Enlarged calf muscles in patients with Duchenne muscular dystrophy are a classic example of muscle pseudohypertrophy.

## Abnormal Movements

Abnormal involuntary movements occur in a host of neurologic conditions. They come in many forms, ranging from tremor to chorea to muscle fasciculations to myoclonic jerks. The only common characteristic is that the movements are spontaneous and not under volitional control. Involuntary movements may be rhythmic or random, fleeting or sustained, predictable or unpredictable. They may occur in isolation or be accompanied by other neurologic signs. Common types include tremor, chorea, athetosis, hemiballismus, dystonia, tics, and dyskinesias.

## Coordination

Coordination and control of fine motor movements are delicate functions that require smooth interactions between the different components of the motor system as well as normal sensory function. The cerebellum is a critical component, and disease of the cerebellum frequently causes impaired coordination in the absence of weakness or other motor abnormalities. But poor coordination may also be a manifestation of corticospinal tract or extrapyramidal disorders.

# CHAPTER 18

# Motor Strength and Power

**M**otor strength and power indicate the capacity of muscles to exert force and expend energy. Decreased strength is weakness, or paresis; absence of muscle contraction is paralysis, or plegia. Weakness may cause loss of the speed, rapidity, or agility of movement and a decrease in the range, or amplitude, of movement before there is loss of power to formal strength testing. Other manifestations of impaired motor function include fatigability, variation in strength on repeated tests, diminished range and rate of movement, loss of coordination, irregularity and clumsiness of motion, tremulousness, loss of associated movements, and lack of ability to carry out skilled acts.

While judgment of the force exerted in either initiating or resisting movement is the major criterion in the evaluation of strength, observation and palpation of either the contraction of the muscle belly or its movement of its tendon may be helpful adjuncts. The contraction of an extremely weak muscle may sometimes be felt when it cannot be seen. In nonorganic weakness, contraction of the apparently weak muscle may be felt when the patient is asked to carry out movements with synergistic muscles, or the antagonists may be felt to contract when the patient is asked to contract the weak muscle. Weakness may be masked when attempts to contract individual weak muscles are accompanied by activation of other muscles to compensate for the loss of power. In these substitution, or "trick," movements, the patient exploits a strong muscle with similar function to compensate for the loss of action of a weak muscle. Careful observation for alterations in normal movement patterns and substitution movements may indicate loss of function. Endurance is the ability to perform the same act repeatedly.

The strength examination assesses primarily voluntary, or active, muscle contraction rather than reflex contraction. Strength may be classified as kinetic—the force exerted in changing position—and static—the force exerted in resisting movement from a fixed position. Strength may be tested in two ways. The patient may place a joint in a certain position, and then hold it there as the examiner tries to move it. Alternately the patient may try to move a joint or contract a muscle against the fixed resistance of the examiner. In most disease processes, both are equally affected, and the two methods can be used interchangeably. Some patients may comprehend and cooperate better with the first method, but having the patient initiate movement may better detect mild weakness. There is disagreement about how the examiner should apply force. Some authorities recommend a slow application of resistance in which the patient and examiner match effort; others contend that a rapid movement by the examiner will better detect mild weakness. With very weak muscles, strength may have to be judged without resistance or only against the resistance offered by gravity.

Many factors may complicate the strength examination and make assessment more difficult, such as fatigue, systemic illness, and failure to understand or cooperate with testing. Other conditions may result in a false or distorted impression of weakness, such as extrapyramidal disease, ataxia, impairment of the range of motion due to pain, spasm, joint ankylosis, or contractures, and psychiatric conditions such as hysteria and malingering. Motor impersistence is the inability to sustain voluntary motor acts that have been initiated on verbal command. The patient is unable to sustain an activity, such as keeping the eyes closed or the hand raised. It may be a form of apraxia, and has been said to occur most often with left hemisphere lesions. Passive movements are often helpful to distinguish loss of range of motion due to contractures from other reasons such as weakness, pain, and muscle spasm. With contracture, a muscle cannot be stretched to its normal limits without considerable resistance and the production of pain. Contractures are particularly common in the calf muscles, drawing the foot downward ("tight heel cords"). In evaluating contractures and deformities, it is important to differentiate between those of neurogenic origin and those due to orthopedic disease, congenital abnormalities, habitual postures, occupational factors, or other factors that cause mechanical difficulty with movement.

Strength may be assessed in absolute terms (e.g., the examiner comparing the patient's power to a belief of what normal should be), or it may be assessed in comparison to the patient's other muscles. The comparison is most often to a homologous muscle on the other side, as in comparing the two biceps muscles. But proximal strength should be commensurate with distal strength in the same patient. A patient with polymyositis may have weakness of the deltoids on both sides, so one deltoid cannot be judged against the other. But the deltoids may be obviously weaker than the wrist extensors, so there is a proximal to distal gradient of increasing strength that is clearly abnormal. The muscles on the dominant side are usually slightly stronger.

In manual muscle testing (MMT), the strength of individual muscles is tested and graded quantitatively using some scale. Strength is most commonly graded using the 5-level MRC (Medical Research Council) scale, which was developed in Britain in World War II to evaluate patients with peripheral nerve injuries (Table 18.1). The MRC scale has been widely applied to the evaluation of strength in general. However, because of the original purpose the scale is heavily weighted toward the evaluation of very weak muscles. So the most commonly used strength grading scale has significant limitations when dealing with many patients.

There is obviously considerable individual variation in muscle power, affecting examiners as well as patients, dependent in part upon size, gender, body build, age, and activity level. A large, young, powerful physician examining a small, old, sick patient may overcall weakness. Conversely, a small, relatively weak physician examining a large, powerful patient may miss significant weakness because of strength mismatch. As a general principle, reliable strength testing should attempt to break a given muscle. By varying the length of lever and the shortening of the muscle permitted, the examiner may give or take mechanical advantage as necessary to compensate for strength mismatch. Many patients

## TABLE 18.1

**The Medical Research Council Scale of Muscle Strength**

| | |
|---|---|
| 0 | No contraction |
| 1 | A flicker or trace of contraction |
| 2 | Active movement with gravity eliminated |
| 3 | Active movement against gravity |
| 4− | Active movement against gravity and slight resistance |
| 4 | Active movement against gravity and moderate resistance |
| 4+ | Active movement against gravity and strong resistance |
| 5 | Normal power |

of different ages, sizes, and strength levels must be examined in this fashion in order to develop an appreciation of the expected strength of a muscle for a given set of circumstances.

## PATTERNS OF WEAKNESS

There are common patterns of weakness. Recognition of a pattern may help greatly in lesion localization and differential diagnosis. Identification of the process causing weakness is further aided by accompanying signs, such as reflex alterations and sensory loss. Table 18.2 reviews the features of upper motor neuron vs. lower motor neuron weakness. Table 18.3 summarizes some common patterns of weakness and their localization.

Weakness may be focal or generalized. When focal, it may follow the distribution of some structure in the peripheral nervous system, such as a peripheral nerve or spinal root. It may affect one side of the body in a "hemi" distribution. A hemi distribution may affect the arm, leg, and face equally on one side of the body, or one or more areas may be more involved than others. The corticospinal tract (CST) preferentially innervates certain muscle groups, and these are often selectively impaired. When weakness is nonfocal, it may be generalized, predominantly proximal, or predominantly distal. Identification of the process causing weakness is further aided by accompanying signs, such as reflex alterations and sensory loss.

### Generalized Weakness

The term generalized weakness implies that the weakness involves both sides of the body, more or less symmetrically. When a patient has truly generalized weakness, bulbar motor functions—such as facial movements, speech, chewing, and swallowing—are involved as well. Weakness of both arms and both legs with normal bulbar function is quadriparesis or tetraparesis. Weakness of both legs is paraparesis. When weakness affects all four extremities, the likely causes include spinal cord disease, peripheral neuropathy, a neuromuscular junction disorder, or a myopathy.

## TABLE 18.2

### Features of Upper Motor Neuron vs. Lower Motor Neuron Weakness

| Feature | Upper Motor Neuron | Lower Motor Neuron |
|---|---|---|
| Weakness distribution | Corticospinal distribution; hemiparesis, quadriparesis, paraparesis, monoparesis, faciobrachial | Generalized, predominantly proximal, predominantly distal or focal. No preferential involvement of corticospinal innervated muscles |
| Sensory loss distribution | Central pattern | None, stocking glove or peripheral nerve or root distribution |
| Deep tendon reflexes | Increased unless very acute | Normal or decreased |
| Superficial reflexes | Decreased | Normal |
| Pathological reflexes | Yes | No |
| Sphincter function | Sometimes impaired | Normal (except for cauda equina lesion) |
| Muscle tone | Increased | Normal or decreased |
| Pain | No | Sometimes |
| Other CNS signs | Possibly | No |

CNS, central nervous system.

## TABLE 18.3

**Common Patterns of Weakness with Lesions at Different Locations in the Neuraxis**

| Location of Lesion | Distribution of Weakness | Sensory Loss | DTRs** | Possible Accompanying Signs |
|---|---|---|---|---|
| Middle cerebral artery | Contralateral arm & face > leg* | Y | Incr | Aphasia, apraxia, visual field deficit, gaze palsy |
| Anterior cerebral | Contralateral leg > arm & face* | Y | Incr | Cortical sensory loss contralateral leg, frontal lobe signs, sometimes incontinence |
| Internal capsule | Contralateral face = arm = leg* | N | Incr | None ("pure motor stroke") |
| Brainstem | Ipsilateral cranial nerve & contralateral body* | Y | Incr | Variable, depending on level |
| Cervical cord (transverse) | Both arms and both legs* | Y | Incr | Bowel, bladder, or sexual dysfunction common |
| Thoracic cord (transverse) | Both legs* | Y | Incr | Bowel, bladder, or sexual dysfunction common |
| Cauda equina | Both legs, asymmetric, multiple root pattern | Y | Decr | Occasional bowel, bladder, or sexual dysfunction; sometimes pain |
| Anterior horn cell | Focal early, generalized late | N | Incr | Atrophy, fasciculations, bulbar weakness |
| Single nerve root | Muscles of the affected myotome | Y | Decr | Pain |
| Plexus | Plexus pattern, complete or partial | Usually | Decr | Pain is common, especially with brachial "plexitis" |
| Mononeuropathy | Muscles of the affected nerve | Usually | Decr | Variable atrophy, variable pain |
| Polyneuropathy | Distal > proximal | Usually | Decr | Variable pain, atrophy late |
| Neuromuscular junction | Bulbar, proximal extremities | N | Normal | Ptosis, ophthalmoparesis, fatigable weakness, fluctuating weakness |
| Muscle | Proximal > distal | N | Normal | Pain uncommon, many potential patterns (limb girdle, facioscapu-lohumeral, etc.), pseudohypertrophy, myotonia |

DTR, deep tendon reflex; Y, yes; N no; Incr, increased; Decr, decreased.
*Extremity weakness in a corticospinal tract distribution.
**With corticospinal lesions, DTRs acutely may be normal or decreased (neural shock).

When spinal cord disease is the culprit and the deficit is incomplete, more severe involvement of those muscles preferentially innervated by the CST can frequently be discerned. Reflexes are usually increased (though in the acute stages they may be decreased or absent); there is usually some alteration of sensation; sometimes a discrete spinal "level"; superficial reflexes disappear; and there may be bowel and bladder dysfunction. Generalized peripheral nerve disease tends to predominantly involve distal muscles, although there are exceptions. There is no preferential involvement of CST innervated muscles; reflexes are usually decreased; sensory loss is frequently present; and bowel and bladder function are not disturbed. With a neuromuscular junction disorder, the weakness is likely to be worse proximally; sensation is spared; reflexes are normal; and there is usually involvement of bulbar muscles, especially with ptosis and ophthalmoplegia. When the problem is a primary muscle disorder, weakness is usually more severe proximally; reflexes are normal; sensation is normal; and with only a few exceptions, bulbar function is spared except for occasional dysphagia. These are generalizations. Some neuropathies may cause proximal weakness, and some myopathies may affect distal muscles; not all patients with a neuromuscular transmission disorder have bulbar involvement.

Motor neuron disease is a special case. Amyotrophic lateral sclerosis (ALS) characteristically involves both the upper and lower motor neurons. It produces a clinical picture of weakness and wasting due to involvement of the lower motor neurons in the anterior horn of the spinal cord, combined with weakness and hyperreflexia due to involvement of the upper motor neurons in the cerebral cortex that give rise to the corticospinal tract. There is upper motor neuron weakness (cerebral cortex pathology) superimposed on lower motor neuron weakness (spinal cord pathology).

### Focal Weakness

Weakness of the arm and leg on one side of the body is hemiparesis. This may range in severity from very mild, manifest only as pronator drift and impairment of fine motor control, to total paralysis. Monoparesis is weakness limited to one extremity, such as the leg contralateral to an anterior cerebral artery stroke. Diplegia is weakness of like parts on the two sides of the body; the term spastic diplegia refers to weakness of both legs that occurs in cerebral palsy; and facial diplegia is weakness of both sides of the face. Spastic weakness of one arm and the opposite leg is referred to as cruciate or crossed paralysis, or hemiplegia alternans. Reflexes—typically increased unless the process is acute—and accompanying sensory loss help identify such focal weakness as central in origin.

Certain patterns of muscle weakness point to a peripheral nerve, plexus, or root lesion. A mononeuropathy, such as a radial nerve palsy, or a spinal root lesion, such as from a herniated disc, causes weakness limited to the distribution of the involved nerve or root. A plexopathy may cause weakness of the entire limb, or weakness only in the distribution of certain plexus components. With such lower motor neuron pathology, reflexes are typically decreased and there is often accompanying sensory loss. Localization of focal weakness due to root, plexus, and peripheral nerve pathology requires intimate familiarity with peripheral neuroanatomy.

With a peripheral nerve lesion, all muscles below the level of the lesion are at risk. When multiple muscles of an extremity are weak in a non-CST distribution, localization depends on recognizing the common innervating structure: root, plexus component, or peripheral nerve.

With lower motor neuron pathology, reflexes are typically decreased, and there is often accompanying sensory loss. Anterior horn cell disease often begins with focal weakness that may simulate mononeuropathy, but it evolves into a more widespread pattern as the disease progresses, culminating in generalized weakness. Except for extraocular muscle involvement in myasthenia gravis, it is rare for a myopathy or neuromuscular junction disorder to cause focal weakness.

## NONORGANIC WEAKNESS

The first step in evaluating weakness is often deciding whether it is organic or nonorganic, i.e., due to a psychiatric disorder. This distinction is not always easy. Patients with nonorganic weakness are commonly thought to have neurologic disease, but just as often patients with real weakness are dismissed as uncooperative, hysterical, or malingering. Coaching is often helpful in improving poor effort, but some patients, in spite of all, will give only erratic and variable effort.

Some things are often useful in distinguishing organic from nonorganic weakness. Patients with bona fide organic muscle weakness will yield smoothly as the examiner defeats the weak muscle. The patient gives uniform resistance throughout the movement. If the examiner decreases his resistance, the patient will begin to win the battle. If the examiner drops the resistance level, the patient with nonorganic weakness will not continue to push or pull. Instead, the patient will also stop resisting so that no matter how little force the examiner applies, there is an absence of follow-through and the patient never overcomes the examiner. When there is nonorganic weakness, resistance is erratic and often collapses abruptly. The muscular contractions are poorly sustained and may give way suddenly, rather than gradually, as the patient resists the force exerted by the examiner. Some patients will give up entirely and allow the muscle or limb to flop; others will provide variable resistance throughout the range of motion with alternating moments of effort and no effort. This pattern of variable strength is referred to as "ratchety," "give way," or "catch and give." It is characteristic of nonorganic weakness. In nonorganic weakness, functional testing may fail to confirm weakness suspected during strength testing. For example, there may be apparent foot dorsiflexion weakness, yet the patient is able to stand on the heel without difficulty. The patient with nonorganic weakness may be calm and indifferent while demonstrating the lack of strength, showing little sign of alarm at the presence of complete paralysis, and smile cheerfully during the examination. If the examiner raises and drops an extremity, a limb with psychogenic paralysis may drop slowly to avoid injury, while an extremity with real weakness would drop rapidly, especially if the paralysis is flaccid.

The Hoover (automatic walking) sign is useful for evaluating suspected nonorganic leg weakness. When a normal supine patient flexes the hip to lift one leg, there is a downward movement of the other leg. The extension counter-movement of the opposite leg is a normal associated movement. An extension movement of one leg normally accompanies flexion of the other leg, as in walking. In organic leg weakness, the downward pressure of the contralateral heel occurs when the patient tries to raise the weak leg, and the examiner can feel the extension pressure by placing a hand beneath the heel that remains on the bed. In nonorganic leg weakness, there is no downward pressure of the contralateral heel, but the extension movement of the "paralyzed" leg may be felt as the good leg is raised (Hoover sign).

## EXAMINATION OF MOTOR STRENGTH AND POWER

Reliable strength testing requires proper patient positioning and avoidance of unwanted movements. Testing may be done in various positions depending on the muscle to be tested and its power. Testing in the seated position suffices under most circumstances. It is important to fix the proximal portion of a limb when the movements of the distal portion are being tested. For instance, when testing forearm pronation strength, the patient must not be allowed to internally rotate the shoulder to compensate for lack of pronation power. When evaluating very weak muscles, gravity must be eliminated to detect residual power. A very weak biceps muscle (MRC grade 2/5), even when it cannot succeed against gravity, may be able to flex the elbow if the arm is raised to shoulder height so that the forearm can be moved horizontally. The wrist and finger drop of radial nerve palsy creates such a mechanical disadvantage for contraction that the patient may appear to have weakness of grip and finger abduction, but these functions are intact when the wrist and fingers are passively extended.

## EXAMINATION OF SPECIFIC MOVEMENTS AND MUSCLES

Many reference sources are available to assist in learning muscle examination techniques. There is some difference regarding the exact innervation of individual muscles among different reference sources, and occasionally there is variable or anomalous innervation. Table 18.4 through Table 18.7

## TABLE 18.4

**Innervation of Muscles Responsible for Movements of the Head and Neck**

| Muscle | Segmental Innervation | Peripheral Nerve |
|---|---|---|
| Sternocleidomastoid | Cranial XI; C (1) 2–3 | Spinal accessory nerve |
| Trapezius | Cranial XI; C (2) 3–4 | Spinal accessory nerve |
| Scalenus anterior | C 4–7 | |
| Scalenus medius | C 4–8 | |
| Scalenus posterior | C 6–8 | |
| Longus capitis | C 1–4 | |
| Longus colli | C 2–6 | |
| Rectus capitis anterior | C 1–2 | Suboccipital nerve |
| Rectus capitis lateralis | C 1 | Suboccipital nerve |
| Rectus capitis posterior | C 1 | Suboccipital nerve |
| Obliquus capitis inferior | C 1 | Suboccipital nerve |
| Obliquus capitis superior | C 1 | Suboccipital nerve |
| Splenius capitis | C 2–4 (1–6) | |
| Splenius cervicis | C 2–4 (1–6) | |
| Semispinalis capitis | C 1–4 | |
| Semispinalis cervicis | C 3–6 | |
| Spinalis cervicis | C 5–8 | |
| Sacrospinalis | C 1–8 | |
| Iliocostalis cervicis | C 1–8 | |
| Longissimus capitis | C 1–8 | |
| Longissimus cervicis | C 1–8 | |
| Intertransversarii | C 1–8 | |
| Rotatores | C 1–8 | |
| Multifidi | C 1–8 | |

Minor innervation indicated by parentheses.

give the most generally accepted spinal cord segment and peripheral nerve innervation of the more important muscles. Table 18.8 and Table 18.9 give the innervation by root.

### Examination of Movements and Muscles of the Neck

The principal neck movements are flexion, extension (retraction), rotation (turning), and lateral bending (tilting, abduction). Many different muscle groups contribute to the various neck movements. Except for the sternocleidomastoid (SCM) and trapezius it is not possible to examine them individually, and the assessment is made of movement (e.g., neck flexion) rather than particular muscles. The SCM is a flexor and rotator of the head and neck; the trapezius retracts the neck and

## TABLE 18.5

**Innervation of Muscles Responsible for Movements of the Shoulder Girdle and Upper Extremity**

| Muscle | Segmental Innervation | Peripheral Nerve |
|---|---|---|
| Trapezius | Cranial XI; C (2) 3–4 | Spinal accessory nerve |
| Levator scapulae | C 3–4 | Nerves to levator scapulae |
| | C 5 | Dorsal scapular nerve |
| Rhomboideus major | C 4–5 | Dorsal scapular nerve |
| Rhomboideus minor | C 4–5 | Dorsal scapular nerve |
| Serratus anterior | C 5–7 | Long thoracic nerve |
| Deltoid | C 5–6 | Axillary nerve |
| Teres minor | C 5–6 | Axillary nerve |
| Supraspinatus | C (4) 5–6 | Suprascapular nerve |
| Infraspinatus | C (4) 5–6 | Suprascapular nerve |
| Latissimus dorsi | C 6–8 | Thoracodorsal nerve |
| Pectoralis major | C 5–T 1 | Lateral and medial anterior thoracic nerves |
| Pectoralis minor | C 7–T 1 | Medial anterior thoracic nerve |
| Subscapularis | C 5–7 | Subscapular nerves |
| Teres major | C 5–7 | Lower subscapular nerve |
| Subclavius | C 5–6 | Nerve to subclavius |
| Coracobrachialis | C 6–7 | Musculocutaneous nerve |
| Biceps brachii | C 5–6 | Musculocutaneous nerve |
| Brachialis | C 5–6 | Musculocutaneous nerve |
| Brachioradialis | C 5–6 | Radial nerve |
| Triceps brachii | C 6–8 | Radial nerve |
| Anconeus | C 7–8 | Radial nerve |
| Supinator | C 6–7 | Radial nerve |
| Extensor carpi radialis longus | C (5) 6–7 | Radial nerve |
| Extensor carpi radialis brevis | C 7–8 | Radial nerve |
| Extensor carpi ulnaris | C 7–8 | Radial nerve |
| Extensor digitorum communis | C 7–8 | Radial nerve |
| Extensor indicis proprius | C 7–8 | Radial nerve |
| Extensor digiti minimi | C 7–8 | Radial nerve |
| Extensor pollicis longus | C 7–8 | Radial nerve |
| Extensor pollicis brevis | C 7–8 | Radial nerve |

*(continued)*

## TABLE 18.5 (Continued)

**Innervation of Muscles Responsible for Movements of the Shoulder Girdle and Upper Extremity**

| Muscle | Segmental Innervation | Peripheral Nerve |
| --- | --- | --- |
| Abductor pollicis longus | C 7–8 | Radial nerve |
| Pronator teres | C 6–7 | Median nerve |
| Flexor carpi radialis | C 6–7 | Median nerve |
| Pronator quadratus | C 7–8 | Median nerve |
| Palmaris longus | C 7–8 | Median nerve |
| Flexor digitorum superficialis | C 7–T 1 | Median nerve |
| Flexor digitorum profundus (radial half) | C 8–T 1 | Median nerve |
| Lumbricales 1 and 2 | C 8–T 1 | Median nerve |
| Flexor pollicis longus | C 7–T 1 | Median nerve |
| Flexor pollicis brevis (lateral head) | C 8–T 1 | Median nerve |
| Abductor pollicis brevis | C 8–T 1 | Median nerve |
| Opponens pollicis | C 8–T 1 | Median nerve |
| Flexor carpi ulnaris | C 7–T 1 | Ulnar nerve |
| Flexor digitorum profundus (ulnar half) | C 8–T 1 | Ulnar nerve |
| Interossei | C 8–T 1 | Ulnar nerve |
| Lumbricales 3 and 4 | C 8–T 1 | Ulnar nerve |
| Flexor pollicis brevis (medial head) | C 8–T 1 | Ulnar nerve |
| Flexor digiti minimi brevis | C 8–T 1 | Ulnar nerve |
| Abductor digiti minimi | C 8–T 1 | Ulnar nerve |
| Opponens digiti minimi | C 8–T 1 | Ulnar nerve |
| Palmaris brevis | C 8–T 1 | Ulnar nerve |
| Adductor pollicis | C 8–T 1 | Ulnar nerve |

Minor innervation indicated by parentheses.

draws it to one side. Other muscles contribute to neck flexion, especially the prevertebral group. Many muscles contribute to neck extension, including the trapezius and the paravertebral muscles. Many of these muscles when contracting unilaterally rotate the spine. The paravertebral musculature is a massive, complex amalgam of individual muscle groups that primarily serve to extend and rotate the neck and trunk.

Neck flexors are tested by having the patient try to place the chin on the chest as the examiner applies extension force to the forehead (Figure 18.1). Extensors are tested by having the patient extend against the examiner's resistance applied to the occiput (Figure 18.2). Neck rotation is accomplished by the contralateral SCM and ipsilateral splenius capitus and trapezius; examination of the SCM and trapezius muscles is discussed in Chapter 15. Neck flexor strength may be tested with the patient sitting or supine, neck extension sitting or prone. Examination of the neck muscles must be done carefully in any patient at risk for cervical spine disease.

## TABLE 18.6

**Innervation of Muscles Responsible for Movements of the Thorax and Abdomen**

| Muscle | Segmental Innervation | Peripheral Nerve |
|---|---|---|
| Diaphragm | C 3–5 | Phrenic nerve |
| Intercostal muscles (internal and external) | T 1–12 | Intercostal nerves |
| Levatores costarum | C 8–T 11 | Intercostal nerves |
| Transversus thoracis | T 2–7 | Intercostal nerves |
| Serratus posterior superior | T 1–4 | Intercostal nerves |
| Serratus posterior inferior | T 9–12 | Intercostal nerves |
| Rectus abdominis | T 5–12 | Intercostal nerves |
| Pyramidalis | T 11–12 | Intercostal nerves |
| Transversus abdominis | T 7–L 1 | Intercostal, ilioinguinal, and iliohypogastric nerves |
| Obliquus internus abdominis | T 7–L 1 | Intercostal, ilioinguinal, and iliohypogastric nerves |
| Obliquus externus abdominis | T 7-L 1 | Intercostal, ilioinguinal, and iliohypogastric nerves |

## TABLE 18.7

**Innervation of Muscles Responsible for Movements of the Lower Extremities**

| Muscle | Segmental Innervation | Peripheral Nerve |
|---|---|---|
| Psoas major | L (1) 2–3 (4) | Nerve to psoas major |
| Psoas minor | L 1–2 | Nerve to psoas minor |
| Iliacus | L 2–3 (4) | Femoral nerve |
| Quadriceps femoris | L 2–4 | Femoral nerve |
| Sartorius | L 2–3 | Femoral nerve |
| Pectineus | L 2–3 | Femoral nerve |
| Gluteus maximus | L 5–S 2 | Inferior gluteal nerve |
| Gluteus medius | L 4–S 1 | Superior gluteal nerve |
| Gluteus minimus | L 4–S 1 | Superior gluteal nerve |
| Tensor fasciae latae | L 4–S 1 | Superior gluteal nerve |
| Piriformis | (L5) S 1–2 | Nerve to piriformis |
| Adductor longus | L 2–4 | Obturator nerve |
| Adductor brevis | L 2–4 | Obturator nerve |
| Adductor magnus | L 2–4 | Obturator nerve |
| Adductor magnus | L 4–5 | Sciatic nerve |

*(continued)*

## TABLE 18.7 (*Continued*)

**Innervation of Muscles Responsible for Movements of the Lower Extremities**

| Muscle | Segmental Innervation | Peripheral Nerve |
|---|---|---|
| Gracilis | L 2–4 | Obturator nerve |
| Obturator externus | L 2–4 | Obturator nerve |
| Obturator internus | L 5–S 1 | Nerve to obturator internus |
| Gemellus superior | L 5–S 1 | Nerve to obturator internus |
| Gemellus inferior | L 5–S 1 | Nerve to quadratus femoris |
| Quadratus femoris | L 5–S 1 | Nerve to quadratus femoris |
| Biceps femoris (long head) | L 5–S 1 | Tibial nerve |
| Semimembranosus | L 5–S 1 | Tibial nerve |
| Semitendinosus | L 5–S 2 | Tibial nerve |
| Popliteus | L 5–S 1 | Tibial nerve |
| Gastrocnemius | S 1–S 2 | Tibial nerve |
| Soleus | S 1–S 2 | Tibial nerve |
| Plantaris | S 1–S 2 | Tibial nerve |
| Tibialis posterior | L 5–S 1 | Tibial nerve |
| Flexor digitorum longus | L 5–S 1 | Tibial nerve |
| Flexor hallucis longus | L 5–S 1 | Tibial nerve |
| Biceps femoris (short head) | L 5–S 2 | Common peroneal nerve |
| Tibialis anterior | L 4–L 5 | Deep peroneal nerve |
| Peroneus tertius | L 5–S 1 | Deep peroneal nerve |
| Extensor digitorum longus | L 5–S 1 | Deep peroneal nerve |
| Extensor hallucis longus | L 5 | Deep peroneal nerve |
| Extensor digitorum brevis | L 5–S 1 | Deep peroneal nerve |
| Extensor hallucis brevis | L 5–S 1 | Deep peroneal nerve |
| Peroneus longus | L 5–S 1 | Superficial peroneal nerve |
| Peroneus brevis | L 5–S 1 | Superficial peroneal nerve |
| Flexor digitorum brevis | S 1–2 | Medial plantar nerve |
| Flexor hallucis brevis | S 1–2 | Medial plantar nerve |
| Abductor hallucis | S 1–2 | Medial plantar nerve |
| Lumbricales (medial 1 or 2) | S 1–3 | Medial plantar nerve |
| Quadratus plantae | S 1–2 | Lateral plantar nerve |
| Adductor hallucis | S 2–3 | Lateral plantar nerve |
| Abductor digiti minimi pedis | S 1–3 | Lateral plantar nerve |
| Flexor digiti minimi brevis | S 2–3 | Lateral plantar nerve |
| Lumbricales (lateral 2 or 3) | S 1–3 | Lateral plantar nerve |
| Interossei | S 2–3 | Lateral plantar nerve |

Minor innervation indicated by parentheses.

## TABLE 18.8

**Major Upper-Extremity Muscles Innervated by Different Roots**

| Root | Muscles Supplied |
|------|------------------|
| C4 | Levator scapulae, rhomboids |
| C5 | Levator scapulae, rhomboids, supraspinatus, infraspinatus, teres major and minor, deltoid, biceps, brachialis, BR, serratus anterior, pectoralis |
| C6 | Supraspinatus, infraspinatus, teres major and minor, deltoid, biceps, brachialis, BR, supinator, serratus anterior, pectoralis, FCR, pronator teres, latissimus dorsi, ECRL (triceps) |
| C7 | Serratus anterior, pectoralis, teres major, latissimus dorsi, triceps, anconeus, pronator teres, FCR, ECRL, EDC, ECU, supinator (EIP, FCU, FDS, FPL, extensor pollicis longus/brevis) |
| C8 | Latissimus dorsi, pectoralis, triceps, anconeus, EDC, ECU, EIP, extensor pollicis longus/brevis, FCU, FDS, FDP, FPL, PQ, APB, APL, OP, AP, ADM, lumbricals, interossei |
| T1 | Pectoralis, FCU, FDS, FDP, FPL, APB, OP, AP, ADM, lumbricals, interossei |

BR, brachioradialis; FCR, flexor carpi radialis; ECRL, extensor carpi radialis longus; EDC, extensor digitorum communis; ECU, extensor carpi ulnaris; EIP, extensor indicis proprius; FCU, flexor carpi ulnaris; FDS, flexor digitorum superficialis; FPL, flexor pollicis longus; FDP, flexor digitorum profundus; PQ, pronator quadratus; APB, abductor pollicis brevis, APL, abductor pollicis longus; OP, opponens pollicis; AP, adductor pollicis; ADM, abductor digiti minimi.

Parentheses signify minor contribution.

## TABLE 18.9

**Major Lower-Extremity Muscles Innervated by Different Roots**

| Root | Muscles Supplied |
|------|------------------|
| L2 | Iliopsoas, sartorius, quadriceps (adductors, gracilis) |
| L3 | Iliopsoas, sartorius, adductors, gracilis, quadriceps |
| L4 | Gracilis, gluteus medius, TFL, quadriceps, adductor magnus, TA (iliopsoas, adductor longus) |
| L5 | Gluteus maximus, internal hamstring, biceps femoris, gluteus medius, TFL, peronei, TA, EHL, EDL, EDB, TP, FDL, EHL (adductor magnus) |
| S1 | Internal hamstring, biceps femoris, gluteus maximus, gastrocnemius, soleus, FDL, FHL, ADMP, AH, EDB, lumbricals (gluteus medius, TFL, peronei, EDL, TP) |
| S2 | Gluteus maximus, gastrocnemius, soleus, AH, ADMP, interossei, lumbricals (internal hamstring, short head of biceps femoris) |
| S3 | Interossei, lumbricals, ADMP |

TFL, tensor fascia lata; TA, tibialis anterior; EHL, extensor hallucis longus; EDL, extensor digitorum longus; EDB, extensor digitorum brevis; TP, tibialis posterior; FDL, flexor digitorum longus; FHL, flexor hallucis longus; ADMP, abductor digiti minimi pedis; AH, abductor hallucis.

Parentheses signify minor contribution.

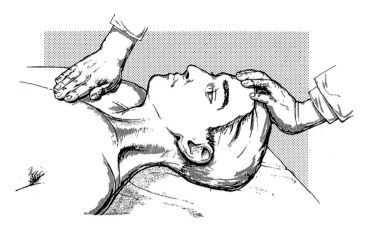

**FIGURE 18.1**  ●   Examination of flexion of the neck. The patient attempts to flex his neck against resistance; the sternocleidomastoid, platysma and other flexor muscles can be seen and palpated.

## Examination of Movements and Muscles of the Upper Extremities

The responsible muscles and their innervation are given in Table 18.5.

### The Shoulder

Movements of the shoulder take place at the sternoclavicular, acromioclavicular, and glenohumeral joints. Because the scapula is firmly connected to the clavicle at the acromioclavicular joint, the two bones tend to move as a unit with the motion taking place primarily at the sternoclavicular joint. Movements of the scapula are elevation, depression, retraction (movement away from the chest wall), protraction (movement toward the chest wall), and rotation. The ventral surface of the scapula is a

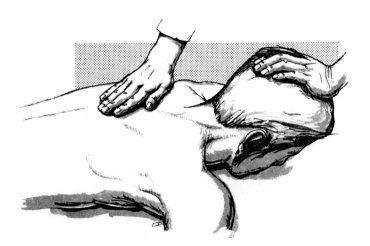

**FIGURE 18.2**  ●   Examination of extension of the neck. The patient attempts to extend his neck against resistance; contraction of the trapezius and other extensor muscles can be seen and felt, and strength of movement can be judged.

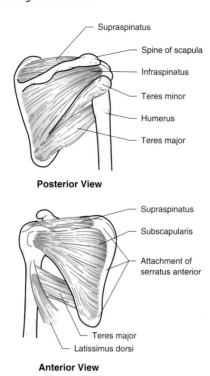

Supraspinatus

Spine of scapula

Infraspinatus

Teres minor

Humerus

Teres major

**Posterior View**

Supraspinatus

Subscapularis

Attachment of
serratus anterior

Teres major

Latissimus dorsi

**Anterior View**

*FIGURE 18.3* ● The muscles of the scapula.

concavity known as the subscapular fossa that is filled mostly with the subscapularis muscle. The serratus anterior lies between the subscapularis and the chest wall and inserts into a thin rim of the scapula along the vertebral border and slightly expanded triangular areas at the superior and inferior angles (Figure 18.3). The serratus runs obliquely from its origination from the upper eight ribs along the lateral chest wall to its attachment to the scapula. The trapezius is a diamond-shaped muscle that attaches widely to the shoulder girdle. The superior fibers insert along the posterior border of the clavicle and scapular spine, the middle and lower fibers along the scapular spine. The upper and middle fibers insert laterally along the scapular spine, the lower fibers more medially (Figure 18.4). The rhomboids (major and minor) arise from the spinous process of the upper thoracic vertebrae, and insert along the medial border of the scapula. The levator scapula originates from the upper cervical vertebra and drops diagonally to insert along the upper medial border of the scapula.

The upper fibers of the trapezius, assisted by the levator scapula, elevate the scapula and the point of the shoulder, and rotate the scapula upward. The middle fibers rotate the scapula upward and assist the rhomboids in retraction. The lower fibers rotate and depress the scapula, and draw it toward the midline. The rhomboids act primarily to retract the scapula, bracing the shoulder backward. The levator scapulae acts with the trapezius to elevate the scapula. The serratus anterior, assisted by the pectoralis minor, protracts the scapula, pulling it anteriorly. It is critical in all functions that involve reaching or pushing forward. The expanded insertion at the inferior angle helps to pull the inferior scapular angle forward around the chest wall. It also, along with the trapezius, rotates the scapula and raises the point of the shoulder to abduct the arm above horizontal. It helps to fix the scapula while other muscles abduct or flex the arm.

Elevation of the scapula, as in shrugging the shoulder, is carried out by the upper trapezius and levator scapulae muscles, assisted by the sternocleidomastoid. The levator scapula is innervated

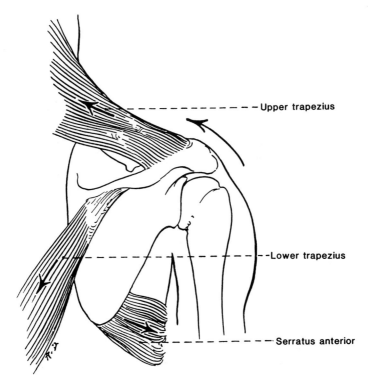

***FIGURE 18.4*** ● Upward rotators of the scapula. (Reprinted with permission from Weibers DO, Dale AJD, Kokmen E, Swanson JW, eds. *Mayo Clinic Examinations in Neurology,* 7th ed. St. Louis: Mosby, 1998.)

by direct branches from C3 and C4 with a contribution from C5 via the dorsal scapular nerve. The levator scapulae draws the scapula upward and rotates it so that the inferior angle approaches the spinal column. Depression of the scapula is carried out primarily by the lower trapezius, pectoralis minor, and subclavius muscles.

   Retraction of the scapula is carried out primarily by the rhomboids and the middle trapezius. The rhomboids also draw the scapulae together, as in standing at attention. The rhomboids are innervated by a twig directly from the C5 nerve root, and not via the brachial plexus. Examination of the rhomboids is important in the differentiation of C5 radiculopathy from upper trunk brachial plexopathy. In protraction of the scapula, the scapula moves forward as in throwing a punch. This movement is carried out primarily by the serratus anterior (long thoracic nerve, C5–C7). The serratus keeps the vertebral border of the scapula applied to the thorax and pulls the scapula forward and laterally. Rotation of the scapula is accomplished by the trapezius, serratus anterior, pectorals, rhomboids, and latissimus dorsi. Normal scapular rotation is essential to efficient shoulder abduction.

### The Scapular Muscles

The rhomboids can be tested by having the patient, with hand on hip, retract the shoulder, against the examiner's attempt to push the elbow forward (Figure 18.5). If the patient braces the shoulders backward as if standing at attention, the bulge of the rhomboids can be seen and palpated along the medial border of the scapula. Another test of rhomboid function is to have the patient place the back of the hand against the small of the back and to push backward with the palm against the examiner's resistance. The rhomboid major contracts vigorously as a downward rotator of the scapula. Lifting the hand off the small of the back is also used to test the subscapularis.

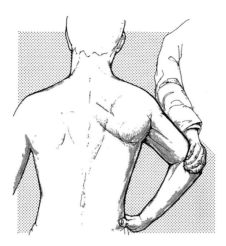

**FIGURE 18.5** ● Examination of the rhomboids. With hand on hip, the patient retracts the shoulder against the examiner's effort to push the elbow forward; the contracting muscles can be seen and palpated.

The different parts of the trapezius must be tested separately. One test of the upper fibers is to have the patient shrug the shoulders against resistance (Figure 15.3). A better test is resisting the patient's attempt to touch the occiput to the acromion. The middle fibers may be tested by having the patient retract the scapula against resistance (Figure 18.6), or having the patient hold the arm horizontally abducted, palm up, and attempting to push the elbow forward. The serratus anterior can be tested by having the patient make movements that involve forward reaching or pushing, and observing for evidence of scapular winging (see next section). The classical test is to have the patient push against a wall, comparing how well the scapulae remain against the chest wall on the two sides (Figure 18.7).

## Winging of the Scapula

Normally, the medial border of the scapula remains close to the chest wall when the arms are raised. However, with weakness of either the serratus anterior or the trapezius, the vertebral border or the entire scapula protrudes posteriorly, away from the thoracic wall. This causes the deformity

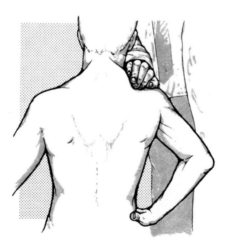

**FIGURE 18.6** ● Examination of the trapezius. On retraction of the shoulder against resistance, the middle fibers of the muscle can be seen and palpated.

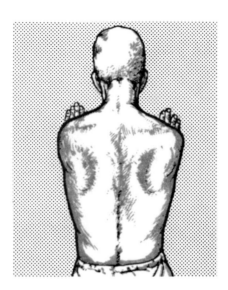

*FIGURE 18.7*  •   Examination of the serratus anterior. The patient pushes against a wall with his arms extended horizontally in front of him; normally, the medial border of the scapula remains close to the thoracic wall.

known as "winging" (Figure 18.8). The trapezius is a rotator and retractor of the scapula and functions primarily during abduction of the arm to the side in the coronal plane of the body. When the trapezius is weak, scapular winging is more apparent on attempted abduction of the arm than on forward elevation. Trapezius winging may be made more conspicuous by having the patient bend

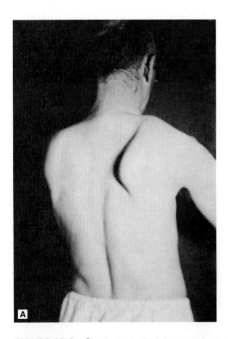

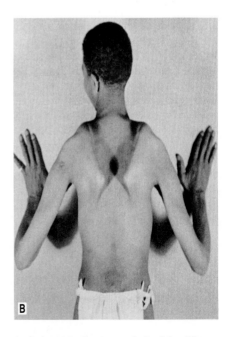

*FIGURE 18.8*  •   "Winging" of the scapula. **A.** Unilateral winging secondary to paralysis of the right serratus anterior. **B.** Bilateral winging in a patient with muscular dystrophy.

forward at the waist so the upper body is parallel to the ground, then raise the arms to the sides, as if beginning a swan dive. This requires strong action by the trapezius to retract the scapula and accentuates the posterior displacement of the shoulder girdle.

The serratus anterior is primarily a protractor of the scapula and functions during forward arm elevation. When the serratus is weak, the inferior angle is shifted medially and the entire vertebral border rides up from the chest wall. Serratus anterior weakness causes winging that is more obvious when trying to elevate the arm in front, in the sagittal plane of the body; it is less obvious when the arms are abducted to the sides. This difference aids in differentiating serratus anterior winging (as from a long thoracic nerve palsy) from the flaring of the scapula that occurs with trapezius weakness (as from a spinal accessory nerve palsy). Serratus winging may be accentuated by having the patient protract the scapula against resistance (Figure 18.7). Scapular winging is also discussed in Chapter 15.

### The Glenohumeral Joint

The principal movements at the glenohumeral joint are abduction, adduction, external and internal rotation, flexion, extension, and elevation of the arm. These movements are best appreciated as taking place in the plane of the body of the scapula rather than in the body as a whole.

The deltoid is the most prominent muscle in the shoulder region. The deltoid has three portions: anterior, middle, and posterior. The middle deltoid and supraspinatus muscles abduct the shoulder. With deltoid contraction, the arm is abducted (raised laterally) to the horizontal plane. Further abduction, or elevation above the horizontal plane, is carried out by the associated action of the trapezius and the serratus anterior, which rotate the scapula and tilt the angle of the glenoid fossa upward.

The major function of the deltoid is tested either by noting the ability of the patient to abduct the arm through the range up to 90 degrees against resistance (Figure 18.9), or to hold the arm in abduction to the horizontal level, either laterally or forward (the elbow may be either flexed or extended), and resist the examiner's attempt to push it down. Testing both sides simultaneously helps the patient maintain balance and also helps in the comparison of strength on the two sides. The supraspinatus helps abduct the shoulder through the first 15 degrees. The muscle belly lies in the supraspinous fossa of the scapula; its contraction can be palpated and sometimes seen when the arm is abducted less than 15 degrees against resistance (Figure 18.10). The supraspinatus, along with the infraspinatus, teres minor, and subscapularis, form the rotator cuff.

The primary adductors of the shoulder are the pectoralis major and latissimus dorsi. On attempts to adduct the horizontally abducted arm against resistance, the contraction of the sternocostal and

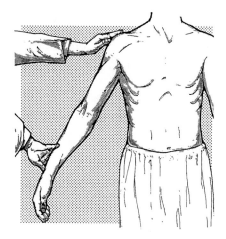

**FIGURE 18.9** ● Examination of the deltoid. The patient attempts to abduct his arm against resistance; the contracting deltoid can be seen and palpated.

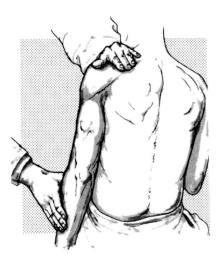

**FIGURE 18.10**  ●   Examination of the supraspinatus. Contraction of the muscle fibers can be felt during early stages of abduction of the arm.

clavicular portions of the pectoralis can be seen and felt (Figure 18.11). The muscle can also be tested by having the patient move the horizontally abducted arm forward, or try to press the hands together with the arms in front, or try to internally rotate the forearms with the elbows at the side and flexed, in a position as if holding a book. The latissimus dorsi adducts, extends, and medially rotates the shoulder and may be tested in various ways (Figure 18.12). The muscle belly can also be felt when the patient coughs or pushes the arm downward and backward.

External rotation of the shoulder is carried out principally by the infraspinatus and teres minor muscles. To test these muscles, the patient attempts to externally rotate the shoulder by turning the forearm laterally and backward against resistance while the elbow is flexed at an angle of 90 degrees and held at the side (Figure 18.13). Internal rotation at the shoulder results primarily from contraction of the subscapularis, the chief internal rotator, and teres major muscles; other muscles also

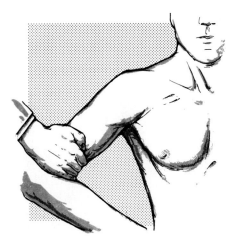

**FIGURE 18.11**  ●   Examination of the pectoralis major. Contraction of the muscle can be seen and felt during attempts to adduct the arm against resistance.

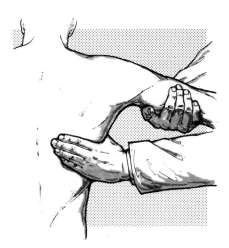

**FIGURE 18.12** ● Examination of the latissimus dorsi. On adduction of the horizontally and laterally abducted arm against resistance, the contracting muscle fibers can be seen and palpated.

contribute. Internal rotation is tested by having the patient move the forearm medially against resistance with the elbow flexed and at the side—the opposite motion from external rotation. Internal rotation can also be tested by having the patient lift the back of the hand off the small of the back against resistance, as is done when testing the rhomboids.

## The Elbow

The principal movements at the elbow are flexion and extension of the forearm at the elbow joint and pronation and supination at the radioulnar joint.

Many muscles contribute to elbow flexion; the primary ones are the biceps brachii, brachialis, and brachioradialis. Which muscle is the prime mover depends on the position of the forearm. The biceps is an elbow flexor and also a strong supinator of the forearm. Its supination power is greatest

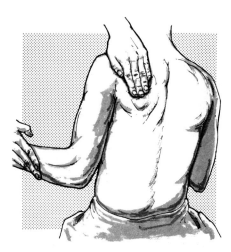

**FIGURE 18.13** ● Examination of the external rotators of the arm. On external rotation of the arm while the elbow is flexed and kept close to the body, the contracting infraspinatus muscle can be seen and palpated.

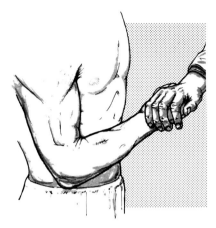

**FIGURE 18.14**  ●  Examination of the biceps brachii. On attempts to flex the forearm against resistance, the contracting biceps muscle can be seen and palpated.

when the forearm is flexed and pronated. Its flexion power is greatest when the forearm is supinated. The brachialis flexes the elbow regardless of forearm position. The brachioradialis acts as an elbow flexor when the forearm is held midway between pronation and supination (thumb up). The brachioradialis acts as a supinator when the forearm is extended and pronated, but as a pronator when the forearm is flexed and supinated.

Biceps and brachialis functions are tested by having the patient attempt to flex the elbow against resistance. The biceps contraction can be seen and felt, but the brachialis is buried (Figure 18.14). The brachioradialis is tested by attempts to flex the semi-pronated forearm (Figure 18.15). When the biceps muscle is weak, the patient may employ trick movements by putting the forearm into mid-pronation and bringing in the brachioradialis, or pulling the elbow backwards. The latter resembles the movement bartenders make when drawing a draft beer and has been called the "bartender's sign."

The triceps brachii is the principal elbow extensor. To test it, place the elbow in a position midway between flexion and extension and have the patient attempt to either extend the elbow or to hold

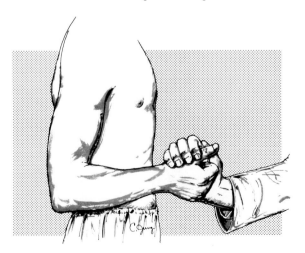

**FIGURE 18.15**  ●  Examination of the brachioradialis. On flexion of the semipronated forearm (thumb up) against resistance, the contracting muscle can be seen and palpated.

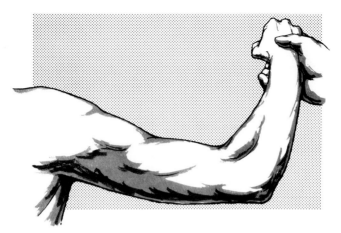

**FIGURE 18.16** ● Extension of the forearm. On attempts to extend the partially flexed forearm against resistance, contraction of the triceps can be seen and palpated.

position against the examiner's resistance (Figure 18.16). The triceps muscle is less powerful when the elbow is fully flexed, and slight weakness may be more easily detected with testing in this position.

Supination of the forearm is done primarily by the supinator muscle, assisted by stronger muscles for movements requiring power. The biceps muscle is the most powerful forearm supinator. Although the supinator is less powerful, it acts through all degrees of flexion and supination. Supination is tested by having the patient supinate against the examiner's resistance. With the forearm in extension, the brachioradialis also participates; with the forearm in flexion, the biceps also participates (Figure 18.17).

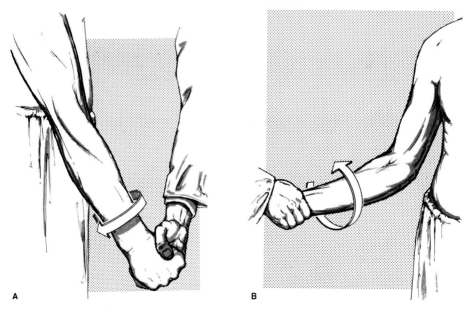

A    B

**FIGURE 18.17** ● Supination of the forearm. **A.** On attempts to supinate the extended forearm against resistance, the contracting brachioradialis can be seen and palpated. **B.** On attempts to supinate the flexed forearm against resistance, the contracting biceps can be seen and palpated.

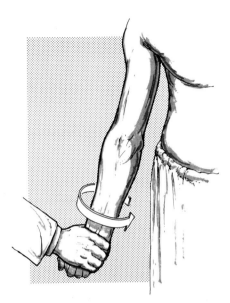

**FIGURE 18.18** ● Pronation of the forearm. On pronation of the forearm against resistance, contraction of the pronator teres can be seen and palpated.

Pronation is brought about primarily by the pronator quadratus (PQ), which is assisted by the much stronger pronator teres (PT) for movements requiring power. To test the PT and PQ, the patient attempts to pronate against resistance (Figure 18.18). To isolate the action of the PQ, pronation should be tested with the elbow extended, when the PT is maximally lengthened and exerts its weakest pull. Flexion of the elbow would signal that the patient is trying to bring the PT into play.

### The Wrist

The principal movements at the wrist are flexion and extension. Flexion of the wrist is carried out primarily by the flexor carpi radialis (FCR) and flexor carpi ulnaris (FCU) muscles. Wrist flexion is tested by having the patient resist the examiner's attempts to extend the wrist (Figure 18.19). Both the FCR and FCU are superficial; their contraction can be seen and felt. The FCR can be

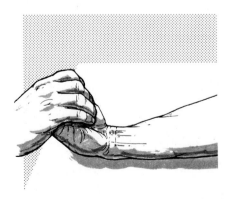

**FIGURE 18.19** ● Flexion at the wrist. On flexion of the hand at the wrist against resistance, the tendon of the flexor carpi radialis can be seen and palpated on the radial side of the wrist, and that of the flexor carpi ulnaris on the ulnar side; the tendon of the palmaris longus can also be seen and palpated.

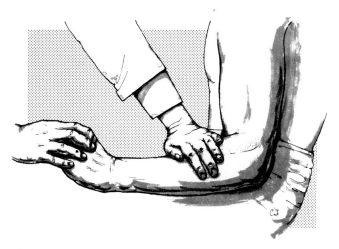

**FIGURE 18.20** ● Extension at the wrist. On attempts to extend the hand at the wrist against resistance, the bellies of the extensors carpi radialis longus, carpi ulnaris, and digitorum communis can be seen and palpated.

tested individually by having the patient flex the wrist toward the radial side against resistance directed toward the thumb. Function of the FCU can be tested by having the patient flex the wrist toward the ulnar side while the examiner presses on the hypothenar region.

Extension (dorsiflexion) of the wrist is executed primarily by the extensor carpi radialis longus (ECRL), extensor carpi radialis brevis, and extensor carpi ulnaris. To test the wrist extensors, the forearm is held in pronation with the wrist partially extended. The patient then resists the examiner's attempts to pull the wrist into flexion (Figure 18.20).

### The Hands and Fingers

The muscles that power the hand can be divided into extrinsics and intrinsics. The extrinsic muscles originate in the forearm and insert on hand structures; the intrinsics originate and insert within the hand. Possible movements include flexion, extension, adduction, abduction, and opposition.

### Flexion of the Fingers

The primary finger flexors are the flexor digitorum superficialis (FDS) and the flexor digitorum profundus (FDP). The FDS tendons pass through the carpal tunnel and then diverge to insert on the palmar surfaces of the middle phalanges. The FDS primarily flexes the proximal interphalangeal (PIP) joints of the four fingers. The tendons of the FDP pass through the carpal tunnel, and then pierce the tendons of the FDS and insert on bases of the distal phalanges. The main action of the FDP is flexion of the distal interphalangeal (DIP) joints.

The flexor digiti minimi brevis flexes and slightly abducts the proximal phalanx of the little finger. Two other muscles acting on the little finger are the abductor digiti minimi (ADM) and the opponens digiti minimi. The palmaris brevis wrinkles the skin over the hypothenar eminence and deepens the hollow of the hand. The palmaris brevis sign is wrinkling of the skin over the hypothenar eminence with small finger abduction in the face of weakness of the ulnar hand intrinsics; it proves the lesion involves the deep palmar branch.

Function of the FDP is tested by having the patient flex the distal phalanges of the individual fingers against resistance while the middle phalanges are fixed (Figure 18.21). The FDS is tested by having the patient flex the fingers at the PIP joints while the proximal phalanges are fixed (Figure 18.22). The patient should try to relax the distal phalanges to eliminate any action of the FDP on the PIP joint. The interossei and lumbricales flex the MCP joints and extend the interphalangeal (IP) joints.

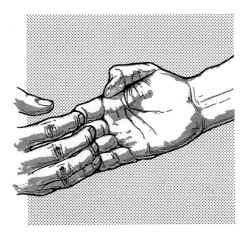

**FIGURE 18.21**  ●  Examination of the flexor digitorum profundus. The patient resists attempts to extend the distal phalanges while the middle phalanges are fixed.

Weakness of these intrinsic hand muscles causes loss of MCP joint flexion and loss of PIP joint extension, together with loss of adduction and abduction of the fingers. The hand assumes a position of rest in which the MCP joints are held in extension and the PIP and DIP joints are flexed (claw hand). Ulnar neuropathy is the most common cause of claw hand (ulnar griffe). Ulnar clawing primarily affects the ring and small fingers because both lumbrical and interosseous function are lost.

### Extension of the Fingers

The long extensors of the fingers include the extensor digitorum communis (EDC), extensor indicis proprius (EIP, aka extensor indicis), and the extensor digiti minimi (EDM). The tendons insert on the dorsal extensor expansions of the first phalanges of the fingers. The primary action of the EDC is extension of the MCP joints, but it can exert some force to extend each joint it crosses. The EIP extends the index finger; the EDM extends the little finger. The interossei and lumbricals also extend the PIP and DIP joints of the fingers.

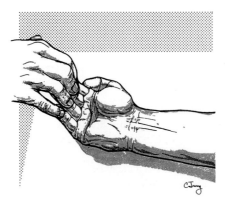

**FIGURE 18.22**  ●  Examination of the flexor digitorum superficialis. The patient resists attempts to straighten the fingers at the first interphalangeal joint.

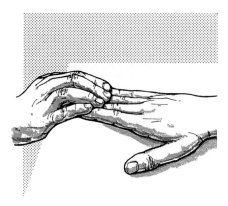

**FIGURE 18.23** ● Examination of the extensor digitorum communis. With hand outstretched and interphalangeal joints held in extension, the patient resists the examiner's attempt to flex the fingers at the metacarpophalangeal joints.

To test the action of the EDC, EIP, and EDM, the patient resists attempts to push the fingers down at the MCP joints with the forearm pronated and the wrist stabilized (Figure 18.23). The extensor function of the lumbricales and interossei is tested by having the patient try to extend the PIP and DIP joints against resistance while the MCP joints are hyperextended and fixed (Figure 18.24).

### The Thumb and Its Muscles

The thumb is capable of movement in many directions. The difference in some of the motions is subtle (e.g., flexion vs. adduction), but the muscle involved and the clinical significance may be marked. Two sets of muscles control thumb motion: those in the forearm (extrinsic thumb muscles), and those that make up the thenar eminence (intrinsic thumb muscles).

The mobility of the opposable thumb requires more elaborate muscle control compared to the other digits. Because the classical anatomical terms describing directions of movement are not easily applied to the thumb, additional directions are designated: palmar, dorsal, ulnar, and radial.

The IP and MCP joints can flex and extend. The carpometacarpal (CMC) joint can move in many directions. In palmar abduction, the thumb moves upward at right angles to the plane of the palm; in

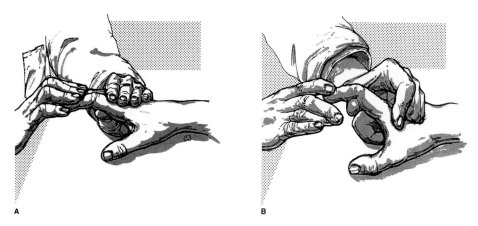

A                                                                        B

**FIGURE 18.24** ● **A** and **B.** Extension of the middle and distal phalanges. The patient attempts to extend the fingers against resistance while the metacarpophalangeal joints are fixed.

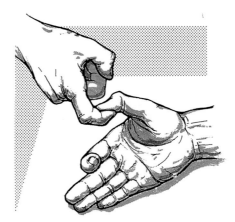

**FIGURE 18.25** ● Examination of the flexor pollicis longus. The patient resists attempts to extend the distal phalanx of the thumb while the proximal phalanx is fixed.

radial abduction, the thumb moves away in the plane of the palm. Ulnar and palmar adduction are movements that touch the first and second metacarpals together. Opposition (anteposition) is the motion of circumduction of the thumb with extended MCP and IP joints; this turns the thumb into semipronation and touches the palmar surface of the tip of the thumb to the palmar surface of the tip of the small finger.

The forearm muscles involved in controlling the thumb are the abductor pollicis longus (APL), extensor pollicis longus (EPL), extensor pollicis brevis (EPB), and flexor pollicis longus (FPL). The APL abducts the thumb and extends it to a slight degree. The EPL extends the terminal phalanx; the EPB extends the proximal phalanx. The FPL flexes the distal phalanx of the thumb. To test the FPL, the patient flexes the distal phalanx of the thumb while the proximal phalanx is flexed and immobilized (Figure 18.25). The EPL is tested by having the patient extend the thumb at the IP joint while the proximal phalanx is immobilized (Figure 18.26). The EPB is tested by having the patient extend the thumb at the MCP joint while the metacarpal bone is immobilized (Figure 18.27).

The muscles that make up the thenar eminence are the abductor pollicis brevis (APB), opponens pollicis (OP), and flexor pollicis brevis (FPB). The APL and APB muscles produce palmar abduction. The OP pronates the thumb, turning the volar thumb surface down, to touch the tip of

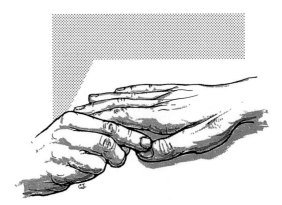

**FIGURE 18.26** ● Examination of the extensor pollicis longus. The patient attempts to resist passive flexion of the thumb at the interphalangeal joint; the tendon can be seen and palpated.

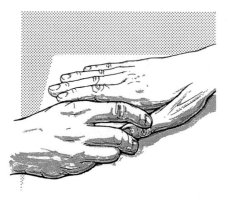

**FIGURE 18.27** ● Examination of the extensor pollicis brevis. The patient attempts to resist passive flexion of the thumb at the metacarpophalangeal joint; the tendon can be seen and palpated.

the thumb to the small finger. The FPB flexes the MCP joint of the thumb. In testing the FPB the patient is asked to flex the MCP joint of the thumb while keeping the IP joint extended.

Abduction of the thumb is carried out in two planes: in the same plane as the palm (radial abduction), and at right angles to the plane of the palm (palmar abduction). To test radial abduction, the thumb is moved outward if the hand is horizontal, and upward if the hand is vertical, against resistance. This movement is executed by the APL and EPB (Figure 18.28). The APB is a thin sheet of muscle lying just medial to the first metacarpal that performs palmar abduction. To test palmar abduction the thumb is moved upward at right angles to the palm, inside the radial margin of the hand, against resistance. It is very easy for both patient and physician to confuse abduction with extension. One trick is to place a pencil or similar object between the thumb and the palm, or radial to the thumb, perpendicular to the palm. The patient then raises the thumb to a point vertically above its original position, keeping it parallel to the pencil with the thumbnail at right angles to the palm (Figure 18.29). In paralysis of abduction the thumb is adducted and rotated, thumbnail parallel rather than perpendicular to the fingernails, falling into the plane of the palm (simian or ape hand).

Opposition of the thumb is tested by having the patient touch the little finger with the thumb (Figure 18.30). With the thumbnail on a plane approximately parallel to the palm, the palmar surface

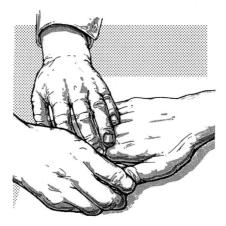

**FIGURE 18.28** ● Radial abduction of the thumb. The patient attempts to abduct the thumb in the same plane as that of the palm; the tendon of the abductor pollicis longus can be seen and palpated.

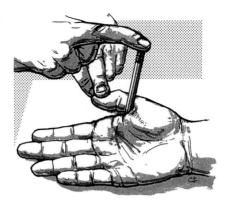

**FIGURE 18.29** ● Palmar abduction of the thumb. The patient attempts, against resistance, to bring the thumb to a point vertically above its original position.

of the tip of the thumb should contact the palmar surface of the tip of the little finger. When the OP is weak, the patient may be able to oppose the thumb to the index or middle finger, but not the little finger. In testing opposition of the little finger by the opponens digiti minimi, the patient moves the extended little finger in front of the other fingers and toward the thumb (Figure 18.31). Opposition of the thumb and little finger may be tested in one maneuver. When both are opposed their extended tips meet and form an arch over the cupped palm (Figure 18.32). The strength of the combined movement may be gauged by the patient's ability to hold onto a piece of paper held between finger and thumb as the examiner tries to pull it free, or the examiner may attempt to pull his finger between the touching tips of the thumb and little finger. The flexors of the thumb and little finger and the short abductor of the thumb probably enter into these movements.

The adductor pollicis adducts the thumb and flexes the first metacarpal. Adduction of the thumb is also carried out in two planes: in the plane of the palm (ulnar adduction), and in a plane at right angles to the palm (palmar adduction). Ulnar adduction is touching the ulnar aspect of the thumb to the radial aspect of the second metacarpal and index finger, thumb in the same plane as the palm, the thumbnail as nearly as possible parallel with the other fingernails, as if to put the hand into salute position. In palmar adduction, the ulnar aspect of the thumb touches the palmar aspect of the second metacarpal and index finger so that the thumb and index finger lie perpendicular to each other, with the thumbnail at right angles to the other fingernails (Figure 18.33). A commonly used test of adduction power in either

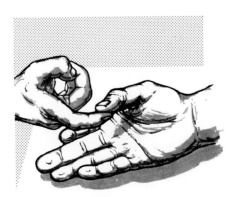

**FIGURE 18.30** ● Examination of the opponens pollicis. The patient attempts, against resistance, to touch the tip of the little finger with the thumb.

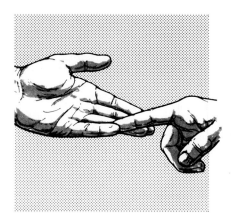

*FIGURE 18.31* ● Examination of the opponens digiti minimi. The patient attempts to move the extended little finger in front of the other fingers and toward the thumb.

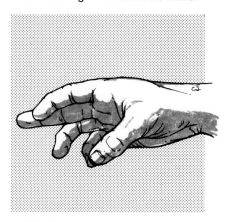

*FIGURE 18.32* ● Opposition of the thumb and little finger.

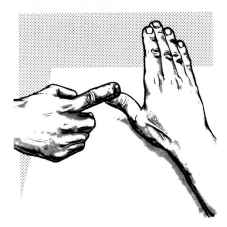

*FIGURE 18.33* ● Palmar adduction of the thumb. The patient, against resistance, attempts to approximate the thumb to the palmar aspect of the index finger; the thumbnail is kept at a right angle to the nails of the other fingers.

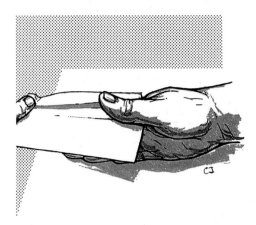

*FIGURE 18.34*  ●  Ulnar adduction of the thumb. The patient attempts to grasp a piece of paper between the thumb and the radial border of the index finger while the thumbnail is parallel to the nails of the other fingers.

of these positions is to have the patient try to hold a piece of paper tightly between thumb and hand as the examiner tries to extract it (Figure 18.34). When thumb adduction is weak, the patient may make a substitution movement, flexing the IP joint with the FPL and trying to secure the paper with the tip of the thumb (Froment sign), a common finding in ulnar neuropathy.

Adduction of the fingers is the movement that brings the fingers tightly together; abduction spreads the fingers apart. Adduction is a function of the volar interossei; abduction is a function of the dorsal interossei. Abduction of the little finger is done by the ADM. Adduction may be tested in several ways. With the fingers abducted and extended, the patient may try to adduct the fingers against resistance (Figure 18.35). The patient may try to clutch a piece of paper between two fingers and resist the examiner's attempts to withdraw it. The examiner may interdigitate his fingers between the patient's and have the patient squeeze as tightly as possible. The usual test of abduction is to have the patient keep the fingers fully extended and spread apart and resist the examiner's attempt to bring them together (Figure 18.36).

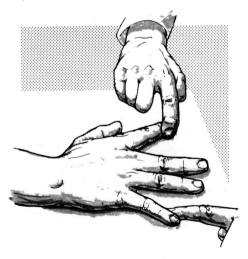

*FIGURE 18.35*  ●  Adduction of the fingers. The patient attempts to adduct the fingers against resistance.

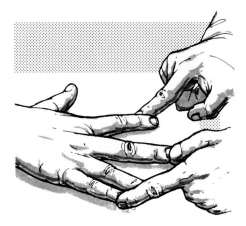

**FIGURE 18.36** ● Examination of the abduction of the fingers. The patient resists the examiner's attempt to bring the fingers together.

## Examination of Movements and Muscles of the Thorax, Abdomen, and Trunk

The actions of the large muscles of the trunk, chest, and abdomen are often combined, and it is difficult to evaluate them individually (Table 18.6). Except for the respiratory muscles, most of these muscles have scant neurologic significance.

### The Muscles of the Thorax, Abdomen, and Spine

The major thoracic muscles consist of the internal and external intercostals, and diaphragm. Muscles attached to the sternum, clavicles, and scapulae act as accessory muscles of respiration. The diaphragm is the principal muscle of respiration. During quiet inspiration, intercostal contraction expands the anteroposterior and transverse diameters of the thorax, and the vertical diameter is increased by the descent of the diaphragm. In deep inspiration, the accessory muscles are brought into action.

Weakness of the intercostal muscles causes adduction of the costal margins and abdominal respiration, with alternate bulging and retraction of the epigastrium as increased diaphragmatic contraction compensates for the intercostal weakness (abdominal breathing). The intercostal spaces may retract during inspiration, and the ribs do not rise and separate. When bilateral paralysis of the diaphragm is present, the excursion of the costal margins is increased and the epigastrium does not bulge during inspiration. The moving shadow caused by retraction of the lower intercostal spaces during inspiration (Litten sign) is absent.

Weakness of the abdominal muscle groups does not often occur in neurologic patients. The abdominal muscles may be tested by having the patient raise the head against resistance (Figure 18.37), cough, or do a sit-up. If the abdominal muscles contract equally in all four quadrants, the umbilicus will not move. If the lower abdominal muscles are paralyzed, as in a T10 myelopathy, the upper abdominal muscles will pull the umbilicus cephalad when the patient raises the head or attempts a sit-up (Beevor sign).

The movements of the spine are flexion, extension, rotation, and lateral bending. The muscles that produce these movements are examined en masse by examining the movements rather than individual muscles. The extensors of the spine are tested by having the prone patient raise the head and shoulders without the assistance of the hands (Figure 18.38). The most common cause of paraspinal weakness is primary muscle disease, particularly muscular dystrophies, especially facioscapulohumeral dystrophy. The flexors of the spine are tested by having the patient rise from recumbent to seated, and then to a standing position without using the hands (Figure 18.39).

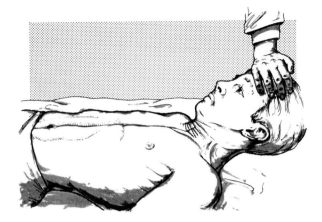

**FIGURE 18.37** ● Examination of the abdominal muscles. The recumbent patient attempts to raise his head against resistance.

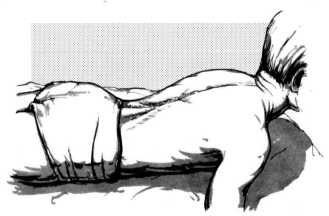

**FIGURE 18.38** ● Examination of the extensors of the spine. The patient, lying prone, attempts to raise the head and upper part of the trunk.

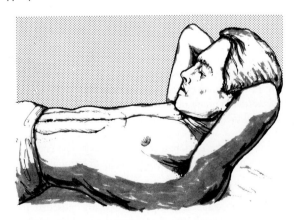

**FIGURE 18.39** ● Examination of the abdominal muscles and flexor muscles of the spine. The patient attempts to rise from a recumbent to a sitting position without the use of the hands.

## Examination of the Movements and Muscles of the Lower Extremities

The movements of the lower extremities are less complex than those of the upper extremities, and there are fewer substitution movements. Table 18.7 lists the pertinent muscles and their innervation.

### The Hip Joint

The movements that take place at the hip are flexion, extension, abduction, adduction, and internal and external rotation. The principal hip flexor is the iliopsoas. The iliopsoas has two parts, the psoas and the iliacus, which have the same function. The psoas arises from both the transverse processes and the bodies of the lumbar vertebra. The intervertebral foramina of L1–L4 lie between these two points of origin, so that the roots that form the lumbar plexus exit into the substance of the muscle and the plexus lies within it. This anatomy accounts for the severe damage to the lumbosacral plexus that commonly occurs with hemorrhage into the psoas muscle. The iliacus portion arises in the iliac fossa.

The two iliopsoas muscles acting together from each side help to maintain an erect posture by balancing the spine and pelvis over the femurs, preventing a backward tilt. When the legs are fixed they flex the trunk and pelvis forward, as in doing a sit-up. Hip flexor strength is tested by having the patient flex the hip against resistance (Figure 18.40). This may be done in the sitting or supine position.

The major hip extensor is the gluteus maximus. The gluteus maximus is important in climbing steps, jumping, and rising from a chair. Hip extensor function is best tested with the patient prone, raising the flexed knee up from the table against downward pressure from the examiner (Figure 18.41). Having the knee flexed minimizes any contribution from the hamstrings. The gluteus maximus can also be tested with the patient lying on the side and extending the hip, or seated and trying to press the raised knee back down as the examiner holds it up, or by testing the ability to stand upright from a stooped position. With hip girdle weakness, particularly in the muscular dystrophies, there is marked weakness of the hip extensors, and the patient arises from a stooped position by using his hands to "climb up the legs" (Gowers maneuver, Figure 20.3).

The primary abductors of the hip are the gluteus medius, gluteus minimus, and tensor fasciae latae (TFL). They also function as internal rotators of the hip. The hip abductors may be tested

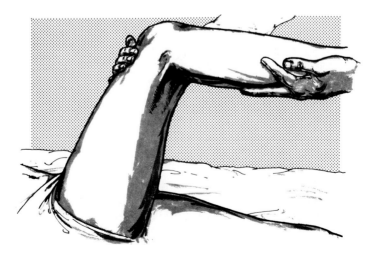

*FIGURE 18.40* ● Examination of the flexors of the thigh. The patient attempts to flex the thigh against resistance; the knee is flexed and the leg rests on the examiner's arm.

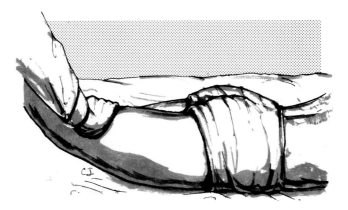

**FIGURE 18.41**  •  Examination of the extensors of the thigh at the hip. The patient, lying prone with the leg flexed at the knee, attempts to extend the thigh against resistance; contraction of the gluteus maximus and other extensors can be seen and palpated.

either supine or sitting by having the patient attempt to hold the lower extremities outward with ankles spread far apart, as the examiner tries to force the ankles together (Figure 18.42). The hip abductors are very important in walking. When the hip abductors are weak there is an exaggerated pelvic swing during the stance phase as the pelvis on the side of the swing leg drops downward (Trendelenburg sign).

Adduction of the hip is principally a function of the three adductors: longus, brevis, and magnus. The adductor magnus is the longest and strongest hip adductor. The adductors can be tested with the patient supine, sitting, or lying on one side. The patient attempts to bring the legs together as the examiner tries to keep them apart (Figure 18.43). As with the abductors, the adductors are so powerful it is helpful to keep the patient's knees extended to give the examiner the advantage of a longer lever.

Internal, or medial, rotation of the hip is carried out principally by the hip abductor muscles (glutei medius and minimus, and TFL), with some contribution from the adductors. To test internal rotation the patient lies supine with the hip and knee flexed, or prone with the knee flexed. He then

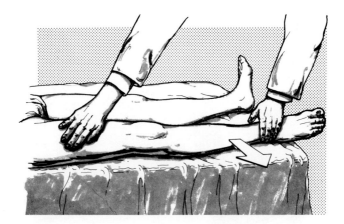

**FIGURE 18.42**  •  Abduction of the thigh at the hip. The recumbent patient attempts to move the extended leg outward against resistance; contraction of the gluteus medius and tensor fasciae latae can be palpated.

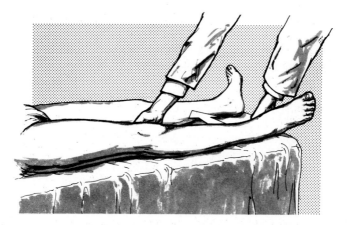

**FIGURE 18.43** ● Examination of adduction of the thigh at the hip. The recumbent patient attempts to adduct the extended leg against resistance; contraction of the adductor muscles can be seen and palpated.

attempts to move the foot laterally against resistance, thus rotating the hip medially (Figure 18.44). Internal rotation can also be tested with the patient supine and the leg extended, rotating the foot medially as if to touch the big toe to the bed. Rotating the foot medially with the knee extended produces the same hip motion as carrying the foot laterally with the knee flexed. With a unilateral CST lesion (e.g., acute stroke), the internal rotators are weak. When the patient lies supine, the involved leg lies externally rotated compared to its fellow. This asymmetry of leg position may be a clue to the presence of a hemiparesis in an obtunded patient.

External, or lateral, rotation of the thigh at the hip is carried out primarily by the gluteus maximus. External rotation is tested by maneuvers similar to those for testing internal rotation, but the patient rotates the hip externally by attempting to carry the foot medially against resistance with the knee flexed.

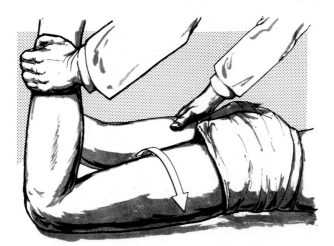

**FIGURE 18.44** ● Examination of internal rotation of the thigh. The patient, lying prone with the leg flexed at the knee, attempts to carry the foot laterally against resistance, thus rotating the thigh medially.

## The Knee Joint

The major movements that take place at the knee joint are flexion and extension. Flexion of the knee is carried out primarily by the hamstring muscles (biceps femoris, semimembranosus, semitendinosus). The hamstrings also act as powerful hip extensors. The knee flexors may be tested with the patient prone (Figure 18.45), supine, or sitting. With the knee in partial flexion the patient resists the examiner's attempts to straighten the knee. The knee flexors are powerful and cannot normally be overcome. Another test is to have the prone patient attempt to maintain both knees flexed at about 45 degrees from horizontal with the feet slightly apart. When the knee flexors are weak on one side, as in a CST lesion, the involved leg will sink, gradually or rapidly (leg drift, leg sign of Barré). Examination of knee flexion with the patient prone makes it easier to see and palpate the muscle contractions and lessens the likelihood of misinterpretation due to simultaneous action of the hip flexors. The sartorius, the longest muscle in the body, has a complex set of actions. It is an abductor, flexor, and lateral rotator of the hip, and a flexor and medial rotator of the knee. The sartorius would be active when trying to look at the bottom of one's foot. The sartorius may be examined by having the patient attempt to flex the knee against resistance with the hip flexed and rotated laterally (Figure 18.46).

The quadriceps femoris is the primary knee extensor. The rectus femoris also crosses the hip, and serves as a hip flexor as well as a knee extensor. The quadriceps may be tested when the patient, sitting or supine, attempts to extend the knee against the examiner's resistance (Figure 18.47). The quadriceps is so powerful it is nearly impossible to overcome in the normal adolescent or adult except by taking extreme mechanical advantage. A sometimes useful technique for testing knee extension is the "barkeeper's hold" (Figure 18.48).

With severe quadriceps weakness, the sitting patient may lean backward when trying to extend the knee, attempting to muster some knee extension force by allowing the rectus femoris to contract across the hip. The patient will have marked difficulty in rising from a kneeling position and in climbing stairs; he can walk backward, but has difficulty walking forward.

## The Ankle Joint

Movements about the ankle joint are plantarflexion, dorsiflexion, eversion, and inversion. Plantar flexion (flexion) of the foot is carried out principally by the gastrocnemius and soleus muscles.

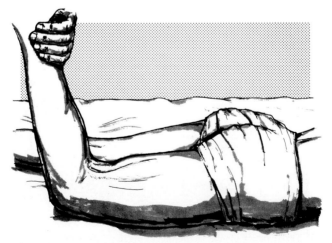

**FIGURE 18.45**  ●  Examination of flexion at the knee. The prone patient attempts to maintain flexion of the leg while the examiner attempts to extend it; the tendon of the biceps femoris can be palpated laterally and the tendons of the semimembranosus and semitendinosus medially.

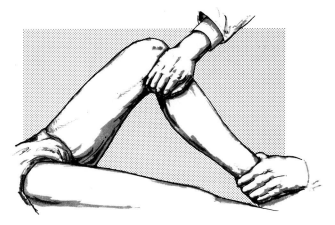

***FIGURE 18.46*** ● Examination of the sartorius. With the thigh flexed and rotated laterally and the knee moderately flexed, the patient attempts further flexion of the knee against resistance.

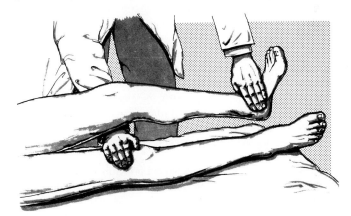

***FIGURE 18.47*** ● Examination of extension of the leg at the knee. The supine patient attempts to extend the leg at the knee against resistance; contraction of the quadriceps femoris can be seen and palpated.

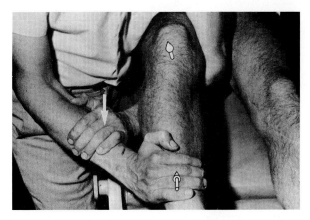

***FIGURE 18.48*** ● The "barkeeper's hold," a powerful move against the quadriceps.
(Reprinted with permission from Wolfe JK. *Segmental Neurology.* Baltimore: University Park Press, 1981.)

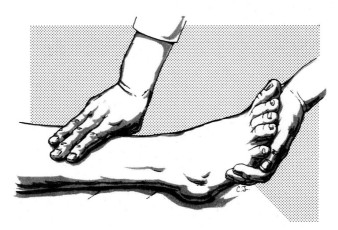

**FIGURE 18.49** ●    Examination of plantar flexion of the foot. The patient attempts to plantar flex the foot at the ankle joint against resistance; contraction of the gastrocnemius and associated muscles can be seen and palpated.

Other muscles cross posterior to the axis of rotation of the ankle, but because of mechanical factors are not very effective plantarflexors. The gastrocnemius also assists in flexing the knee. The gastrosoleus raises the heel, as in walking, and inverts the foot.

The function of these muscles is tested manually by having the patient plantar flex the ankle as the examiner offers resistance by pressure against the sole of the foot (Figure 18.49). The plantarflexors of the ankle are among the most powerful muscles in the body. They cannot normally be defeated by hand and arm strength alone, even when the examiner takes maximal mechanical advantage. A better test of plantarflexor strength is to have the patient stand on tiptoe. Normally, a patient can easily support the entire body weight on one tiptoe, hop on one foot, and even do multiple toe raises on one foot.

Dorsiflexion (extension) of the ankle is carried out primarily by the tibialis anterior muscle, assisted by the extensors digitorum longus and hallucis longus. The foot dorsiflexors are tested by having the patient pull the foot up against the examiner's resistance (Figure 18.50). The dorsiflexors are powerful and cannot normally be overcome, even with maximal effort from the examiner. Dorsiflexion may also be tested by having the patient stand on the heels, raising the toes as high as possible. The toes on the weak side cannot be lifted as far.

Inversion at the ankle is elevation of the inner border of the foot to turn the sole medially. Inversion is tested by having the patient attempt to invert the ankle against resistance (Figure 18.51). Weakness of ankle inversion is a key clinical sign indicating that a foot drop is due to L5 radiculopathy and not peroneal neuropathy at the knee.

Eversion, or lateral deviation, is elevation of the outer border of the foot to turn the sole laterally. This movement is carried out by the peronei longus, brevis, and tertius and the extensor digitorum longus. To test these muscles, the patient attempts to evert the ankle against resistance applied to the lateral border of the foot (Figure 18.52).

### Muscles of the Foot and Toes

The function of individual foot and toe muscles is not so clearly defined as in the hand, and muscle testing cannot be carried out with as much detail. The principal movements are extension (dorsiflexion) and flexion (plantarflexion) of the toes. With plantar flexion there is cupping of the sole. Abduction and adduction of the toes are minimal.

The toe extensors are the extensors digitorum longus (EDL) and brevis (EDB) and the extensors hallucis longus (EHL) and brevis.

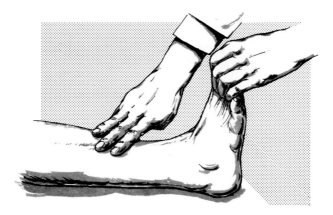

*FIGURE 18.50*  ●  Examination of dorsiflexion (extension) of the foot. The patient attempts to dorsi-flex the foot against resistance; contraction of the tibialis anterior can be seen and palpated.

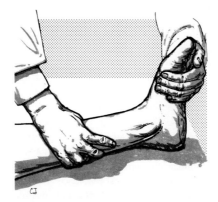

*FIGURE 18.51*  ●  Examination of inversion of the foot. The patient attempts to raise the inner border of the foot against resistance; the tendon of the tibialis posterior can be seen and palpated just behind the medial malleolus.

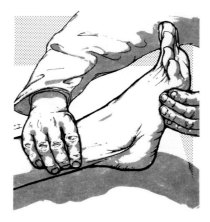

*FIGURE 18.52*  ●  Examination of eversion of the foot. The patient attempts to raise the outer border of the foot against resistance; the tendons of the peronei longus and brevis can be seen and palpated just above and behind the lateral malleolus.

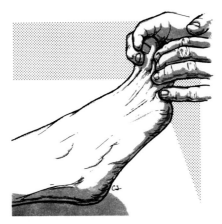

**FIGURE 18.53** ● Examination of dorsiflexion (extension) of the toes. On attempts to dorsiflex the toes against resistance, the tendons of the extensors digitorum and hallucis longus and the belly of the extensor digitorum brevis can be seen and palpated.

The long toe extensors extend the metatarsophalangeal (MTP) and IP joints and dorsiflex the ankle joint. The EDB aids the EDL in extending the four medial toes. Dorsiflexion of the toes against resistance may be used as a test for the function of these muscles. The tendons of the long extensors and the belly of the EDB can be palpated during this maneuver (Figure 18.53). The EDB normally forms a prominent bulge on the dorsolateral aspect of the foot. Its most medial and largest belly is the extensor hallucis brevis. When the EHL is severely weak in the absence of severe weakness of the other foot and toe extensors, the patient may have a "toe drop" rather than a "foot drop."

Flexion of the toes is carried out by the flexors digitorum and hallucis longus, flexors digitorum and hallucis brevis, and some of the intrinsic muscles of the sole of the foot. These muscles are tested by having the patient flex the toes against resistance (Figure 18.54). Testing of the intrinsic muscles of the sole of the foot is difficult and not clinically useful. These muscles may be tested together by asking the patient to cup the sole of the foot (Figure 18.55).

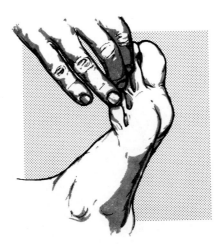

**FIGURE 18.54** ● Examination of flexion of the toes. The patient attempts to flex the toes against resistance.

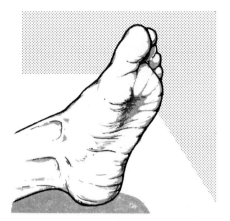

*FIGURE 18.55* ● Cupping of the sole of the foot.

## EXAMINATION FOR SUBTLE HEMIPARESIS

The motor examination is not concluded just with the formal strength assessment. Patients with mild CST lesions may have normal strength to routine testing, but the neurologic deficit may be brought out using ancillary maneuvers. The most important of these is the examination for pronator drift (Barré sign). With the patient's upper extremities outstretched to the front, palms up and with the eyes closed, observe the position of each extremity (Figure 18.56). The patient should hold this position for at least 20 to 30 seconds. In normals, the palms will remain flat, the elbows straight, and the limbs horizontal. Any deviation from this position will be similar on the two sides.

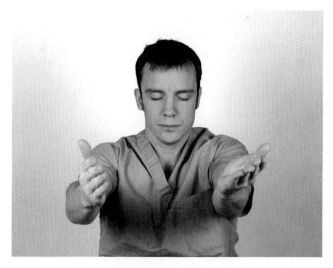

*FIGURE 18.56* ● Technique for testing for pronator drift. In the presence of a corticospinal tract lesion the selectively weakened muscles are the shoulder abductors and external rotators, the supinators, and the elbow extensors. These muscles are overcome by their antagonists to cause pronation, elbow flexion, and downward drift. This is an illustration of mild pronator drift of the right upper extremity. Patients with mild corticospinal tract lesions may demonstrate a pronator drift, or have an abnormal arm or finger roll test in the absence of clinically detectable weakness to formal strength testing.

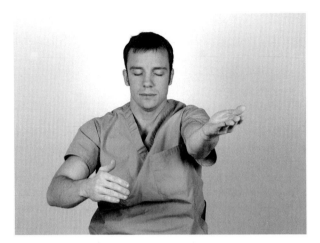

**FIGURE 18.57** ● Moderate drift with further development of the posture.

The patient with a mild CST deficit may demonstrate "pronator drift," to varying degrees. With mild drift there is slight pronation of the hand and slight flexion of the elbow on the abnormal side. With more severe drift there is more prominent pronation and obvious flexion of the elbow, and there may be downward drift of the entire arm (Figure 18.57). Because of the innervation pattern of the CST, the minimally weak CST innervated muscles are overcome by the non-CST muscles. With a mild CST lesion, the minimally weak muscles in the upper extremity are the extensors, supinators, and abductors. These are overcome by the uninvolved and therefore stronger muscles: the pronators, biceps, and internal rotators of the shoulder. As these overcome the slightly weakened CST innervated muscles, the hand pronates, the elbow flexes, and the arm drifts downward. The tendency to pronation and flexion in mild hemiparesis has also been attributed to subtle hypertonicity in the pronator and flexor muscle groups. Imagine what would occur if this motion continued to the extreme: the hand would become hyperpronated, the elbow fully flexed, and the shoulder internally rotated, i.e., the position of spastic hemiparesis (Figure 18.58). The abnormal

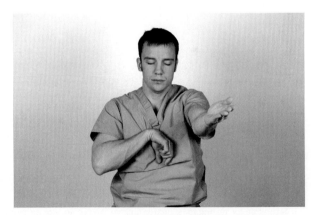

**FIGURE 18.58** ● Further development of pronator drift, with the evolution of severe drift to show how marked weakness of the corticospinal innervated muscles produces the posture of spastic hemiparesis. The pathophysiologic basis for pronator drift and for the upper-extremity posture of fully developed spastic hemiparesis and for the upper-extremity posture of decorticate rigidity is the same; it is only a matter of degree. A mild corticospinal tract lesion results in mild pronator drift; a severe lesion results in spastic hemiparesis.

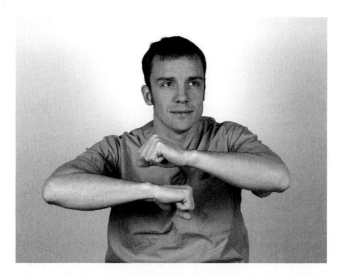

**FIGURE 18.59** ● Testing for a corticospinal tract lesion using arm roll. The involved extremity tends to have a lesser excursion as the forearms roll about each other, so that the normal extremity tends to rotate around the abnormal extremity, which tends to remain relatively fixed. Patients with mild corticospinal tract lesions may have an abnormal arm roll test in the absence of clinically detectable weakness to formal strength testing.

upper limb positions in minimal pronator drift and in severe spastic hemiparesis are due to the same underlying phenomenon: strong non-CST muscles overcome variably weak CST muscles involved by the disease process. Another sign occasionally useful is the digiti quinti sign. With the hands outstretched in drift position, the small finger on the hemiparetic side may be abducted more than on the normal side. The examination for pronator drift is a very important part of the neurologic examination. Abnormal drift can occasionally occur with lesions elsewhere in the nervous system. Cerebellar disease may cause drift to some degree but the movement is outward and usually slightly upward. In parietal lobe lesions, there may be "updrift," with the involved arm rising overhead without the patient's awareness, ostensibly because of loss of position sense.

Other useful maneuvers include examination of forearm roll, finger roll, and rapid alternating movements. Abnormal forearm rolling is a sensitive indicator of neurologic pathology. To test it, the patient is instructed to make fists, to hold the forearms horizontally so that the fists and distal forearms overlap with the palms pointed more or less toward the umbilicus, and then to rotate the fists around each other, first in one direction and then the other (Figure 18.59). Normal patients will have about an equal excursion of both forearms so that the fists and forearms roll about each other symmetrically. With a unilateral corticospinal lesion, the involved side does not move as much as the normal side, so the patient will appear to plant or fix one forearm and to rotate the opposite forearm around it. Finger roll is an even more sensitive version of the same test. The patient is asked to extend the forefingers from the clenched fists and to rotate the fingers around each other, moving just the fingers. Again, the finger on the abnormal side will move less than its fellow.

Normal fine motor control requires functional integrity of both the CST and the cerebellum. Testing for rapid alternating movements is part of the cerebellar examination, but the primary function of the CST is to provide discrete, fractionated movements to the distal extremities. Either CST or cerebellar disease may interfere with fine motor control of distal muscles. Normal fine motor control also requires intact proprioceptive pathways. Traditionally, different tests have been done to look for CST signs than for cerebellar signs, but both involve rapid alternating movements. This test is also referred to as assessment of alternate motion rate, but in fact more than the rate of motion provides useful information. Fine motor control can be tested in numerous ways, most advantageously by comparing the dexterity and precision of the two hands while performing rapid, repetitive movements, making allowance of course for hand dominance. The patient may be asked to repetitively, and as quickly as possible, touch the tip of the index finger to the tip of the thumb, as in making the OK sign. Any finger can be used, but the index and small fingers are favorites. The movements will be slower and less agile on the abnormal side. This test is often done by having the patient touch the IP joint rather than the tip of the thumb. Other tests requiring a high level of coordination include quickly touching the tip of each finger in turn to the thumb, flicking the fingers as if flicking off water, doing one-handed clapping, and making quick, small finger movements as if playing a piano. Fine motor control of the foot can be assessed by having the patient do rapid, repetitive foot taps, on the floor if standing, against the examiner's palm if supine.

# CHAPTER 19

# Muscle Tone

**M**uscle tone has been defined as the tension in the relaxed muscle, or the resistance to passive movement when voluntary contraction is absent. Because of resting tone, normal muscles have slight resistance to passive movement even in the relaxed state. The inherent attributes of muscle tissue—such as viscosity, elasticity, and extensibility—contribute to resting tone. Even apparently relaxed muscle fibers have a constant slight fixed tension by which they hold their resting position, resist changes in length, prevent undue mobility at joints, and are in position to contract when necessary. Resting muscle tone is greatest in the anti-gravity muscles that maintain the body in an erect position.

## EXAMINATION OF TONE

Tone is difficult to assess. The determination of tone is subjective and prone to interexaminer variability. There are no methods that can measure tone quantitatively. The determination is based solely on the clinical judgment of the examiner; accurate assessment of tone requires clinical experience. It is difficult to separate slightly increased tone from poor relaxation in a tense or apprehensive patient. Tone is especially difficult to evaluate in infants, where there may be wide variations in apparent tone on different examinations, in either health or disease.

The examination of tone requires a relaxed and cooperative patient. Small talk may help the patient relax. Simple observation may reveal an abnormality of posture or resting position that indicates an underlying change in tone. Muscle palpation is sometimes useful, but well-muscled individuals may have firm muscles despite normal resting tone, while in other individuals the muscles may feel flabby despite an underlying hypertonicity. Muscles may have a firm consistency to palpation because of edema, inflammation, spasm due to pain, or pseudohypertrophy.

The most important part of the examination of tone is determination of the resistance of relaxed muscles to passive manipulation as well as the extensibility, flexibility, and range of motion. Abnormalities of tone are more easily detected in extremity than in trunk muscles. The limb is moved passively, first slowly and through a complete range of motion, and then at varying speeds. The examiner may shake the forearm to and fro and note the excursions of the patient's hand, or brace a limb and then suddenly remove the support, or note the range of movement of a part in response to a slight blow. Bilateral examination of homologous parts helps compare for differences in tone on the two sides of the body.

Tone should be assessed by both slow and rapid motion and through partial and full range of motion, documenting the distribution, type, and severity of any abnormality. Certain specific maneuvers may be helpful in evaluation of abnormal tone.

## The Babinski Tonus Test

The arms are abducted at the shoulders, and the forearms are passively flexed at the elbows. With hypotonicity there is increased flexibility and mobility, and the elbows can be bent to an angle more acute than normal. With hypertonicity there is reduced flexibility and passive flexion cannot be carried out beyond an obtuse angle.

## The Head-Dropping Test

The patient lies supine without a pillow, completely relaxed, eyes closed and attention diverted. The examiner places one hand under the patient's occiput and with the other hand briskly raises the head, and then allows it to drop. Normally the head drops rapidly into the examiner's protecting hand, but in patients with extrapyramidal rigidity there is delayed, slow, gentle dropping of the head because of rigidity affecting the flexor muscles of the neck. When meningismus is present there is resistance to and pain on flexion of the neck.

## Pendulousness of the Legs

The patient sits on the edge of a table, relaxed with legs hanging freely. The examiner either extends both legs to the same horizontal level and then releases them, or gives both legs a brisk, equal backward push. If the patient is completely relaxed and cooperative, there will normally be a swinging of the legs that progressively diminishes in range and usually disappears after six or seven oscillations. In extrapyramidal rigidity, there is a decrease in swing time, but usually no qualitative change in the response. In spasticity, there may be little or no decrease in swing time, but the movements are jerky and irregular, the forward movement may be greater and more brisk than the backward, and the movement may assume a zigzag pattern. In hypotonia, the response is increased in range and prolonged beyond the normal. In all of these maneuvers a unilateral abnormality will be more apparent.

## The Shoulder-Shaking Test

The examiner places her hands on the patient's shoulders and shakes them briskly back and forth, observing the reciprocal motion of the arms. With extrapyramidal disease, there will be a decreased range of arm swing on the affected side. With hypotonia, especially that associated with cerebellar disease, the excursions of the arm swing will be greater than normal.

## The Arm-Dropping Test

The patient's arms are briskly raised to shoulder level, and then dropped. In spasticity, there is a delay in the downward movement of the affected arm, causing it to hang up briefly on the affected side; with hypotonicity the dropping is more abrupt than normal. A similar maneuver may be carried out by lifting and then dropping the extended legs of the recumbent patient.

## Hand Position

Hypotonicity, especially that associated with cerebellar disease or Sydenham chorea, may cause the hands to assume a characteristic posture. With the arms and hands outstretched, there is flexion at the wrists and hyperextension of the fingers ("spooning"), accompanied by moderate overpronation. With the arms raised overhead the overpronation is exaggerated with the palms turned outward. This overpronation phenomenon differs from the pronator drift sign, in which the overpronation is due to weakness of corticospinal innervated muscles or increased tone in the pronator muscles.

## MYOTATIC IRRITABILITY, MYOEDEMA, AND TENDERNESS

In addition to the inspection, palpation, and resistance to passive motion used in the assessment of tone, it is sometimes useful to observe the reaction to direct percussion of the muscle belly. The idiomuscular contraction is the brief and feeble contraction of a muscle belly after it is tapped with a percussion hammer, causing a slight depression at the site of the stimulus. The contraction involves only those fibers tapped directly. This is different from the reaction to muscle stretch, as in elicitation of the deep tendon or muscle stretch reflexes. Direct muscle percussion causes a contraction in normal muscles, even when the deep tendon reflex (DTR) is absent. Myotatic irritability has been defined as both the response to direct percussion as well as the ability of a muscle to contract in response to sudden stretch.

The response to direct muscle percussion in normal muscle is very slight, and in most muscles is seen or felt with difficulty. The reaction may be more pronounced in wasting diseases, such as cachexia and emaciation, and in some diseases of the lower motor neuron. Hyperexcitability to such stimulation occurs in tetanus, tetany, and certain electrolyte disturbances. Occasionally, after a muscle is percussed with a reflex hammer, a wave of contraction radiates along the muscle away from the point of percussion. A small ridge or temporary swelling may persist for several seconds at the point of stimulation. This stationary muscle mounding is known as myoedema. There is no accompanying electrical muscle activity. The idiomuscular contraction causes a slight depression, myoedema a rounding up. The mechanism of myoedema is poorly understood, but it is probably a normal physiological phenomenon. Its presence alone does not indicate a neuromuscular disorder but the response may be exaggerated in some circumstances, most notably hypothyroid myopathy. Myotonia is a persisting contraction following mechanical stimulation of muscle that is quite different from myoedema.

During muscle palpation, muscle tenderness may sometimes be elicited. Muscle tenderness on squeezing the muscle belly, or even with very slight pressure, may cause exquisite pain. Widespread muscle tenderness to palpation may occur with inflammatory myopathy, especially polymyositis and dermatomyositis, in some neuropathies, and in acute poliomyelitis. Focal muscle tenderness occurs with trauma or overexertion of muscles.

## ABNORMALITIES OF TONE

Pathologic conditions may cause an increase or decrease in tone. In addition, there are different varieties of hypotonicity and hypertonicity. Hypotonicity may develop from disease of the motor unit, the proprioceptive pathways, cerebellar lesions, and in the choreas. The muscle may be flaccid, flabby, and soft to palpation. The involved joints offer decreased resistance to passive movement. The excursion of the joint may be increased with an absence of the normal "checking" action on extreme passive motion. If the involved extremity is lifted and allowed to drop, it falls abruptly. A slight blow causes it to sway through an excessive excursion. The DTRs are usually decreased or absent when hypotonia is due to a lesion involving the motor unit or proprioceptive pathways.

### Hypotonia

When hypotonia is due to disease of the motor unit, there is invariably some degree of accompanying weakness. The hypotonia that results from central processes (e.g., cerebellar disease) does not cause weakness; muscle power is preserved even though hypotonia is demonstrable on examination. Infantile hypotonia (floppy baby syndrome) is a common clinical condition in which there is generalized decrease in muscle tone, typically affecting a neonate. There are numerous causes, both central and peripheral. Tone may also be decreased when disease affects the muscle spindle afferent system. Hypotonicity may occur with various types of cerebellar disease, but is never as severe as that which occurs with diseases of the lower motor neuron. Cerebellar hypotonia is not associated with weakness and the reflexes are not lost, although they may be pendular; there are no pathologic reflexes. Muscle tone is of course decreased in deep sleep, coma, and other states of impaired consciousness. Sudden attacks of impaired muscle tone in an awake patient occur in akinetic epilepsy and in cataplexy. In akinetic epilepsy the attacks of sudden loss of muscle tone occur spontaneously, and the patient falls to the ground. In cataplexy the attacks are typically precipitated by sudden strong emotions, such as laughing. Cataplexy is usually a component of narcolepsy. Sleep paralysis is a state common in narcolepsy, in which a patient has diffusely decreased tone and is unable to move immediately after awakening from sleep. The hemiparesis that is present acutely following hemispheric stroke may be associated with hypotonia (cerebral or neural "shock"), which gradually evolves into hypertonia with the passage of time. Some conditions may cause abnormal joint laxity, which may be confused with muscle hypotonia (e.g., Ehlers-Danlos syndrome).

## Hypertonia

Hypertonia occurs under many circumstances. It is a routine feature of lesions that involve the corticospinal tract after the acute stage. It can occur with diffuse cerebral disorders, with disease involving the extrapyramidal system, with disease of spinal cord interneurons (e.g., stiff person syndrome), and even with muscle disorders in continuous muscle fiber activity syndromes.

## Extrapyramidal Rigidity

Extrapyramidal rigidity is a diffuse increase in muscle tone to passive movement that occurs primarily with lesions that involve the basal ganglia. There is a fairly constant level of increased tone that affects both agonist and antagonist and is equally present throughout the range of motion at a given joint. Both flexor and extensor muscles are involved, with resistance to passive movement in all directions. The increased tone is equally present from the beginning to the end of the movement and does not vary with the speed of the movement. This type of rigidity is referred to as "lead-pipe." The involved muscles may be firm and tense to palpation. After being placed in a new position, the part may remain there, causing the limbs to assume awkward postures.

In cogwheel rigidity there is a jerky quality to the hypertonicity. As the part is manipulated, it seems to give way in a series of small steps as if the limb were attached to a heavy cogwheel or ratchet. The jerky quality of the resistance may be due to tremor superimposed on lead-pipe rigidity. Cogwheel rigidity is most commonly encountered in Parkinson disease and other parkinsonian syndromes. It appears first in proximal muscles and then spreads distally. Any muscle may be affected, but there is predominant involvement of neck and trunk muscles and the flexor muscles of the extremities. The rigidity of extrapyramidal disease may be brought out by the head-dropping, shoulder-shaking, and similar tests. The rigidity on one side may be exaggerated by active movements of the contralateral limbs.

In extrapyramidal disease, there is usually associated hypokinesia and bradykinesia, but no real paralysis. With repeated active movements there is a gradual decrease in speed and amplitude. This may be brought out by having the patient rapidly open and close the eyes or mouth, open and close the hand, or oppose finger and thumb. Patients also have loss of associated movements. Patients may also show slowness of starting and limitation of the amplitude of movement, loss of pendulousness of the arms and legs, inability to carry out rapid repeated movements or to maintain two simultaneous voluntary movements, and impairment of associated movements, such as swinging of the arms when walking.

Paratonia is an alteration in tone to passive motion that is often a manifestation of diffuse frontal lobe disease. It has been divided into inhibitory paratonia and facilitory paratonia. Gegenhalten is a form of rigidity in which the resistance to passive movement seems proportional to the vigor with which the movement is attempted. The resistance of the patient increases in proportion to the examiner's efforts to move the part; the harder the examiner pushes, the harder the patient seems to push back. It seems as though the patient is actively fighting, but the response is involuntary. It is said that the severity of gegenhalten can be judged by the loudness of the examiner's exhortations to relax. In the limb placement test, the examiner passively lifts the patient's arm, instructs the patient to relax, releases the arm, and notes whether or not it remains elevated. The arm remaining aloft, in the absence of parkinsonism or spasticity, indicates paratonia. In facilitory paratonia, the patient cooperates too much. The patient actively assists the examiner's passive movements, and the limb may continue to move even after the examiner has released it.

## Spasticity

Spasticity is due to lesions involving the corticospinal pathways. The hypertonicity to passive movements differs from that of rigidity because it is not uniform throughout the range of movement, and it varies with the speed of movement. In addition, rigidity tends to affect all muscles to about the same degree, whereas the hypertonia of spasticity varies greatly from muscle to muscle. In spasticity, if the passive movement is made slowly, there may be little resistance. But if the movement is made quickly, there will be a sudden increase in tone partway through the arc, causing a catch or a block as though the muscle had impacted a stop. The relationship of the hypertonus to the speed of movement is a key feature distinguishing spasticity from rigidity. In the upper extremity it is useful to look for spasticity involving the pronator muscles. With the patient's elbow flexed to about 90 degrees and the forearm fully pronated, the examiner slowly supinates the patient's hand. Unless spasticity is severe, there will be little or no resistance to this slow movement. If, after several slow repetitions, the examiner supinates the patient's hand very quickly, there will be sudden resistance at about the midrange of movement, referred to as a "pronator catch." The catch will then relax, and the supination movement can be completed. When hypertonus is severe, this maneuver may elicit pronator clonus.

A similar slow then rapid motion technique can be used to detect lower-extremity spasticity. With hands behind the knee, the examiner slowly flexes and extends the knee of the supine and relaxed patient. With adequate relaxation the foot remains on the bed. After several slow repetitions, from the position of full extension, the examiner abruptly and forcefully pulls the knee upward. When tone is normal, the foot will scoot back, remaining in contact with the bed. When there is spasticity, the foot flies upward in a kicking motion (spastic kick). In the heel- or foot-dropping test, the examiner holds the patient's leg flexed at the knee and hip, one hand behind the knee, the other supporting the foot. The foot is suddenly released. Normally its descent is smooth, but when there is spasticity in the quadriceps muscle the foot may hang up and drop in a succession of choppy movements.

Spastic muscles may or may not feel firm and tense to palpation. The range of movement of spastic extremities, and the degree of hypertonicity, often vary between examinations. No devices for quantitating spasticity exist, and clinical evaluation remains the most useful tool. The Ashworth scale is used to quantitate spasticity on a scale from 1 (no increase in muscle tone) to 5 (affected part rigid in flexion or extension). In the presence of spasticity, the DTRs are exaggerated and pathologic reflexes such as the Babinski and Chaddock signs can often be elicited. Clonus is often present. There may be abnormal associated movements.

Upper motor neuron weakness is often accompanied by sustained contraction of specific groups of muscles. With hemiparesis or hemiplegia, spasticity is most marked in the flexor and pronator muscles of the upper and the extensor muscles of the lower extremity; this causes a posture of flexion of the arm and extension of the leg, the characteristic distribution in cerebral hemiplegia (Figure 19.1). The arm is adducted, flexed at the elbow, and the wrist and fingers are flexed; there may be forced grasping. The lower extremity is extended at the hip, knee, and ankle, with inversion and plantar flexion of the foot; there may be marked spasm of the hip adductors. There is more passive resistance to extension than to flexion in the upper extremities, and to flexion than to extension in the lower extremities. With bilateral lesions the increased tone of the hip adductors causes a scissors gait, in which one leg is pulled toward the other as each step is taken. Although spasticity in the lower extremities usually affects the extensors most severely, in some patients with severe myelopathy or extensive cerebral lesions, there is marked hypertonicity in the flexor muscles, drawing the legs into a position referred to as paraplegia in flexion.

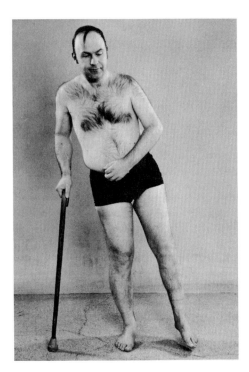

**FIGURE 19.1** ● Left hemiparesis of 15 years' duration. The patient circumducts his left leg as he begins walking.

## Catatonic Rigidity

The abnormal muscle tone in catatonia is in many respects similar to extrapyramidal rigidity and may be physiologically related. There is a waxy or lead-pipe type of resistance to passive movement that may be accompanied by posturing, bizarre mannerisms, and evidence of psychosis. It may be possible to mold the extremities into any position, in which they remain indefinitely.

## Decerebrate and Decorticate Rigidity

Decerebrate rigidity is characterized by marked rigidity and sustained contraction of the extensor muscles of all four extremities; in decorticate rigidity there is flexion of the elbows and wrists with extension of the legs and feet. Similar generalized rigidity with neck extension can occur with severe meningismus (opisthotonos), as well as in the tonic phase of a generalized seizure.

## Voluntary Rigidity

Various muscle groups may be consciously tensed or braced to protect against injury or in response to pain. It is often difficult to differentiate between tension that is truly volitional and that which is unconscious or involuntary, especially when related to excitement, alarm, pain, or fatigue. Tense, apprehensive individuals may show increased muscular tension at all times, and may have exaggerated tendon reflexes. The reflex exaggeration is one of range of response, and the latent period is not shortened. Conversely, the reflexes may be suppressed because the semivoluntary contraction prevents normal movement.

## Involuntary Rigidity

Rigidity that is involuntary, reflex, or nonorganic may resemble voluntary rigidity. Rigidity of psychogenic origin may be bizarre and may simulate any type of hypertonicity. Hysterical rigidity may simulate decerebration or catatonia. It may be extreme, with neck retraction and opisthotonos, the body resting with only the head and heels upon the bed (arc de cercle).

## Reflex Rigidity

Muscles may develop reflex rigidity, or spasm, in response to afferent impulses, particularly pain. Muscle spasm is a state of sustained involuntary contraction accompanied by muscle shortening. The abnormal contraction is visible and palpable. Common examples of reflex muscle spasm are the board-like abdomen of acute abdominal disorders, rigidity of the neck and back in meningitis, and the localized spasm in the extremities following trauma. Reflex rigidity may follow other sensory stimuli, such as cold. Muscle contracture may follow prolonged spasm. In some metabolic myopathies (e.g., McArdle disease), painful muscle cramps and spasms are brought on by exercise; the muscle cramp is a physiologic form of contracture due to abnormal metabolism, and is not accompanied by electrical activity.

## Myotonia

Myotonia is a disorder of the muscle membrane that can occur in many different conditions. Tone is usually normal when the muscles are relaxed, but contraction produces a temporary involuntary tonic perseveration of muscle contraction with slow relaxation. Sudden movements may cause marked spasm and inability to relax. In grip myotonia, the patient has difficulty letting go of an object after gripping it strongly. The myotonia usually decreases with repetition of the movement (warm-up phenomenon). In rare instances the myotonia increases with repetitive movement (paradoxical myotonia). Percussion myotonia is elicited by tapping on the muscle. Percussion over the thenar eminence produces a prolonged tonic abduction and opposition movement lasting several seconds, over which the patient has no control. Tapping over the extensor digitorum communis to the middle finger causes the finger to snap into extension, after which it slowly falls over a much longer period of time than normal. Percussion myotonia can also be elicited over other muscles. Oblique elimination with a penlight may help to make the slowly disappearing depression or dimple more visible. Percussion of a tongue blade placed transversely on edge across the tongue may produce a segmental myotonic contraction that constricts the tongue circumferentially (napkin-ring sign).

# CHAPTER 20

# Muscle Volume and Contour

A search for evidence of muscle atrophy or hypertrophy is an important part of the motor examination. There is normally an appreciable individual variation in muscular development, but noteworthy changes in the size or shape of individual muscles or muscle groups, especially when focal or asymmetric, may be significant.

Muscle atrophy (amyotrophy) causes a decrease in muscle volume or bulk, and is usually accompanied by changes in shape or contour. Neurologic conditions likely to cause muscle atrophy are primarily those that affect the anterior horn cell, the nerve root(s), the peripheral nerve, or the muscle. Neuromuscular junction disorders do not cause muscle atrophy. Atrophy may also result from such things as disuse or inactivity, immobilization, tendonotomy, muscle ischemia, malnutrition, endocrine disorders, and normal aging.

Muscle hypertrophy is an increase in the bulk, or volume, of muscle tissues. It may result from excessive use of the muscles (physiologic hypertrophy) or occur on a pathologic basis. Hypertrophied muscle is not necessarily stronger than normal. Persistent abnormal muscle contraction may cause hypertrophy. Patients with myotonia congenita have a diffuse muscularity without significant increase in strength. Patients with dystonia may develop hypertrophy of the abnormally active muscle. In cervical dystonia (spasmodic torticollis), it is common to see hypertrophy of one sternomastoid muscle. Muscular dystrophies, especially Duchenne dystrophy, often cause pseudohypertrophy of muscle, with enlargement due to infiltration of the muscle with fat and connective tissue without an actual increase in muscle fiber size or number.

## EXAMINATION OF MUSCLE VOLUME AND CONTOUR

There is a great deal of individual variation in muscular development, in part constitutional and in part due to training, activity, and occupation. Certain individuals have small or poorly developed muscles, while others show outstanding muscular development. The sedentary, the elderly, and those with chronic disease may have small muscles without evidence of wasting or atrophy. Athletes may develop physiologically hypertrophic muscles. In normal individuals, the dominant side may exhibit an increase in the size of the muscles, even of the hand and foot. The appraisal of bulk and contour should be correlated with the other parts of the motor examination, especially with the evaluation of strength and tone.

Muscle volume and contour may be appraised by inspection, palpation, and measurement. Inspection generally compares symmetric parts on the two sides of the body, noting any flattening, hollowing, or bulging of the muscle masses. A useful technique for comparing extremities is to look down the long axis. Hold the patient's arms outstretched and close together, comparing "down the barrel" from fingertips to shoulders for any asymmetry.

Palpation assesses muscle bulk, contour, and consistency. Normal muscles are semi-elastic and regain their shape at once when compressed. When hypertrophy is present, the muscles are firm and hard; in pseudohypertrophy they appear enlarged but may feel doughy or rubbery on palpation. Atrophic muscles are often soft and pulpy in consistency. When degenerated muscles have undergone fibrotic changes, they may be hard and firm. Those infiltrated or replaced by fat may feel pliant and flabby.

Measurements may be very useful in assessing atrophy or hypertrophy. A pronounced difference in muscle size may be recognized at a glance, especially when confined to one side of the body, one extremity, or one segment of a limb. Slight differences are more difficult to detect, and measurements with a tape measure or calipers may be necessary. Measurements should be made from fixed points or landmarks, and the sites—such as the distance above or below the olecranon, anterior superior iliac spine, or patella—recorded. The extremities should be in the same position and in comparable states of relaxation. It may also be valuable to measure the length of the limbs.

Atrophy or hypertrophy may be limited to an individual muscle, to muscles supplied by a specific structure (e.g., a nerve or root), to those muscles supplied by certain spinal cord segments, or to one half of the body; or it may be multifocal or generalized. In atrophy related to arthritis and disuse there may be a pronounced decrease in volume with little change in strength. In myopathies, on the other hand, there is often little atrophy in spite of a striking loss of power.

## ABNORMALITIES OF VOLUME AND CONTOUR
### Muscular Atrophy

Muscular atrophy may be caused by many processes. Neurogenic atrophy follows disease of the anterior horn cell, root, or peripheral nerve. Atrophy due to other neurologic processes, such as the hemiatrophy associated with congenital hemiplegia, is not typically considered neurogenic atrophy even though it is related to nervous system disease. The term neurogenic atrophy as commonly used implies disease affecting some part of the lower motor neuron. Myogenic atrophy is that due to muscle disease, such as muscular dystrophy. As a generalization, when weakness and wasting are comparable the process is more likely to be neurogenic; when the weakness is disproportionately greater than the wasting the process is more likely to be myopathic. When a muscle appears wasted but is not weak the cause is likely to be non-neurologic, such as disuse.

### Neurogenic Atrophy

When a lesion completely disrupts the lower motor neuron or its peripheral processes, the affected muscle lies inert and flaccid, and no longer contracts voluntarily or reflexively. Muscle fibers decrease in size, causing wasting or atrophy of the entire muscle mass. Without timely reinnervation the muscle may become fibrotic, with an increase in connective tissue and fatty infiltration. The more abrupt or extreme the interruption of nerve supply, the more rapid is the wasting. The atrophy may either precede or follow other signs, such as weakness. In rapidly progressing diseases weakness precedes atrophy, but in slowly progressive diseases the atrophy may precede appreciation of weakness. If the pathologic process is confined to the anterior horn cells or the spinal cord, the neurogenic atrophy is segmental in distribution. Some conditions cause rapid destruction of the anterior horn cells and atrophy in the distribution of the affected spinal cord segments that develops within a short period of time (e.g., poliomyelitis).

In more slowly progressive disorders of the motor neuron (e.g., amyotrophic lateral sclerosis [ALS]), there is a gradual but widespread degeneration of the brainstem motor nuclei and anterior horn cells, causing progressive muscular atrophy that may appear before weakness is evident

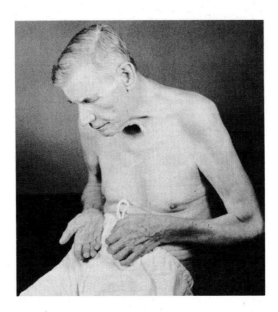

**FIGURE 20.1**  ●  A patient with amyotrophic lateral sclerosis, showing advanced atrophy of the muscles of the hands and shoulders.

(Figure 20.1). The distribution of the atrophy is important. To make a diagnosis of motor neuron disease, it is necessary to demonstrate widespread denervation in a multiple nerve, multiple root distribution. Eventually the disease becomes widespread, but it often begins segmentally in one limb.

Particular groups of muscles are often affected. In classical ALS and in progressive spinal muscular atrophy (SMA) of the Aran-Duchenne type, atrophy is usually first seen in the distal musculature, then spreads up the limbs to the proximal parts. In hereditary motor neuron syndromes, the involvement is often proximal. The proximal distribution and slow progression in SMA type 3 (juvenile proximal SMA, Kugelberg-Welander disease) may simulate muscular dystrophy. Segmental atrophy may also follow focal spinal cord lesions involving the anterior horn cells (e.g., syringomyelia). The rapidity of the progress depends upon the type of pathologic change.

Involvement of nerve roots, plexus elements, or peripheral nerves leads to atrophy of the muscles supplied by the diseased or injured component. With severe lesions involving a peripheral nerve or nerve plexus, atrophy may develop within a short period of time. Lesions involving single nerve roots usually do not cause much atrophy, because most muscles are innervated from more than one level. Marked wasting in a disease that appears consistent with radiculopathy suggests multiple root involvement. In generalized peripheral neuropathy, weakness and wasting are usually greatest in the distal portions of the extremities. The amount of atrophy depends on the severity and chronicity of the neuropathy. The hereditary peripheral neuropathy, Charcot-Marie-Tooth disease (peroneal muscular atrophy), typically causes marked atrophy in a characteristic distribution involving the lower legs (inverted champagne bottle deformity, Figure 20.2). Because of interruption of autonomic pathways, diseases of the lower motor neuron may be associated with trophic changes in the skin and subcutaneous tissues.

Upper motor neuron lesions in adults are usually not followed by atrophy of the paralyzed muscles except for some generalized loss of muscle volume and secondary wasting because of disuse, which is seldom severe. With lesions dating from birth or early childhood, there may be a failure of growth of the contralateral body. Such congenital hemiatrophy may involve one side of the face or the face and corresponding half of the body.

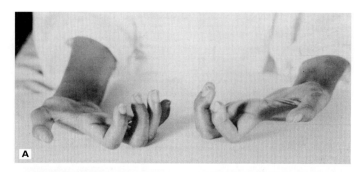

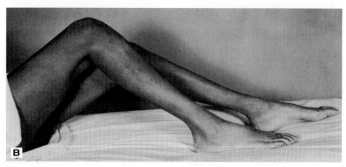

*FIGURE 20.2* ● A patient with Charcot-Marie-Tooth disease (peroneal muscular atrophy), showing wasting of distal muscles and contractures of the hands and feet.

## Other Varieties of Muscular Atrophy

Myogenic, or myopathic, atrophy occurs as a result of primary muscle disease. In some conditions there may be prominent wasting without much weakness. In most of these, the primary pathologic change is type 2 fiber atrophy. Wasting with little weakness occurs in disuse, aging, cachexia, and some endocrine myopathies. Weakness out of proportion to wasting occurs in inflammatory myopathy, myasthenia gravis, and periodic paralysis.

Muscle wasting is common in muscular dystrophy, and the distribution of the wasting parallels the weakness. In dystrophinopathies, the weakness and atrophy primarily involve the pelvic and shoulder girdle muscles (Figure 20.3). As the disease progresses there is increasing wasting of all muscles of the shoulders, upper arms, pelvis, and thighs. In the face of all of the atrophy, certain muscles—particularly the calf muscles—are paradoxically enlarged due to pseudohypertrophy. The limb-girdle syndromes also primarily involve the pelvic and shoulder girdles. In facioscapulohumeral dystrophy, the atrophy predominates in the muscles of the face, shoulder girdles (especially the trapezius and periscapular muscles), and upper arms, especially the biceps (Figure 20.4). Involvement is often asymmetric and occasionally there is pseudohypertrophy of the deltoid and other shoulder muscles. Some myopathies cause striking weakness and atrophy involving certain muscles or muscle groups.

Disuse atrophy follows prolonged immobilization of a part of the body. It may be rapid in onset and can sometimes simulate neurogenic atrophy. The degree of muscle wasting is greater than the degree of weakness, which may be minimal or absent. Muscle atrophy may accompany malnutrition, weight loss, cachexia, and other wasting diseases. The loss of muscle mass is typically greater than the degree of accompanying weakness.

Endocrine dysfunction of various types may lead to atrophy and other changes in muscle. In thyrotoxic myopathy atrophy is particularly prone to involve the shoulder girdle and may lead to

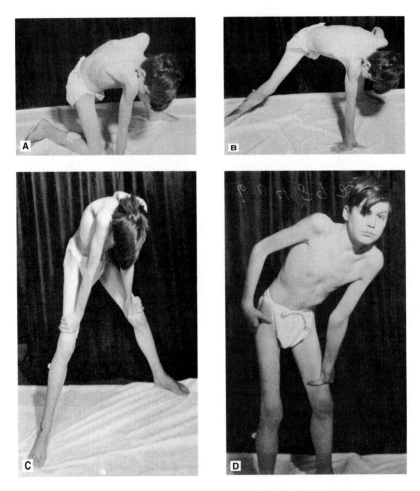

**FIGURE 20.3** ● A patient with muscular dystrophy, showing wasting of the musculature in the shoulders and thighs; weakness and atrophy of the glutei cause difficulty in assuming the erect position, and the patient "climbs up on his thighs" (Gowers maneuver) in order to stand erect.

scapular winging. Myopathy due to excess corticosteroids, exogenous or endogenous, may be associated with muscle wasting. Muscle wasting also occurs with diabetes. Distal weakness and atrophy are common in diabetic distal axonopathy. Diabetic amyotrophy is a common syndrome of bilateral but asymmetric weakness and atrophy that involves the pelvic and thigh muscles due to radiculoplexopathy. It is usually associated with severe pain.

Congenital hypoplasia or absence of a muscle may be mistaken for atrophy. Almost any muscle may be congenitally absent, but some are particularly prone, including the depressor angulii oris, palmaris longus, trapezius, peroneus tertius, and anterior abdominal muscles (prune belly syndrome).

## Muscular Hypertrophy and Pseudohypertrophy

Enlarged muscles are encountered less frequently than atrophy. In true muscle hypertrophy the muscle is enlarged, in pseudohypertrophy the muscle appears enlarged because it is replaced by fat and fibrous tissue. Except for physiologic hypertrophy due to exercise, pseudohypertrophy is

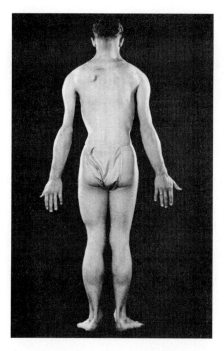

**FIGURE 20.4** ● A patient with scapulohumeral muscular dystrophy, showing atrophy of the muscles of the shoulders and upper arms.

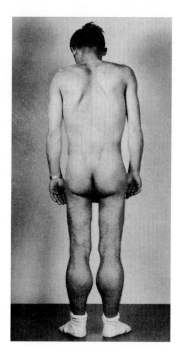

**FIGURE 20.5** ● A patient with muscular dystrophy, showing pseudohypertrophy of the calf muscles.

encountered more commonly than true hypertrophy. Pseudohypertrophy is common in some forms of muscular dystrophy. Muscle biopsy reveals severe myopathy, with fatty and connective tissue infiltrations. Pseudohypertrophy is common in Duchenne and Becker dystrophy; an alternate term for Duchenne dystrophy is pseudohypertrophic muscular dystrophy. Certain muscles, particularly the calf muscles and the infraspinatus, are often strikingly enlarged due to pseudohypertrophy (Figure 20.5). Comparing the circumference of the calf to the knee is most informative. In the early stages of the disease, the enlarged muscles may feel firm and hard and remain strong, and there may actually be an element of true hypertrophy. With progression, they develop a soft doughy or rubbery feeling.

Muscle hypertrophy is common in myotonia congenita, especially the dominant form (Thomsen disease), because of the excessive contraction. These patients may have the impressive muscularity of a bodybuilder; although they may appear strong and muscular, strength is normal or there is even slight weakness. Muscle enlargement, either true hypertrophy or pseudohypertrophy, occurs as an occasional feature in other neuromuscular disorders. Muscle enlargement may be a manifestation of hypothyroidism. Muscle enlargement may also occur due to interstitial infiltrates, as in sarcoidosis and amyloidosis. Loss of body fat may lend the appearance of muscle enlargement.

# CHAPTER 21

# Abnormalities of Movement

**M**ovement disorders may involve any portion of the body. They usually result from disease involving various parts of the motor system, and the etiologies are many. The character of the movement depends on both the site of the lesion and the underlying pathology. Movement disorders disrupt motor function not by causing weakness but by producing either abnormal, involuntary, unwanted movements (hyperkinetic movement disorders), or by curtailing the amount of normal free flowing, fluid movement (hypokinetic movement disorders).

## HYPOKINETIC MOVEMENT DISORDERS

The archetype of hypokinetic movement disorders is Parkinson disease (PD). Other disease processes may produce a similar clinical picture, characterized by decreased movement and rigidity; these have been grouped together as the akinetic-rigid syndromes. About 80% of the instances of akinetic-rigid syndrome are due to PD (Table 21.1). The terms parkinson syndrome or parkinson plus are sometimes used to designate such other disorders, and the features that resemble PD are referred to as parkinsonism, or parkinsonian. Parkinsonism is a clinical diagnosis appropriate in the presence of resting tremor, bradykinesia, rigidity, and impaired postural reflexes. Parkinson disease is but one cause of parkinsonism, and it must be differentiated from other conditions that may have some of its typical features as a component of another disorder.

### Parkinson Disease

Parkinson disease is due to a degeneration of neurons in the dopaminergic nigrostriatal pathway. It is the second most common movement disorder behind essential tremor. Cardinal manifestations include bradykinesia, rigidity, tremor, an expressionless face, and postural instability. Asymmetry is characteristic. The disease often begins asymmetrically; the signs may be so lateralized as to warrant the designation of hemi-PD, and some asymmetry usually persists even when the disease is well established. The major manifestations vary from case to case.

Parkinson disease causes marked hypertonia, or rigidity, which principally affects the axial muscles and the proximal and flexor groups of the extremities, causing an increased tone to passive movement. The rigidity has a rhythmic quality referred to as cogwheel rigidity, presumably due to the superimposition of the tremor. Cogwheeling may be brought out as the examiner passively moves an elbow or wrist by having the patient grit the teeth, look at the ceiling, or use the opposite hand to make a fist, trace circles in the air, or imitate throwing a ball. The rigidity is present evenly throughout the range of movement, without the ebb at the extremes of the range that occurs in spasticity.

## TABLE 21.1

### The Differential Diagnosis of Parkinson Disease

Parkinson disease
Parkinsonian syndromes
   Progressive supranuclear palsy
   Multisystem atrophy
   Olivopontocerebellar degeneration (sporadic form)
   Striatonigral degeneration
   Shy-Drager syndrome
   Diffuse Lewy body disease
   Corticobasal degeneration
   Drug-induced parkinsonism
   Dopa responsive dystonia
Other non-Parkinson akinetic-rigid syndromes
Huntington disease (rigid or juvenile form)
Wilson disease
Essential tremor
Depression
Arthritis, polymyalgia, fibromyalgia

In PD, there is a paucity of movement and a slowing of movements. Strictly speaking, akinesia means an absence of movement, bradykinesia a slowness of movement, and hypokinesia a decreased amount or amplitude of movement, but the term bradykinesia is often used to encompass all three. There is loss of associated and automatic movements, with masking of the face, infrequent smiling and blinking, and loss of swinging of the arms in walking (Figure 21.1).

Patients with PD have poor balance, a tendency to fall, and difficulty walking. The gait abnormality is stereotypical: slow and shuffling with a reduced stride length, sometimes markedly so, a stooped flexed posture of the body and extremities, reduced arm swing, and a tendency to turn "en-bloc." Impaired postural reflexes lead to a tendency to fall forward (propulsion), which the patient tries to avoid by walking with increasing speed but with very short steps, the festinating gait. Falls are common. If a patient, standing upright, is gently pushed either backward or forward, she cannot maintain balance and will fall in the direction pushed. Facial immobility and lack of expressiveness is a common feature of PD (hypomimia, masked face). A decreased rate of blinking, accompanied by slight eyelid retraction, causes patients to have a staring expression (reptilian stare). The voice is typically soft, breathy, monotonous, and tremulous. Other common manifestations include hyperhidrosis, greasy seborrhea, micrographia, somnolence, difficulty turning over in bed, blepharospasm, and apraxia of eyelid opening. Oculogyric crisis, forced involuntary eye deviation, usually upward, is a feature of postencephalitic PD and can occur in drug-induced parkinsonism, but it does not happen in idiopathic PD. Other common manifestations include foot dystonia, "striatal toe," an exaggerated glabellar tap reflex (Myerson sign), and impaired handwriting (especially micrographia). Advancing disease is characterized by increasing gait difficulty, worsening of tremor and bradykinesia, motor fluctuations related to levodopa therapy, behavioral changes, cognitive impairment, hallucinations, intractable drooling, and sleep impairment. The impairment of cognition in PD is extremely variable, ranging from minimal involvement to profound dementia. Some degree of cognitive blunting may occur in 20% to 40% of patients. Early, prominent, and non-visual hallucinations raise the possibility of dementia with Lewy bodies.

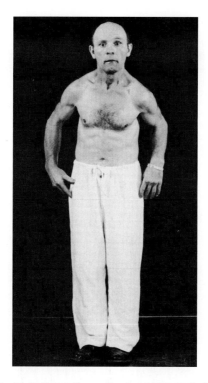

*FIGURE 21.1* ● A patient with Parkinson disease, showing rigidity, masked facies, and typical posture.

The diagnosis of PD is predominantly clinical, and differential diagnosis essentially is between other conditions causing tremor, of which essential tremor is the commonest, and other akinetic-rigid syndromes. Clinical features that favor PD include prominent rest tremor, asymmetric signs, preservation of balance and postural reflexes in the early stages of the disease, and a good response to levodopa replacement therapy. The other degenerative disorders with parkinsonian features typically produce other neurologic signs, such as gaze limitation, cerebellar signs, pyramidal signs, severe dementia, apraxia and other parietal lobe signs, or dysautonomia, although these other manifestations may not be apparent early in the course. Certain drugs can induce a reversible condition that mimics PD. The most common agents that cause drug-induced parkinsonism are antipsychotics, especially the high-potency piperazine compounds such as haloperidol. Some of the other conditions important in the differential diagnosis of PD include multiple system atrophy, progressive supranuclear palsy, corticobasal degeneration, and diffuse Lewy body disease.

Wilson disease (hepatolenticular degeneration) is a rare, autosomal recessive disorder due to abnormal copper deposition in the brain. The usual age of onset is between the ages of 10 and 20, and major manifestations include tremor, rigidity, dystonia and abnormal involuntary movements of various types, dysarthria, dementia, parkinsonian features, spasticity, cerebellar signs, and psychiatric abnormalities (anxiety, depression, psychosis). Kayser-Fleischer rings are crescents of green-brown discoloration of the cornea due to copper deposits in Descemet membrane; these are essentially always present in patients with neurologic involvement but may not be visible without a slit lamp. Hallervorden-Spatz syndrome, or neurodegeneration with brain iron accumulation type-1, is a rare, autosomal recessive disorder associated with macroscopic rust-brown discoloration of the globus pallidus and substantia nigra due to iron deposition. The clinical phenotype is variable but usually includes rigidity, involuntary movements, ataxia, and dystonia.

## TABLE 21.2

**Abnormal Involuntary Movements as a Spectrum of Movements**

| Regular/Predictable | Intermediate | Fleeting/Unpredictable |
|---|---|---|
| Tremor | Most dystonias | Fasciculations |
| Hemiballism | Myokymia | Myoclonus |
| Palatal myoclonus | Athetosis | Chorea |
| | Tic | Dyskinesias |
| | Stereotypy | |
| | Myorhythmia | |

## HYPERKINETIC MOVEMENT DISORDERS

Hyperkinesia refers to increased movement. Hyperkinesias are abnormal involuntary movements that occur in a host of neurologic conditions. Hyperkinesias come in many forms, ranging from tremor to chorea to muscle fasciculations to myoclonic jerks. Any level of the motor system, from the motor cortex to the muscle itself, may be involved in their production. The only common characteristic is that the movements are spontaneous and, for the most part, not under volitional control. They may be rhythmic or random, fleeting or sustained, predictable or unpredictable, and may occur in isolation or accompanied by other neurologic signs. Table 21.2 summarizes some of these features.

In the examination of abnormal movements, the following should be noted: (a) the part of the body involved; (b) the extent or distribution of the movement; (c) the pattern, rhythmicity, and regularity; (d) the course, speed, and frequency; (e) the amplitude and force of the movement; (f) the relationship to posture, rest, activity, various stimuli, fatigue, and time of day; (g) the response to heat and cold; (h) the relationship to the emotional state; (i) the degree that movements are suppressible by attention or the use of sensory tricks; and (j) the presence or absence of the movements during sleep. In general, involuntary movements are increased by stress and anxiety and decrease or disappear with sleep. Truly involuntary movements must be separated from complex or bizarre voluntary movements, such as mannerisms or compulsions.

## TREMOR

A tremor is a series of involuntary, relatively rhythmic, purposeless, oscillatory movements. The excursion may be small or large, and may involve one or more parts of the body. A simple tremor involves only a single muscle group; a compound tremor involves several muscle groups and may have several elements in combination, resulting in a series of complex movements. A tremor may be present at rest or with activity. Some tremors are accentuated by having the patient hold the fingers extended and separated with the arms outstretched. Slow movements, writing, and drawing circles or spirals may bring tremor out.

Tremors may be classified in various ways: by location, rate, amplitude, rhythmicity, relationship to rest and movement, etiology, and underlying pathology. Other important factors may include the relationship to fatigue, emotion, self-consciousness, heat, cold, and the use of medications, alcohol, or street drugs. Tremor may be unilateral or bilateral and most commonly involves distal parts of the extremities—the fingers or hands—but may also affect the arms, feet, legs, tongue, eyelids, jaw, and head, and may occasionally seem to involve the entire body. The rate may be slow, medium, or fast. Oscillations of 3 to 5 Hz are considered slow, 10 to 20 Hz rapid. Amplitude may be fine, coarse, or medium. Tremor may be constant or intermittent, rhythmic or relatively nonrhythmic, although a certain amount of rhythmicity is implied in the term tremor. Irregular "tremor" may be due to myoclonus.

The relationship to rest or activity is the basis for classification into two primary tremor types: rest and action. Resting (static) tremors are present mainly during relaxation (e.g., with the hands in the lap), and attenuate when the part is used. Rest tremor is seen primarily in PD and other parkinsonian syndromes. Action tremors appear when performing some activity. Action tremors are divided into subtypes: postural, kinetic, task-specific, and isometric. Only when they are very severe are action tremors present at rest. Postural tremors become evident when the limbs are maintained in an antigravity position (e.g., arms outstretched). Common types of postural tremor are enhanced physiologic tremor and essential tremor (ET). Kinetic tremor appears when making a voluntary movement, and may occur at the beginning, during, or at the end of the movement. The most common example is an intention (terminal) tremor. Intention tremor is a form of action tremor seen primarily in cerebellar disease. The tremor appears when precision is required to touch a target, as in the finger-nose-finger or toe-to-finger test. It progressively worsens during the movement. Approaching the target causes the limb to shake, usually side-to-side perpendicular to the line of travel, and the amplitude of the oscillation increases toward the end of the movement. Some tremors fall into more than one potential classification. Most tremors are accentuated by emotional excitement, and many normal individuals develop tremor with anxiety, apprehension, and fatigue.

Physiologic tremor is present in normal individuals. The frequency varies from 8 to 12 Hz, averaging about 10 Hz in the young adult, somewhat slower in children and older persons. The visible tremor brought out in normal persons by anxiety, fright, and other conditions with increased adrenergic activity is accentuated or enhanced physiologic tremor. A typical example of enhanced physiologic tremor is that seen in hyperthyroidism. The tremor involves principally the fingers and hands, and may be fine and difficult to see. Similar tremor occurs due to the effects of alcohol, nicotine, caffeine, amphetamines, ephedrine, and other stimulants (Table 21.3).

## TABLE 21.3

### Some Drugs that Cause Tremor

Sympathomimetics (epinephrine, pseudoephedrine, isoproteronol, metaproteronol, albuterol, terbutaline, ritodrine)
Aminoglycoside antibiotics (amikacin, kanamycin, tobramycin)
Methylxanthines (aminophylline, theophylline)
Amphetamines
Anticholinergics
Antihistamines
Bupropion
Carisoprodol, orphenadrine (centrally acting muscle relaxants)
Antipsychotics
Cyclosporine
Benzodiazepines (diazepam, oxazepam)
Selective serotonin reuptake inhibitors (SSRIs)
Other antidepressants (mirtazapine, amoxapine, trazodone, clomipramine)
Lithium
Thyroid supplements
Antiarrhythmics (mexiletine, amiodorone, quinidine)
Opioid antagonists (naloxone)
Phenytoin
Tramadol
Valproic acid
Vasopressin
Yohimbine

Essential tremor is often of medium amplitude and rate but may be coarse when severe. The intention tremor of multiple sclerosis (MS) and cerebellar disease is usually of medium amplitude and may vary in degree from mild to severe; it may be coarse and irregular, especially when associated with ataxia. Coarse tremors occur in a variety of disease states, and are usually slow. Parkinsonian tremor is one of the most characteristic. Coarse tremor also occurs in Wilson disease and other extrapyramidal syndromes. The tremor of general paresis and alcoholism may also be coarse, especially if the movements are diffuse, as in delirium tremens. Psychogenic tremor and the tremor associated with midbrain and cerebellar disease may also be coarse and slow. Two of the commonest causes of tremor are PD and ET.

## Parkinsonian Tremor

Resting, static, or nonintention tremor occurs most frequently in diseases of the basal ganglia and extrapyramidal pathways. The most characteristic tremor of this type is seen in PD and the various parkinsonian syndromes. The tremor of PD is fairly rhythmic, gross, from 2 to 6 Hz, and may involve the hands, feet, jaw, tongue, lips, and pharynx, but not the head. It is typically a resting tremor that lessens during voluntary movement and disappears in sleep. The tremor fluctuates, increasing in amplitude but not rate when the patient becomes excited. The tremor often is more apparent when the patient is walking. The movement in the hand characteristically consists of alternate contractions of agonist and antagonist, involving the flexors, extensors, abductors, and adductors of the fingers and thumb, together with motion of the wrist and arm. As a result there is a repetitive movement of the thumb on the first two fingers, together with the motion of the wrist, producing the classical pill-rolling. The tremor may be unilateral at onset; it may even begin in a single digit, but in most cases eventually becomes bilateral.

## Essential Tremor

Essential tremor is the most common of all movement disorders, and is often familial. Senile tremor is ET occurring during senescence with a negative family history. Essential tremor is higher in frequency and lower in amplitude than the tremor of PD. There is a postural and action tremor that tends to affect the hands, head, and voice. It is made worse by anxiety. A common problem is differentiating the tremor of early PD from ET. The tremor of PD is most prominent at rest, while that of ET occurs with a sustained posture, such as with the hands outstretched, or on action. Parkinsonian tremor may persist with hands outstretched but usually damps, at least momentarily, when making a deliberate movement, whereas ET usually worsens with any attempt at a precise action. The ET patient may have great difficulty sipping water from a cup, but the PD patient may do so without spilling a drop. The head and voice are often involved with ET, only rarely with PD, although the tremor in PD may involve the lips and jaw. Alcohol and beta blockers often improve ET but have no effect on parkinsonian tremor.

# CHOREA

Chorea is characterized by involuntary, irregular, purposeless, random, nonrhythmic hyperkinesias. The movements are spontaneous, abrupt, brief, rapid, jerky, and unsustained. Individual movements are discrete, but they are variable in type and location, causing an irregular pattern of chaotic, multiform, constantly changing movements that seem to flow from one body part to another. The movements may at times appear purposeful to a casual observer, but they are actually random and aimless. They are present at rest but are increased by activity, tension, emotional stress, and self-consciousness. The patient may be able to temporarily and partially suppress the movements, and they disappear in sleep.

The distribution of the choreic movements is variable. They may involve one extremity, one half of the body (hemichorea), or be generalized. They occur most characteristically in the distal parts of the upper extremities, but may also involve the proximal parts, lower extremities, trunk, face, tongue, lips, and pharynx. When asked to hold the hands outstretched, there may be constant random movements of individual fingers (piano-playing movements). If the patient holds the examiner's finger in her fist, there are constant twitches of individual fingers (milkmaid grip). The patient may try to incorporate a spontaneous, involuntary movement into a semi-purposeful movement in order to mask the chorea (parakinesia). If a choreic movement suddenly makes a hand fly upward, the patient may continue the movement and reach up and scratch her nose. In addition to the abnormal movements, there is hypotonia of the skeletal muscles, with decreased resistance to passive movement. The outstretched hands are held with hyperextension of the fingers with flexion and dorsal arching of the wrist (spooning). Motor impersistence—the inability to sustain a contraction—frequently accompanies chorea. The patient is frequently unable to hold the tongue out for any length of time; when asked to do so, the tongue shoots out, then jerks back quickly (snake, darting, flycatcher, or trombone tongue). The blink rate is increased. Many disorders may cause chorea, among them Huntington disease and Sydenham chorea.

## Huntington Disease

Huntington disease (HD, Huntington chorea) is an autosomal dominant, neurodegenerative condition that is inexorably progressive and ultimately fatal. The onset is usually between the ages of 35 and 50, and the typical course is from 15 to 20 years. Patients are usually reduced to a vegetative state about 10 to 15 years after onset.

The chorea is accompanied by progressive intellectual deterioration. The abnormal movements may affect the larger muscle groups and the proximal extremities, causing repeated shrugging of the shoulder or flail-like movements of the arm and twisting and lashing movements that lie between those of chorea and athetosis. Facial grimacing may be marked. Movements of the fingers and hands are often accentuated as the patient walks. Pronounced chorea of the arms and legs when walking may lead to a bizarre, prancing gait. Cognitive impairment usually begins at about the same time as the abnormal movements, but may precede it, and progresses in tandem. Most patients also develop psychiatric abnormalities, particularly personality changes and mood disorders.

## Other Forms of Chorea

Sydenham chorea occurs in childhood and adolescence in relationship to streptococcal infection, and has become a rarity in developed countries. Chorea gravidarum occurs during pregnancy. Chorea can be seen as a manifestation of many systemic illnesses, such as systemic lupus erythematosus, hyperthyroidism, nonketotic hyperglycemia, and others. Chorea may be a transient side effect of many medications. It may be a persisting feature of past or present exposure to psychoactive drugs as part of the syndrome of tardive dyskinesia.

## ATHETOSIS

In athetosis, the hyperkinesias are slower, more sustained, and larger in amplitude than those in chorea. They are involuntary, irregular, coarse, somewhat rhythmic, and writhing or squirming in character. They may involve the extremities, face, neck, and trunk. In the extremities they affect mainly the distal portions, the fingers, hands, and toes. The movements are characterized by any combination of flexion, extension, abduction, pronation, and supination, often alternating and in varying degrees (Figure 21.2). They flow randomly from one body part to another, and the direction of movement changes randomly. The affected limbs are in constant motion. The movements can often be brought out or intensified by voluntary activity of another body part (overflow phenomenon). They disappear in sleep. Voluntary movements are impaired, and coordinated action may be difficult or impossible. Athetosis is usually congenital, the result of perinatal injury to the basal ganglia. Choreoathetosis refers to movements that lie between chorea and athetosis in rate and rhythmicity, and may represent a transitional form. Slow athetoid movements begin to blend with dystonia. Pseudoathetosis (sensory athetosis) is a term used to describe similar undulating

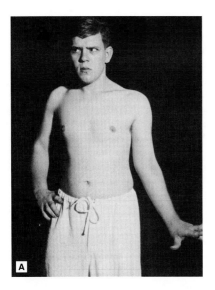
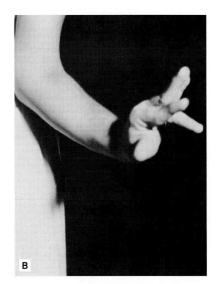

*FIGURE 21.2*  ●  A patient with congenital unilateral athetosis.

and writhing movements of the extremities due to loss of position sense as a result of a parietal lobe lesion, or peripheral deafferentation due to such conditions as tabes dorsalis, posterolateral sclerosis, and peripheral nerve disease (Figure 21.3). The movements are more marked when the eyes are closed and are usually unassociated with an increase in muscle tone.

## DYSTONIA

Dystonia refers to spontaneous, involuntary, sustained muscle contractions that force the affected parts of the body into abnormal movements or postures, sometimes with co-contraction of agonists and antagonists. Dystonia often affects the extremities, neck, trunk, eyelids, face, or vocal cords. It may be either constant or intermittent, and generalized, segmental, focal, multifocal, or in a hemi-distribution. Dystonic movements are patterned, tending to recur in the same location,

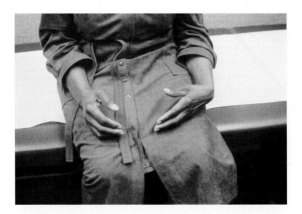

*FIGURE 21.3*  ●  Pseudoathetosis of the hand in a patient with a parietal lobe lesion.

in contrast to the random and fleeting nature of chorea. The speed of dystonia varies widely, from slow, sustained, and cramp-like (athetotic dystonia) to quick and flicking (myoclonic dystonia). Action dystonia occurs when carrying out a voluntary movement. As in athetosis, overflow may occur, with the dystonia brought out by use of another part of the body.

Generalized dystonia causes involuntary movements similar in many respects to athetosis, but involving larger portions of the body, often producing distorted postures of the limbs and trunk. The movements are slow, bizarre, and sometimes grotesque, with an undulating, writhing, twisting, turning character, and a tendency for the contraction to be sustained at the peak of the movement (torsion dystonia, torsion spasm). The term dystonia is sometimes used to describe the postures or positions assumed by the patient, as well as for the hyperkinesia itself.

The focal dystonias are disorders causing involuntary contractions in a limited distribution. A relatively common form of focal dystonia is cervical dystonia (spasmodic torticollis), which affects the neck, and sometimes the shoulder, muscles producing either a sustained or jerky turning of the head to one side, often with some element of head tilt. "Torti" implies a twisting or turning movement; less common variants of cervical dystonia include retrocollis (extension movement) and anterocollis (flexion movement). In the beginning the twisting and turning may be intermittent or present only in paroxysms (spasmodic), but later in the course of the syndrome there is persistent contraction of the involved muscles with resulting deviation of the head. Many if not most patients with cervical dystonia learn they can straighten their head by placing a hand or finger somewhere on the face, or performing some other maneuver to provide sensory stimulation or light counterpressure (geste antagoniste, sensory trick, counterpressure sign, Figure 21.4).

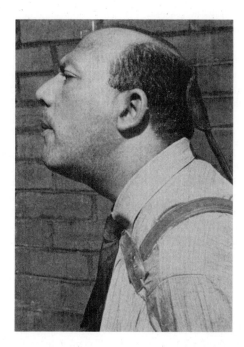

*FIGURE 21.4* ● This patient with cervical dystonia causing retrocollis keeps a wooden spoon inserted into his suspenders to keep light counterpressure on the back of his head (geste antagoniste, sensory trick). (Reprinted with permission from Haymaker W. Bing's *Local Diagnosis in Neurological Disease.* C. V. Mosby, St. Louis, 1969.)

Writer's cramp is a focal dystonia of the hand or forearm muscles brought on by use of the part, most frequently by writing. There are a number of other focal, occupational, or task-specific dystonias related to specific activities. Blepharospasm (upper facial dystonia) causes involuntary closure of both eyes. Oromandibular dystonia involves the mouth, lips, and jaw. The combination of blepharospasm and oromandibular dystonia constitutes Meige (Brueghel) syndrome. Spasmodic dysphonia is dystonia of the vocal cords.

## HEMIBALLISMUS

Hemiballismus (hemiballism) refers to a dramatic neurologic syndrome of wild, flinging, incessant movements that occur on one side of the body, usually due to infarction or hemorrhage in the region of the contralateral subthalamic nucleus. The ballistic movements of hemiballismus resemble those of chorea but are more pronounced. The clinical distinction between severe hemichorea and hemiballismus becomes arbitrary. Like chorea, hemiballistic movements are involuntary and purposeless, but they are much more rapid and forceful and involve the proximal portions of the extremities. When fully developed, there are continuous, violent, swinging, flinging, rolling, throwing, flailing movements of the involved extremities. The movements are ceaseless during the waking state and disappear only with deep sleep. They are usually unilateral, and involve one entire half of the body.

## DYSKINESIAS

All hyperkinetic movements are technically dyskinesias, but the term is often used to encompass complex involuntary movements that do not neatly fit into another category. Dyskinesia is used most often to refer to abnormal involuntary movements related to drugs. Dyskinesias are a common dose-related complication of the treatment of PD with levodopa and dopamine agonists. Orofacial dyskinesias are involuntary movements of the mouth, face, jaw, or tongue that may consist of grimacing, pursing of the mouth and lips, "fish-gaping" movements, and writhing movements of the tongue. Tardive dyskinesias are involuntary movements that usually develop in patients who have received phenothiazines or related compounds. The movements typically involve primarily the mouth, tongue, and jaw with incessant chewing, smacking, licking, and tongue-thrusting movements that are difficult to eradicate.

## MYOCLONUS

The term myoclonus has been used for several differing motor phenomena. In general, myoclonus may be defined as single or repetitive, abrupt, brief, rapid, lightning-like, jerky, arrhythmic, asynergic, involuntary contractions involving portions of muscles, entire muscles, or groups of muscles. The movements are quicker than chorea. Myoclonus is seen principally in the muscles of the extremities and trunk, but the involvement is often multifocal, diffuse, or widespread. It may involve the facial muscles, jaws, tongue, pharynx, and larynx. There may be successive or simultaneous involvement of many muscles. Myoclonus may appear symmetrically on both sides of the body; such synchrony may be an attribute unique to myoclonus. The sudden, shock-like contractions usually appear in paroxysms at irregular intervals, during either the resting or active state, and may be activated by emotional, mental, tactile, visual, and auditory stimuli. Myoclonic movements often affect entire muscles or muscle groups, producing clonic movements of the extremities. They may be so violent as to cause an entire limb to be suddenly flung out, and may even throw the patient to the ground. Myoclonus may also be subtle, a quick flick of a finger or foot.

Myoclonic movements may occur in a variety of conditions, and their significance varies. Sleep starts and hiccups are physiologic forms of myoclonus that occur in normals. Myoclonus is frequently encountered in epilepsy. Massive myoclonic spasms of infancy are characterized by frequent, sudden, violent jerking attacks with flexion of the neck and trunk and adduction or abduction and extension of the arms and legs (infantile spasms, West syndrome. The progressive myoclonic epilepsies are a group of disorders that cause both generalized seizures and myoclonus. Patients with juvenile myoclonic epilepsy have generalized tonic-clonic seizures that are associated with frequent myoclonic jerks predominantly affecting the arms, especially on awakening. The condition is familial, with both dominant and recessive forms, and is relatively benign.

Myoclonus occurs without prominent seizures in a number of conditions, including metabolic disorders (especially uremic and anoxic encephalopathy), Creutzfeldt-Jakob disease, Alzheimer disease, and Huntington disease. Opsoclonus refers to random, chaotic, lightning-fast eye movements. Opsoclonus accompanied by myoclonus may occur as a postinfectious encephalopathy or as a paraneoplastic syndrome, especially due to occult neuroblastoma. Action myoclonus occurs with use of the involved limb. A syndrome of action or intention myoclonus may develop as a sequel to cerebral anoxia.

Myoclonus is typically arrhythmic and diffuse, but the term has also been applied to rhythmic and localized motor phenomena. Palatal myoclonus is characterized by involuntary, rhythmic movements of the soft palate and pharynx, sometimes of the larynx, eye muscles, and diaphragm, and occasionally of other muscles. The movements are generally not influenced by drugs or sleep. Palatal myoclonus occurs with lesions involving the connections between the inferior olivary, dentate, and red nuclei. Palatal myoclonus is also referred to as palatal microtremor. Tremors are due to alternating agonist-antagonist contractions, rhythmic myoclonus to contraction-relaxation cycles of an agonist. In addition, tremors usually disappear in sleep and these palatal movements do not. Whether palatal myoclonus is best characterized as rhythmic myoclonus or a tremor remains unclear.

## ASTERIXIS

Seen primarily in metabolic encephalopathy, particularly hepatic encephalopathy, asterixis is an inability to sustain normal muscle tone. With the arms outstretched and wrists extended, "like stopping traffic," the lapse in postural tone may cause the hands to suddenly flop downward, then quickly recover, causing a slow and irregular flapping motion. When severe, the entire arm may drop.

## TICS AND RELATED MOVEMENTS

The hyperkinesias discussed to this point have been involuntary movements. In another type of abnormal movement the patient has some degree of awareness of the movement, but must make a movement in response to the urge of some compelling inner force. The patient experiences tension and restlessness, which are temporarily relieved by making a particular movement. Such movements have been called "unvoluntary." Examples include tics, akathisia, stereotypies, compulsions, and restless legs.

Tics (habit spasms) are quick, irregular but repetitive movements that are more often seen in children than adults. A tic may be defined as a coordinated, repetitive, seemingly purposeful act involving a group of muscles in their normal synergistic relationships. Tics are stereotyped, recurrent movements that may seem purposeful but are relatively involuntary. Patients are able to suppress the movements temporarily with concentration, but they quickly return when attention is diverted to some other task. Voluntary suppression causes a sense of intolerable mounting tension and an urge to move that is temporarily relieved by indulgence in a tic. Tics are exaggerated by emotional strain and tension; they cease during sleep.

Patients affected with Gilles de la Tourette syndrome (maladie des tics) have multifocal tics, compulsive behavior, imitative gestures, stereotyped movements, grunts and groans, and evidence of regressive behavior. Tics are very common and usually benign; patients with Tourette syndrome have exaggerated, complex tics, which together with the other features of the disease can be very disabling. The large repertoire of tics and the combination of motor and vocal tics distinguish Tourette syndrome from ordinary tics.

Patients suffering from akathisia experience an inner restlessness and urge to move that causes them to remain in almost constant motion. It occurs most often as a result of treatment with major psychotropic drugs. A stereotypy is a repetitive, purposeless but often seemingly purposeful, involuntary, patterned motor activity. Common foot shaking and other mannerisms are examples of simple stereotypies. More complex stereotypies may involve ritualistic behavior, such as the compulsions of obsessive-compulsive disorder. Stereotypies most commonly occur in psychiatric disorders, but may also be a part of neurologic disorders, such as tardive dyskinesia and Tourette syndrome. Hyperekplexia refers to disorders characterized by an excessive startle response in the absence of other evidence of neurologic disease, sometimes accompanied by echolalia, automatic behavior, or automatic obedience. Colorful names have been used for variants of the condition described in different geographic regions (jumping Frenchmen of Maine, latah, myriachit).

Except for palatal myoclonus, involuntary movements generally do not occur during sleep. There are some disorders, however, that occur primarily during sleep. Restless legs syndrome is a common disorder causing unpleasant and difficult-to-describe sensations in the legs that are temporarily relieved by movement. The symptoms commonly occur at night as the patient is drifting off to sleep. Many affected individuals get up and walk around to obtain respite.

## FASCICULATIONS

Fasciculations are fine, rapid, flickering or vermicular twitching movements due to contraction of a bundle, or fasciculus, of muscle fibers. They are usually not extensive enough to cause movement of joints, except occasionally the digits. They vary in size and intensity, from so faint and small as to only slightly ripple the surface of the overlying skin, to coarse and impossible to overlook. They are random, irregular, fleeting, and inconstant. At times they are abundant; at other times they require a careful search. Fasciculations always seem to strike where the examiner is not looking, and are usually seen from the corner of the eye. Fasciculations are brought out by fatigue and cold. When assessing fasciculations, the patient should be warm, comfortable, and completely relaxed. Good light is necessary in order to visualize fasciculations; oblique lighting is best. Many patients are unaware of fasciculations; others may see or feel them, or both. Fasciculations continue in sleep. Fasciculations are a characteristic feature of motor neuron disease. They serve as a very useful marker for the disease, and the diagnosis should remain circumspect when fasciculations are not demonstrable. Fasciculations of small hand muscles in chronic anterior horn cell disease, particularly spinal muscular atrophy, may cause small amplitude, subtle finger twitches called minipolymyoclonus (polyminimyoclonus), which are of course not real myoclonus. Although fasciculations are most characteristic of motor neuronopathies, they can occur in any chronic denervating process, including radiculopathy and peripheral neuropathy. Except for thyrotoxicosis, myopathies generally do not cause fasciculations. Fasciculations unaccompanied by atrophy or weakness do not necessarily indicate the presence of a serious disease process. About 70% of the population, especially health care workers, have occasional benign fasciculations.

## MYOKYMIA

Myokymia refers to involuntary, spontaneous, localized, transient, or persistent quivering movements that affect a few muscle bundles within a single muscle but usually are not extensive enough to cause movement at a joint. The movements are somewhat coarser, slower, and undulating ("worm-like"), usually more prolonged, and involve a wider local area than fasciculations. They usually are not affected by motion or position, and they persist during sleep. Myokymia often occurs in normal individuals, causing persistent, focal twitching of a muscle, most commonly the orbicularis oculi. Myokymia usually occurs in isolation, without evidence of an accompanying neurologic disease. Myokymia occurs in a variety of disease states. It may be generalized or focal/segmental. Focal myokymia is much more common than generalized myokymia. Myokymia sometimes occurs in the facial muscles in patients with MS or other lesions of the brainstem or cranial nerves. Focal limb myokymia is particularly characteristic of radiation damage to a nerve or plexus. Generalized myokymia (Isaacs syndrome) causes generalized muscle stiffness and persistent contraction because of underlying continuous muscle fiber activity.

## SPASMS

Spasms are involuntary contractions of a muscle or group of muscles. The tonic contraction may cause either alteration of position or limitation of movement. They may occur in almost any muscle. A painful, tonic, spasmodic muscular contraction is often spoken of as a cramp. Spasms that limit movement may be defensive or protective. Spasms are often of reflex origin, due to peripheral irritation affecting either muscles or nerves. Pain is a common cause of defensive spasm and reflex rigidity. Carpopedal spasm is a common manifestation of tetany and hyperventilation.

# The Sensory Examination

# CHAPTER 22

# Overview of the Sensory Examination

Thehe sensory system places the individual in relationship to the environment. Every sensation depends on impulses that arise by stimulation of receptors, or end-organs. These impulses are carried to the central nervous system (CNS) by sensory nerves, and then conveyed through fiber tracts to higher centers for conscious recognition, reflex action, or other consequences of sensory stimulation. In this section, only general somatic sensory modalities are considered; the special senses—smell, vision, taste, hearing, and vestibular sensation—are discussed with the cranial nerves that mediate them.

The sensory system consists of exteroceptive, interoceptive, and proprioceptive components. Exteroceptive sensation provides information about the external environment, including somatosensory functions and special senses. The interoceptive system conveys information about internal functions, blood pressure, or the concentration of chemical constituents in bodily fluids. Proprioception senses the orientation of the limbs and body in space.

Sensory systems may function on a conscious or unconscious level. Unconscious visceral sensory systems help regulate the internal environment. The monitoring of limb position in space has both a conscious component—the posterior column pathways—and an unconscious component—the spinocerebellar pathways. The conscious somatosensory system has two components: the position/vibration/fine discriminatory touch system and the pain/temperature/crude touch system. The different sensory modalities are carried over peripheral nerve fibers that vary in size, diameter, and myelination, and over central fiber tracts that vary in location as they travel through different parts of the nervous system. Fine touch, position, and vibration from the body are carried over the posterior column/medial lemniscus system. These sensations from the head and face are processed by the trigeminal principal sensory nucleus in the pons. Pain and temperature from the body are carried over the spinothalamic tracts, and from the head and face over the spinal tract and nucleus of the trigeminal.

## Dermatomes

Sensory nerve roots supply cutaneous innervation to specific dermatomes. The dermatome innervation of the extremities is complex, in part due to the migration of the limb buds during embryonic development. As a result, the C4-C5 dermatomes abut T1-T2 on the upper chest, and the L1-L2 dermatomes are close to the sacral dermatomes on the inner aspect of the thigh near the genitalia. The generally available dermatomal charts are primarily derived from three sources: Head and Campbell, Foerster, and Keegan and Garrett, who all used very different approaches. Figure 26.5 shows the dermatome distributions as depicted by Keegan and Garrett.

## CLINICAL EXAMINATION

Sensory function is divided clinically into primary modalities and secondary or cortical modalities. The primary modalities include touch, pressure, pain, temperature, joint position sense, and vibration. The cortical or secondary modalities are those that require synthesis and interpretation of primary modalities by the sensory association area in the parietal lobe. These include two-point discrimination, stereognosis, graphesthesia, tactile localization, and others. When the primary modalities are normal in a particular body region, but the cortical modalities are impaired, a parietal lobe lesion may be responsible. Itch and tickle sensations are closely allied to pain; they are probably perceived by the same nerve endings and are absent following procedures used for the relief of pain.

Many terms have been used, not always consistently, to describe sensory abnormalities. The definition of esthesia is perception, feeling, or sensation (Gr. *aesthesis* "sensation"). Algesia refers to the sense of pain (Gr. *algos* "pain"). Hypalgesia is a decrease, and analgesia (or analgesthesia) an absence, of pain sensation. The combining form "algia" refers to any painful condition. Hypesthesia is a decrease, and anesthesia an absence, of all sensation. Paresthesia is an abnormal sensation; dysesthesia (Gr. *dys* "bad") is an abnormal, unpleasant, or painful sensation. Table 22.1 summarizes some of the definitions.

Sensory abnormalities may be characterized by an increase, decrease, absence, or perversion of sensation. An example of increased sensation is pain—an unpleasant or disagreeable feeling that results from excessive stimulation of certain sense organs, fibers, or tracts. Perversions of sensation take the form of paresthesias, dysesthesias, and phantom sensations. Impairment and loss of sensation result from decreased acuity of the sensory organs or receptors, impaired conduction in sensory fibers or tracts, or dysfunction of higher centers causing impairment in the powers of perception or recognition.

The sensory examination is performed to discover whether areas of absent, decreased, exaggerated, or perverted sensation are present, and to determine the type of sensation affected, the degree of abnormality, and the distribution of the abnormality. Findings may include loss, decrease, or increase of one or more types of sensation; dissociation of sensation with loss of one modality type but not of others; loss of ability to recognize differences in degrees of sensation; misinterpretations (perversions) of sensation; or areas of localized hyperesthesia. More than one of these may occur simultaneously.

The sensory examination is arguably the most difficult and tedious part of the neurologic examination. Some examiners prefer to assess sensory functions early in the course of the examination, when the patient is most likely to be alert and attentive. Fatigue causes faulty attention and slowing of the reaction time, and the findings are less reliable when the patient has become weary during the examination. Others argue the routine sensory examination is the most subjective and least useful part of the neurologic examination, and prefer to leave it until the end. Since the results depend largely on subjective responses, the full cooperation of the patient is necessary if conclusions are to be accurate. Occasionally, objective evidence, such as withdrawal of the part

## TABLE 22.1

**Generally Accepted Definitions of Commonly Used Terms Regarding the Sensory System and Abnormalities of Sensation**

| Term | Definition |
|------|-----------|
| Allodynia | Increase in sensibility to pain; pain in response to a stimulus not normally painful |
| Alloesthesia (allesthesia) | Perception of a sensory stimulus at a site other than where it was delivered; tactile allesthesia is feeling something other than at the site of the stimulus; visual allesthesia is seeing something other than where it actually is |
| Analgesia (alganesthesia) | Absence of sensibility to pain |
| Astereognosis | Absence of spatial tactile sensibility; inability to identify objects by feel |
| Anesthesia | Absence of all sensation |
| Dysesthesias | Unpleasant or painful abnormal perverted sensations, either spontaneous or after a normally nonpainful stimulus (e.g., burning in response to touch); often accompany paresthesias |
| Hypalgesia | Decrease in sensibility to pain |
| Hyperalgesia | Increase in sensibility to pain; pain in response to a stimulus not normally painful |
| Hyperpathia | Increase in sensibility to pain; pain in response to a stimulus not normally painful |
| Kinesthesia | The sense of movement |
| Pallesthesia | Vibratory sensation (decreased, hypopallesthesia; absent, apallesthesia) |
| Paresthesias | Abnormal spontaneous sensations experienced in the absence of specific stimulation (feelings of cold, warmth, numbness, tingling, burning, prickling, crawling, heaviness, compression, or itching) |

stimulated, wincing, blinking, and changes in countenance, may aid in the delineation of areas of sensory change. Pupillary dilation, tachycardia, and perspiration may accompany painful stimulation. Keenness of perception and interpretation of stimuli differ in individuals, in various parts of the body, and in the same individual under different circumstances.

For a reliable sensory examination, the patient must understand the procedure and be ready and willing to cooperate. Accurate communication is vital. The purpose and method of testing should be explained in simple terms, so that the patient understands the expected responses. During the examination the patient should be warm, comfortable, and relaxed. The best results are obtained when the patient is lying comfortably in a warm, quiet room. Obtaining patient confidence is important. Satisfactory results cannot be obtained when the patient is suspicious, in pain, uncomfortable, fearful, confused, or distracted by sensations such as noise or hunger. If the patient is in pain or discomfort, or if he has recently been sedated, the examination should be postponed. The areas under examination should be uncovered but it is best to expose the various parts of the body as little as possible. The patient's eyes should be closed or the areas under examination shielded to eliminate distractions and to avoid misinterpretation of stimuli. Homologous areas of the body should be compared whenever possible.

The detail and technique used for the sensory examination depend on the history. For example, a patient with no sensory complaints referred for evaluation of headache or vertigo requires only a screening examination. A patient who is seen for possible carpal tunnel syndrome, radiculopathy, peripheral neuropathy, or a suspected parietal lobe lesion requires a very different approach.

The examiner should first determine whether the patient is aware of subjective changes in sensation or is experiencing abnormal spontaneous sensations. Sensory symptoms may be divided into negative symptoms, lack of sensation, and positive symptoms, abnormal sensory discharges such as paresthesias and dysesthesias. Positive and negative symptoms may occur together. Inquire whether the patient has noticed pain, paresthesias, or loss of feeling; whether any part of the body feels numb, dead, hot, or cold; whether he has perceived sensations such as tingling, burning, itching, "pins and needles," pressure, distention, formication, or feelings of weight or constriction. If such symptoms are present, determine their type and character, intensity, distribution, duration, and periodicity, as well as exacerbating and relieving factors. Spontaneous pain must be differentiated from tenderness. Pain and numbness may exist together, as in thalamic pain and peripheral neuropathy. The patient's manner of describing the pain or sensory disturbance and the associated affective responses, the nature of the terms used, the localization, and the precipitating and relieving factors may aid in differentiating between organic and nonorganic disturbances. Nonorganic abnormalities are often associated with inappropriate affect (either excessive emotionality or indifference), are often vague in character or location, and reactions to them are not consistent with the degree of disability.

If the patient has no sensory symptoms, testing can be done rapidly, bearing in mind the major sensory nerve and segmental supply to the face, trunk, and extremities. In certain situations, more careful sensory testing is required. If there are specific sensory symptoms; motor symptoms such as atrophy, weakness, or ataxia; or if any areas of sensory abnormality are detected on the survey examination; or if the clinical situation suggests the likelihood of sensory abnormalities; then detailed sensory examination should be performed. The presence of trophic changes, especially painless ulcers and blisters, is also an indication for careful sensory testing, since these may be the first manifestations of a sensory disorder of which the patient is unaware. In patients with limited cooperation, it may be desirable to examine the areas of sensory complaint first and then survey the rest of the body.

The simpler the method of examination, the more satisfactory the conclusions. Explain to the patient what is to be done and demonstrate in an area expected to be normal what the stimulus feels like. Then have the patient close his eyes and begin the testing. The subject should be asked to tell the type of stimulus perceived and its location, with the examiner taking care not to suggest responses. Responses are normally prompt, and a consistent delay in answering may indicate an abnormal delay in perception. There are two general screening patterns: side to side and distal to proximal. The side-to-side screening should usually compare the major dermatomes and peripheral nerve distributions, although more abbreviated screening may be appropriate in certain clinical circumstances. Distal to proximal testing is appropriate when peripheral neuropathy is part of the differential diagnosis. The distribution of abnormalities can be drawn on the skin with a marker and recorded on a chart, indicating areas of change in the various modalities by horizontal, vertical, or diagonal lines, stippling, or different colors. A key helps to explain the meaning of the various symbols and colors, as does a note regarding the cooperation and insight of the patient and an estimate of the reliability of the examination. Sensory charts are helpful for comparison with the results of subsequent examinations in following the course of the patient's illness, and for comparison with the results of other examiners.

Accuracy in localization of pain, temperature, and tactile stimuli is also informative. Tactile localization is a sensitive test of sensory function; there may be loss of localization before there is a detectable change in sensory threshold. Tactile localization is most accurate on the palmar surfaces of the fingers, especially the thumb and index finger. The patient should name or point to the area stimulated, comparing responses on the two sides of the body.

The results of the sensory examination may at times seem unreliable and confusing. The process can become tedious, and the findings difficult to interpret. Sensory changes due to suggestion are notoriously frequent in emotionally labile individuals, but suggestion can produce nonorganic findings in patients with organic disease. Care must be taken in drawing conclusions. To obtain reliable results, it may be necessary to postpone the sensory examination if the patient has become fatigued, or to repeat the testing at a later time. The sensory examination should always be repeated at least once to confirm the findings. Sensory testing, more than any other part of the neurologic examination, requires patience and detailed observation for reliable interpretation.

The following are some of the difficulties that may be encountered in performing the sensory examination. The uncooperative patient may be indifferent to the sensory examination or object to the use of painful stimuli. The overly cooperative patient, on the other hand, may make too much of small differences and report changes that are not present. Some areas of the body, such as the antecubital fossae, the supraclavicular fossae, and the neck, are more sensitive than others; apparent sensory changes in these regions may lead to fallacious conclusions. The last in a series of identical stimuli may be interpreted as the strongest. Even though pain sensibility is absent, a patient may still be able to identify a sharp stimulus with a pin. Occasionally in syringomyelia, with lost pain but preserved tactile sensibility, the patient may recognize the pin point in an analgesic area and give confusing and inconsistent responses. Sensory findings are difficult to evaluate in individuals with low intellectual endowment, language difficulties, or a clouded sensorium, but it may be necessary to carry out the examination despite these obstacles. In patients with altered mental status or a decreased sensorium, pain may be tested grossly by pricking or pinching the skin, comparing responses on the two sides of the body. In such patients, it may only be possible to determine whether or not the patient reacts to painful stimuli in various parts of the body. A child may be fearful of testing, requiring assurance at the outset that the examination will be brief and not actually painful. In young children, it is often best to delay sensory testing until the end of the examination, particularly when even mildly uncomfortable, yet threatening, stimuli are applied. This may also hold true for some apprehensive adults.

# CHAPTER 23

# The Exteroceptive Sensations

**E**xteroceptive sensations originate in peripheral receptors in response to external stimuli and changes in the environment. There are four main types of general somatic sensation: pain, thermal or temperature sense, light touch or touch-pressure, and position sense or proprioception.

## PAIN AND TEMPERATURE SENSATION

There are many methods for testing superficial pain sensation. A simple and commonly used method, as reliable as any, is to use a common safety pin bent at right angles so its clasp may serve as a handle. The instrument should be sharp enough to create a mildly painful sensation, but not so sharp as to draw blood. A hypodermic needle is far too sharp unless its point has been well blunted against some hard surface. A broken wooden applicator stick is often used, and is usually satisfactory provided the shards are sharp. Adequately sharp ends can be obtained by holding the stick at the very ends while breaking it. Disposable sterile devices, sharp on one end and dull on the other, are commercially available. While it is not necessary for the stimulating instrument to be sterile, whatever is used must be discarded after use on a single patient to avoid the risk of transmitting disease from accidental skin puncture. A helpful trick is to hold the pin or shaft of the applicator stick lightly between thumb and fingertip, and let the shaft slide between fingertip and thumb tip with each stimulation. This helps insure more consistent stimulus intensity than putting a fingertip on the end of the instrument and trying to control the force with the hand or wrist. Experience teaches how to gauge the intensity of the applied stimulus and the expected reaction to it.

It is best to do the examination with the patient's eyes closed. The patient should be asked to judge whether the stimulus feels as sharp on one side as on the other. Always suggest the stimuli should be the same, as by language such as, "Does this feel about the same as that?" Avoid such language as "Does this feel any different?" or "Which feels sharper?" Suggesting there should be a difference encourages some patients to overanalyze and predisposes them to spurious findings and a tedious, often unreliable examination. A commonly used technique is asking the patient to compare one side to the other in monetary or percentage terms, for example, "If this (stimulating the apparently normal side) side is a dollar's worth (or 100%), how much is this (stimulating the apparently abnormal side) worth?" The overanalytical but neurologically normal patient often responds with an estimate on the order of "95 cents," while the patient with real, clinically significant sensory loss is more apt to respond with "5 cents" or "25 cents." Delivering alternately sharp and dull stimuli, as with the sharp and blunt ends of a safety pin, and instructing the patient to reply "sharp" or "dull" is frequently useful but may not detect subtle sensory loss only detectable in comparison with an uninvolved area. Slight changes can sometimes be demonstrated in a cooperative patient by asking her to indicate the alterations in sensation when a pinpoint is drawn lightly over the skin. A cooperative patient with a discrete distribution of sensory loss may be able to map out the involved area quite nicely if instructed how to proceed and left alone for a short time with tools and a marking instrument. The affected area can then be compared with a figure showing sensory distributions.

The latent time in the response to stimulation is eliminated and the delineation more accurate if the examination proceeds from areas of lesser sensitivity to those of greater sensitivity, rather than the reverse. If there is hypalgesia, move from areas of decreased sensation to those of normal sensation; if there is hyperalgesia, proceed from the normal to the hyperalgesic area. There may be a definite line of demarcation between the areas of normal and abnormal sensation, a gradual change, or at times a zone of hyperesthesia between them. It is occasionally useful to move from the normal to the numb area. In myelopathy, a spinal sensory level that is the same going from rostral to caudal as from caudal to rostral suggests a very focal and destructive lesion; when the two levels are far apart the lesion is usually less severe. If testing is done too rapidly, the area of sensory change may be misjudged. Applying the stimuli too close together may produce spatial summation; stimulating too rapidly may produce temporal summation. Either of these may lead to spurious findings. If stimulation is too rapid, or if conduction is delayed, a given response may refer to a previous stimulation. Stimuli should be applied at irregular intervals to avoid patient anticipation. If the patient knows when to expect a stimulus, a seemingly normal response can occur even from an anesthetic area. Include control stimuli from time to time, especially if the patient is comparing sharp and dull (e.g., using the dull end of the pin while asking if it is sharp), to be sure the patient has understood the instructions and is paying attention.

Temperature sensation may be tested with test tubes containing warm and cool water, or by using various objects with different thermal conductivity. Ideally, for testing cold the stimuli should be 5°C to 10°C (41°F to 50°F), and for warmth, 40°C to 45°C (104°F to 113°F). The extremes of free-flowing tap water are usually about 10°C and 40°C. Temperatures much lower or higher than these elicit pain rather than temperature sensations. Normally, it is possible to detect a difference of about 1°C in the range around 30°C. The tubes must be dry, as dampness may be interpreted as cold. The tines of a tuning fork are naturally cool and work well for giving a quick impression of the ability to appreciate coolness. The tines quickly warm with repeated skin contact; applying the tines alternately and waving the fork in the air between stimuli helps prevent this warming. Holding the tines under cold running tap water may also be helpful. Some examiners warm one tine deliberately by rubbing, and then test the ability to discriminate between the warm side and the cool side of the fork. This technique has limited practicality because the cool side warms so rapidly with skin contact. The latency for detecting temperature is longer than for other sensory modalities and the application of the stimulus may need to be extended.

In the general examination, it is sufficient to determine whether the patient can distinguish hot and cold stimuli. It may be useful in some circumstances, such as the detection of mild peripheral neuropathy, to determine whether the patient is able to differentiate between slight variations in temperature. This is best done with special devices for testing temperature sensation quantitatively. In most instances, heat and cold sensibility are equally impaired. Rarely, one modality may be involved more than the other; the area of impaired heat sensibility is usually the larger. Pain and temperature sensibility are usually involved equally with lesions of the sensory system, and it is rarely necessary to test both. Testing temperature may be useful when the patient does not tolerate pinprick stimuli, has confusing or inconsistent responses to pain testing, or to help map an area of sensory loss. In some instances the deficit is more consistent with temperature testing than with pinprick. Temperature testing may not be very reliable in patients with circulatory insufficiency or vasoconstriction causing acral coolness.

## TACTILE SENSATION

There are many methods available for evaluating tactile sensation. Light touch can be tested with a wisp of cotton, tissue paper, a feather, a soft brush, light stroking of the hairs, or even using a very light touch of the fingertip. Some appreciation of light touch may be obtained by noting the responses to the blunt end of the stimulus used to test pinprick.

More detailed and quantitative evaluation can be accomplished using Semmes-Weinstein filaments, an aesthesiometer, or von Frey hairs. These methods employ filaments of different thicknesses to deliver stimuli of varying, graded intensity. For routine testing, simple methods suffice. It is enough to determine whether the patient recognizes and roughly localizes light touch stimuli and differentiates intensities. The stimulus should not be heavy enough to produce pressure on subcutaneous tissues. Ask the patient to say "now" or "yes" on feeling the stimulus, or to name or point to the area stimulated. Allowance must be made for the thicker skin on the palms and soles and the especially sensitive skin in the fossae. Similar stimuli are used for evaluating discriminatory sensory functions such as tactile localization and two-point discrimination. It is best to avoid hairy skin because the sensory stimulation due to hair motion may be confused with the test stimulus; hairy skin is exceptionally sensitive to touch. Two-point discrimination is considered both a delicate tactile modality and a more complex sensation requiring cortical interpretation.

# CHAPTER 24

# The Proprioceptive Sensations

The proprioceptive sensations arise from the deeper tissues of the body, principally from the muscles, ligaments, bones, tendons, and joints. Proprioception has both a conscious and an unconscious component. The conscious component travels with the fibers subserving fine, discriminative touch; the unconscious component forms the spinocerebellar pathways. The conscious proprioceptive sensations that can be tested clinically are motion, position, vibration, and pressure.

## SENSES OF MOTION AND POSITION

The sense of motion consists of an awareness of motion of various parts of the body. The sense of position, or posture, is awareness of the position of the body or its parts in space. These sensations depend on impulses arising as a result of motion of the joints and of lengthening and shortening of the muscles. Motion and position sense are usually tested together, by passively moving a part and noting the patient's appreciation of the movement and recognition of the direction, force, and range of movement; the minimum angle of movement the patient can detect; and the ability to judge the position of the part in space. In the lower extremity, testing usually begins at the metatarsophalangeal joint of the great toe, in the upper extremity at one of the distal interphalangeal joints. If these distal joints are normal there is no need to test more proximally. Testing is done with the patient's eyes closed. It is extremely helpful to instruct the patient, eyes open, about the responses expected before beginning the testing. No matter the effort, nonsensical replies are frequent. The examiner should hold the patient's completely relaxed digit on the sides, away from the neighboring digits, parallel to the plane of movement, exerting as little pressure as possible to eliminate clues from variations in pressure. If the digit is held dorsoventrally, the grip must be firm and unwavering so that the pressure differential to produce movement provides no directional clue. The patient must relax, and not attempt any active movement of the digit that may help to judge its position. The part is then passively moved up or down, and the patient is instructed to indicate the direction of movement from the last position (Figure 24.1). Even when instructed that the response is two alternatives, forced choice, up or down, some patients cannot be dissuaded from reporting the absolute position (e.g., down), even if the movement was up from a down position; a surprising number insist on telling the examiner the digit is "straight" when it is moved into that position. It is often useful simply to ask the patient to report when he first detects movement, then move the digit up and down in tiny increments, gradually increasing the excursion until the patient is aware of the motion. Quick movements are more easily detected than very slow ones. Healthy young individuals

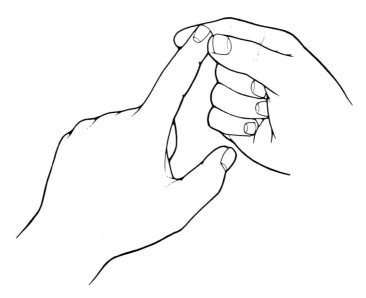

*FIGURE 24.1* ● Method of testing position sense; done similarly with toe.

can detect great toe movements of about 1 mm; in the fingers virtually invisible movements at the distal interphalangeal joint are accurately detected. There is some rise in the threshold for movement and position sense with advancing age.

Minimal impairment of position sense causes first loss of the sense of position of the digits, then of motion. In the foot these sensations are lost in the small toes before they disappear in the great toe; in the hand involvement of the small finger may precede involvement of the ring, middle, or index finger, or thumb. Loss of small movements in the midrange is of dubious significance, especially in an older person. Loss of ability to detect the extremes of motion of the great toe is abnormal at any age. Errors between these two extremes require clinical correlation. If the senses of motion and position are lost in the digits, one should examine more proximal joints, such as ankle, wrist, knee, or elbow. Abnormality at such large joints is invariably accompanied by significant sensory ataxia and other neurologic abnormalities.

Position sense may also be tested by placing the fingers of one of the patient's hands in a certain position (e.g., the "OK" sign) while his eyes are closed, and then asking him to describe the position or to imitate it with the other hand. The foot may be passively moved while the eyes are closed, and the patient asked to point to the great toe or heel. With the hands outstretched and eyes closed, loss of position sense may cause one hand to waver or droop. One of the outstretched hands may be passively raised or lowered, and the patient asked to place the other extremity at the same level. One hand may be passively moved, with eyes closed, and the patient asked to grasp the thumb or forefinger of that hand with the opposite hand. Abnormal performance on these latter tests does not indicate the side of involvement when a unilateral lesion is present. Loss of position sense may cause involuntary, spontaneous movements (pseudoathetosis, Figure 21.3). Reduction in the ability to perceive the direction of passive skin movement may indicate impairment of position sense superficial to the joint. Such impairment is usually associated with joint-sense deficit as well. In the pinch-press test, the patient is asked to tell if the examiner is lightly pinching or pressing the skin. Neither stimulus should be sufficiently intense to cause pain. The methods available for evaluating the senses of motion and position are all relatively crude, and there may be functional impairment not adequately brought out by the testing procedures.

Normal coordination requires intact proprioceptive sensory function in order to keep the nervous system informed about the moment-to-moment position of the limbs and body in space. Patients with severe proprioceptive deficits may have ataxia and incoordination which closely resemble those seen in cerebellar disease, except that they are much worse when the eyes are closed. The incoordination due to proprioceptive loss is referred to as sensory ataxia. The ataxia and incoordination are significantly influenced by vision. Visual input allows for conscious correction of errors and permits the patient to compensate to some degree for the proprioceptive loss. There may be some degree of incoordination with eyes open, but performance is significantly degraded with eyes closed. The incoordination may be apparent on the tests usually employed for cerebellar function, such as finger to nose and heel to shin. When trying to stand and walk, the patient with sensory ataxia may not be aware of the position of his feet or the posture of his body. He may walk fairly well with eyes open, but with eyes closed he staggers and may fall. Although the standing posture with eyes open is stable, with eyes closed there is a tendency to sway and fall. The Romberg test explores for imbalance due to proprioceptive sensory loss. The patient is able to stand with feet together and eyes open but sways or falls with eyes closed; it is one of the earliest signs of posterior column disease. The gait of sensory ataxia and the Romberg sign are discussed in more detail in Chapter 44. A classic disease causing sensory ataxia, now seldom seen, is tabes dorsalis. Sensory ataxia is currently more likely to be encountered in patients with severe peripheral neuropathy (especially if it involves large fibers), dorsal root ganglionopathy, or vitamin $B_{12}$ deficiency.

## SENSE OF VIBRATION (PALLESTHESIA)

Vibratory sensation is the ability to perceive the presence of vibration when an oscillating tuning fork is placed over certain bony prominences. For clinical purposes, it can be considered a specific type of sensation, but more probably results from a combination of other sensations. Bone may act largely as a resonator. The oscillations of the tuning fork invoke impulses that are coded so that one cycle of the sinusoidal wave produces one action potential. The frequency of action potentials in the afferent nerve fiber signals the vibration frequency. The intensity of vibration is related to the total number of sensory nerve fibers activated.

Impulses are relayed with the proprioceptive and tactile sensations through large, myelinated nerve fibers, and enter the spinal cord through the medial division of the posterior root. Vibration has been traditionally considered to ascend the spinal cord with other proprioceptive impulses in the dorsal columns, but likely other pathways are involved. Fibers in the dorsolateral funiculus may be the most important pathway subserving vibratory sensation in man. Loss of position sense and vibration sense do not always parallel one another, and in some clinical conditions one is affected much more and much earlier than the other. Divergence of the position sense and vibration sense pathways may partially explain the occasional dissociation between changes in position sense and vibration sense. In subacute combined degeneration it is not uncommon for vibration loss to be much worse than position sense loss, conversely for tabes dorsalis.

A tuning fork of 128 Hz, with weighted ends, is most frequently used. Sensation may be tested on the great toes, the metatarsal heads, the malleoli, the tibia, anterior superior iliac spine, sacrum, spinous processes of the vertebrae, sternum, clavicle, styloid processes of the radius and ulna, and the finger joints. It is possible to test vibration perceived from the skin by testing on the pads of the fingertips, or even on the skin overlying muscle and other tissues. Both the intensity and duration of the vibration perceived depend to a great extent on the force with which the fork is struck and the interval between the time it is set in motion and the time of application.

For clinical testing, the tuning fork is struck and placed on a bony prominence, usually the dorsum of the great toe interphalangeal joint initially, and held there until the patient no longer feels the vibration. A frequent problem is failure to adequately instruct the patient in the desired response. The novice examiner strikes the tuning fork, touches it to the patient's great toe, and says, "Do you feel that?" A deceptive problem lies in the definition of "that." A patient with absent vibratory sensation may feel the touch of the handle of the tuning fork, misinterpret it as the "that" inquired about, and respond affirmatively. Thus very gross defects in vibratory sensibility may be completely missed. Always set the fork in motion, touch it to some presumably normal body part and tell the patient "this is vibrating or buzzing," then dampen the tines, reapply the stimulus, and tell the patient "this is just touching," or something similar that clearly differentiates the nature of the two stimuli, and then proceed with the testing. With normal vibratory sensation, the patient can feel the fork over the great toe until it has almost stopped vibrating. If vibration is impaired, when the fork is no longer perceptible distally it is moved to progressively more proximal locations until a level is found that is normal. It is also important to compare vibratory sensibility at homologous sites on the two sides. Sensing the vibration briefly when moving to one side after vibration has ceased on the other side is not abnormal; it probably has to do with sensory adaptation. Consistent asymmetry of vibratory sensation is abnormal. It is important to include occasional control applications, striking the fork so the patient hears the hum, and then quickly grabbing and damping the tines before applying the handle. The patient who then claims to feel the vibration has not understood the instructions. Occasional peripheral neuropathy patients with constant tingling in the feet may think they feel a vibration even when the fork is silent.

The threshold for vibratory perception is normally somewhat higher in the lower than in the upper extremities. There is progressive loss of vibratory sensibility with advancing age, and the sensation may be entirely absent at the great toes in the elderly. The best control is an approximately age-matched normal, such as the patient's spouse. If patient and examiner are about the same age, the examiner can compare the patient's perception of vibration with his own.

Vibration is a sensitive modality because the nervous system must accurately perceive, transmit, and interpret a rapidly changing stimulus. An early physiologic change due to demyelination is prolongation of the nerve refractory period, which causes an inability of the involved fiber to follow a train of impulses. An example is the flicker fusion test, no longer used, in which a patient with optic nerve demyelination perceives a strobe as a steady light on the involved side at a frequency when it is still flickering on the normal side. The ability to follow a train of stimuli is one of the first functions impaired when there is demyelination in the nervous system, either peripheral or central. Testing vibratory sensibility measures this functional ability, and loss of vibratory sensation is a sensitive indicator of dysfunction of the peripheral nervous system or the posterior columns, especially when there is any degree of demyelination. It is common for vibratory sensation to be impaired out of proportion to other modalities in patients with multiple sclerosis.

Vibratory sensation can be quantitated fairly simply by noting where the patient can perceive it and for how long (e.g., "absent at the great toes and first metatarsal head, present for 5 seconds over the medial malleoli [128 Hz fork]"). If the patient returns having lost vibration over the malleoli, then the condition is progressing. If on follow-up, vibration is present for 12 seconds over the malleoli and can now be perceived for 3 seconds over the metatarsal heads, then the patient is improving.

Vibratory sensation may be impaired or lost in lesions of the peripheral nerves, nerve roots, dorsal root ganglia, posterior columns, and lesions involving the medial lemniscus and other central connections. In patients with posterior column or peripheral nerve disease, vibratory sensation is lost in the lower extremities much earlier than in the upper. The finding of a normal vibratory threshold in the distal lower extremities usually obviates the need for testing proximally or in the upper extremities, absent specific symptoms involving these areas. A moderate decrease in vibratory perception in the lower extremities or a difference between the lower and the upper extremities may be clinically significant. Marked vibratory loss distally (e.g., the toe), with a transition to normal more proximally (e.g., the knee), is more consistent with peripheral neuropathy. Impaired vibration from posterior column disease is more likely to be uniform at all sites in the involved extremities. Occasionally, in localized spinal cord lesions, a "level" of vibration sensory loss may be found on testing over the spinous processes. Because bone is such an efficient resonator, occasional patients with severe deficits to vibration in the distal lower extremities may feel transmitted vibrations in the hip and pelvis. When vibration seems more intact than it should, ask the patient where he feels the sensation.

## PRESSURE SENSATION

Pressure or touch-pressure sensation is closely related to tactile sense, but involves the perception of pressure from the subcutaneous structures rather than light touch from the skin. It is also closely related to position sense and is mediated via the posterior columns. Pressure sense is tested by a firm touch on the skin or by pressure on deep structures (muscle masses, tendons, nerves), using finger pressure or a blunt object. The patient should both detect and localize the pressure. Strong pressure over muscles, tendons, and nerves tests deep pain sensibility.

## DEEP PAIN SENSE OR PRESSURE PAIN

Pain originating from the deeper tissues of the body is more diffuse and less well localized than superficial pain. The pathways for deep pain are the same as for superficial pain. Deep pain may be tested by squeezing muscles, tendons, or the testicles; by pressing on superficial nerves or on the eyeballs, or by pushing a finger interphalangeal joint into extreme, forced hyperflexion. Firm pressure on the base of a nail with a hammer or tuning fork handle also hurts a great deal. Loss of deep pain sensibility is a classic finding in tabes dorsalis. The response to superficial or deep pain stimulation may be simply delayed before it is lost.

# CHAPTER 25

# Cerebral Sensory Functions

Cerebral sensory functions are those which involve the primary sensory areas of the cortex to perceive the stimulus, and the sensory association areas to interpret the meaning of the stimulus and place it in context. These functions are also referred to as secondary or cortical modalities. The term combined sensation describes perception that involves integration of information from more than one of the primary modalities for the recognition of the stimulus. Cortical sensory processing is primarily a function of the parietal lobes. The parietal lobe functions to analyze and synthesize the individual varieties of sensation, to correlate the perception of the stimulus with memory of past stimuli that were identical or similar, and with knowledge about related stimuli to interpret the stimulus and aid in discrimination and recognition. The parietal cortex receives, correlates, synthesizes, and refines the primary sensory information. It is not concerned with the cruder sensations, such as recognition of pain and temperature, which are subserved by the thalamus. The cortex is important in the discrimination of the finer or more critical grades of sensation, such as the recognition of intensity, the appreciation of similarities and differences, and the evaluation of the gnostic, or perceiving and recognizing, aspects of sensation. It is also important in localization, in the recognition of spatial relationships and postural sense, in the appreciation of passive movement, and in the recognition of differences in form and weight and of two-dimensional qualities. These elements of sensation are more than simple perceptions, and their recognition requires integration of the various stimuli into concrete concepts as well as calling forth engrams. Cortical sensory functions are perceptual and discriminative, rather than the simple appreciation of information from the stimulation of primary sensory nerve endings. The cortical modalities of greatest clinical relevance include stereognosis, graphesthesia, two-point discrimination, sensory attention, and other gnostic or recognition functions. The loss of these varieties of combined sensation may be considered a variety of agnosia, or the loss of the power to recognize the meaning of sensory stimuli. The primary modalities must be relatively preserved before concluding that a deficit in combined sensation is due to a parietal lobe lesion. Only when the primary sensory modalities are normal can the unilateral failure to identify an object by feel be termed astereognosis, and be attributed to a central nervous system (CNS) lesion. A patient with severe carpal tunnel syndrome and numb fingers may not be able to identify a small object by feel; this finding is not astereognosis anymore than the inability to recognize sound from a deaf ear is auditory agnosia or the inability to recognize objects visually from a blind eye is visual agnosia.

Stereognosis is the perception, understanding, recognition, and identification of the form and nature of objects by touch. Inability to do this is astereognosis. Astereognosis can be diagnosed only if cutaneous and proprioceptive sensations are intact; if these are significantly impaired, the primary impulses cannot reach consciousness for interpretation. There are several steps in object recognition. First, the size is perceived, followed by appreciation of shape in two dimensions, form in three dimensions, and finally identification of the object. These steps may be analyzed individually. Size perception is tested by using objects of the same shape but different sizes; shape perception with objects of simple shape (circle, square, triangle), cut out of stiff paper or plastic; and form perception by using solid geometric objects (cube, pyramid, ball). Finally, recognition is evaluated by having the patient identify only by feel simple objects placed in his hand (e.g., key, button, coin, comb, pencil, safety pin, paper clip). For more refined testing the patient may be asked to differentiate coins, identify letters carved from wood or fiberboard, or count the number of dots on a domino. Obviously, stereognosis can be tested only in the hands. If weakness or incoordination prevents the patient from handling the test object, the examiner may rub the patient's fingers over the object. When stereognosis is impaired, there may be a delay in identification, or a decrease in the normal exploring movements as the patient manipulates the unknown object. Stereognosis testing normally compares the two hands, and any deficit will be unilateral. Inability to recognize objects by feel with either hand, if the primary modalities are intact, is tactile agnosia. Recognition of texture is a related type of combined sensation in which the patient tries to recognize similarities and differences between objects of varying textures, such as cotton, silk, wool, wood, glass, and metal.

Graphesthesia (traced figure discrimination) is the ability to recognize letters or numbers written on the skin with a pencil, dull pin, or similar object. It is a fine, discriminative variety of cutaneous sensation. Testing is often done over the finger pads, palms, or dorsum of the feet. Letters or numbers about 1 cm in height are written on the finger pads, larger elsewhere. Easily identifiable, dissimilar numbers should be used (e.g., 3 and 4 rather than 3 and 8). It really does not seem to matter whether the numbers are written as the patient would "read" them or "upside down"; and, despite the temptation, it is not necessary to "erase" between stimuli. Loss of this sensory ability is known as agraphesthesia or graphanesthesia. Even minimal impairment of primary sensory modalities may cause agraphesthesia. A related function is the ability to tell the direction of movement of a light scratch stimulus drawn for 2 cm to 3 cm across the skin (tactile movement sense, directional cutaneous kinesthesia), which may be a sensitive indicator of function of the posterior columns and primary somatosensory cortex. Loss of graphesthesia or the sense of tactile movement with intact peripheral sensation implies a cortical lesion, particularly when the loss is unilateral.

Two-point, or spatial, discrimination is the ability to differentiate, eyes closed, cutaneous stimulation by one point from stimulation by two points. The best instrument for testing is a two-point discriminator designed for the purpose. Commonly used substitutes are electrocardiogram calipers, a compass, or a paper clip bent into a "V," adjusting the two points to different distances. There are two types of two-point discrimination: static and moving. To test static two-point, the test instrument is held in place for a few seconds on the site to be tested. Either one-point or two-point stimuli are delivered randomly, and the minimal distance that can be discerned as two points is determined. Accurate instructions are vital. It is best to start with a two-point stimulus, points relatively far apart ("this is two points"), then a single point ("this is one point"), and then two points close together ("this is two so close it feels like one"). Then one- and two-point stimuli are varied randomly, bringing the points closer and closer until the patient begins to make errors. The result is taken as the minimum distance between two points that can be consistently felt separately. This distance varies considerably in different parts of the body. Normal two-point discrimination is about 1 mm on the tip of the tongue, 2 mm to 3 mm on the lips, 2 mm to 4 mm on the fingertips, 4 mm to 6 mm on the dorsum of the fingers, 8 mm to 12 mm on the palm, 20 mm to 30 mm on the back of the hand, and 30 mm to 40 mm on the dorsum of the foot. Greater separation is necessary for differentiation on the forearm, upper arm, torso, thigh, and leg. The findings on the two sides of the body must always be compared. For moving two-point, the technique is the same except the instrument is drawn slowly across the test area. To test moving two-point on a finger pad, the discriminator would be pulled from the crease of the distal interphalangeal joint toward the tip of the finger over several seconds. Discrimination for two moving points is slightly better than for two stationary points. Moving two-point tests the rapidly adapting mechanoreceptors, and may have some advantages in the management of patients with peripheral nerve injuries.

Two-point discrimination requires keen tactile sensibility. The pathway is mainly through the posterior columns and medial lemniscus. Loss of two-point discrimination with preservation of other discriminatory tactile and proprioceptive sensation may be the most subtle sign of a lesion of the opposite parietal lobe.

Sensory extinction or inattention is loss of the ability to perceive two simultaneous sensory stimuli. Testing for tactile extinction uses double simultaneous light touch stimuli at homologous sites on the two sides of the body. Extinction occurs when one of the stimuli is not felt. Extinction can also be done on one side, touching the face and hand simultaneously. In general the more rostral area is the dominant one; when face and hand are stimulated, there is extinction of the hand percept (the face-hand test). It may be normal to extinguish the hand stimulus. The most subtle abnormality is for a hand stimulus on the normal side to extinguish a face stimulus on the abnormal side, but such testing pushes the limit of usefulness of the technique. The severity of extinction can be approximately quantitated by increasing the intensity of the stimulus on the abnormal side. Using one fingertip on the normal side, a patient with mild extinction will extinguish a two-fingertip stimulus on the abnormal side, but a one-fingertip/three-fingertip set will be felt as bilateral stimuli. With severe extinction, it may require a whole hand stimulus or even a firm squeeze on the abnormal side for the patient to appreciate that the stimulation was bilateral. Similar testing can be done with pinprick.

Tactile extinction is most likely to occur with a lesion of the parietal lobe, but has been reported with lesions involving the thalamus or sensory radiations. Double simultaneous stimulation above and below the presumed level of a spinal cord lesion in which there is relative but not absolute sensory loss may aid in demonstrating the level of the lesion. If only the upper stimulus is perceived, the lower is moved more rostrally until the intensity of both is equal; this may indicate the segmental level of the lesion.

Autotopagnosia (somatotopagnosia, body-image agnosia) is inability to identify body parts, orient the body, or understand the relation of individual parts—a defect in the body scheme. The patient may have complete loss of personal identification of one limb or one half of the body. He may drop his hand from the table onto his lap and believe that some other object has fallen, or feel an arm next to his body and not be aware that it is his own. Lack of awareness of one-half of the body is referred to as agnosia of the body half. Finger agnosia is an inability to name or recognize fingers. Finger agnosia occurs most commonly as part of Gerstmann syndrome (finger agnosia, agraphia, acalculia, and right-left disorientation). Anosognosia is an absence of awareness, or denial of the existence, of disease. It is often used more or less synonymously with somatotopagnosia to refer to patients who deny the existence of hemiplegia or fail to recognize the paralyzed body parts as their own. Anosognosia is most often found in lesions of the right parietal lobe. These disorders are discussed in more detail in Chapter 7.

# CHAPTER 26

# Sensory Localization

**D**iminution or loss of sensation may occur because of lesions involving the peripheral nerves, nerve roots, spinal cord, brainstem, or higher centers of the brain, as may abnormal sensations, such as pain or paresthesia. Localization depends on the pattern and distribution of the sensory abnormality.

The primary modalities may be impaired because of disease involving peripheral nerve, spinal root, or sensory pathways within the central nervous system (CNS). When the primary modalities are normal in a particular body region, but the cortical modalities are impaired, a parietal lobe lesion may be responsible. When some primary modalities are involved more than others, the sensory loss is said to be "dissociated." The pathways conveying pain and temperature (the spinothalamic tracts) run in a different location than the pathways conveying touch, pressure, position, and vibration (the posterior columns and medial lemniscus). After running divergently through much of their central course, the sensory pathways converge again as they approach the thalamus and remain together in the thalamocortical projections. When the pathways are close together, such as in the peripheral nerve, spinal root, or thalamus, disease processes tend to affect all primary modalities to an approximately equal degree. When the pathways are remote from each other, such as in the spinal cord and brainstem, a disease process may affect one type of sensation and not another, producing dissociated sensory loss. A common example of dissociated sensory loss is lateral medullary stroke, or Wallenberg syndrome. There is a very characteristic pattern of sensory loss, which only involves pain and temperature and completely spares light touch. The pain and temperature loss involves the ipsilateral face because of involvement of the spinal tract of cranial nerve V, and the contralateral body because of damage to the lateral spinothalamic tract, sparing the light touch pathways that are running in the midline in the medial lemniscus. A classic but not common cause of dissociated sensory loss is syringomyelia. The pain and temperature sensory fibers crossing in the anterior commissure are affected; light touch sensory fibers running in the posterior columns are well removed from the site of the pathology and remain intact. As a result, syringomyelia characteristically causes sensory loss to pain and temperature with preservation of light touch. Anterior spinal artery stroke is another example of dissociated sensory loss. The infarction involves the anterior two-thirds of the cord, sparing the posterior columns, which are perfused by the posterior spinal arteries. The patients have dense motor deficits and dense sensory loss to pain and temperature, but normal touch, pressure, position, and vibration. Patients with Brown-Séquard syndrome have extreme dissociation of modalities, with loss of pain and temperature on one side of the body and loss of touch, pressure, position, and vibration on the other side of the body.

In contrast, disease processes affecting a peripheral nerve trunk or a spinal root tend to involve all of the sensory fibers traveling in that nerve or root. The sensory loss involves all modalities. Occasionally, generalized polyneuropathies may have a predilection for large or small fibers, and can cause some differential involvement of pain and temperature as opposed to touch and pressure. These neuropathies are uncommon and tend to be generalized. When there is marked sensory dissociation affecting one body region, the pathology is virtually always going to be in the CNS, specifically in those regions where the different sensory pathways run in widely divergent locations.

The other consideration in elucidating the cause of sensory loss, in addition to the modalities involved, is the distribution of the abnormality. Deficits in a "hemi" distribution obviously suggest CNS disease, likely involving either the cortex or the thalamus. Crossed deficits, affecting the face on one side and the body on the opposite side, suggest brainstem disease. Deficits involving both sides of the body below a certain level (e.g., T5) suggest spinal cord disease. A spinal cord level with "sacral sparing" suggests intraparenchymal spinal cord pathology rather than a myelopathy due to external pressure. Deficits due to generalized peripheral nerve disease typically involve the most distal body regions in a "stocking-glove" distribution. Sensory loss due to dysfunction of a peripheral nerve, nerve root, or nerve plexus follows the innervation pattern of that particular structure. Figure 26.1 depicts some of the commonly seen patterns of sensory loss. In hemi-distribution sensory loss there is a certain amount of side-to-side crossing or overlap of innervation along the anterior midline, which is greater on the trunk than on the face. Because of this midline overlap, organic sensory loss usually stops short of the

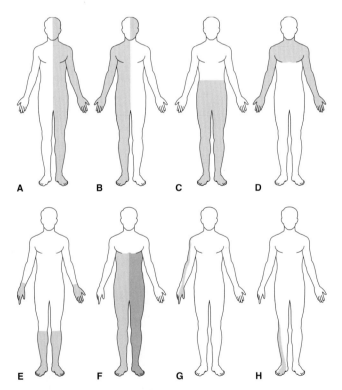

*FIGURE 26.1*  ●  Some common patterns of sensory loss. **A.** Hemisensory loss due to a hemispheric lesion. **B.** Crossed sensory loss to pain and temperature due to a lateral medullary lesion. **C.** Midthoracic spinal cord level. **D.** Suspended, dissociated sensory loss to pain and temperature due to syringomyelia. **E.** Distal, symmetric sensory loss due to peripheral neuropathy. **F.** Crossed spinothalamic loss on one side with posterior column loss on the opposite side due to Brown-Sequard syndrome. **G.** Dermatomal sensory loss due to cervical radiculopathy. **H.** Dermatomal sensory loss due to lumbosacral radiculopathy.

midline, while nonorganic sensory loss may "split the midline" (see further on). Sacral sensation is not tested as part of a routine neurologic examination. In some instances, sensation in the saddle distribution should be examined (e.g., when a conus medullaris or cauda equina lesion is a possibility; when there is evidence of a myelopathy; or when there is bladder, bowel, or sexual dysfunction).

Sensory function and motor activity are interdependent, and severe motor disabilities may occur because of impaired sensation. This is particularly evident with parietal lobe lesions, but motor dysfunction may also occur with lesions involving the posterior roots, peripheral nerves, posterior columns of the spinal cord, or the other central sensory pathways. Conversely, motor dysfunction may affect sensory discrimination. When equal weights are placed in a patient's hands, she may underestimate the weight on the side with cerebellar dysfunction and overestimate it on the side with extrapyramidal dysfunction.

Diminution or perversion of sensation may occur with pathology involving the sensory receptors, but this does not often arise in primary neurologic illnesses. Pain and pruritus due to skin irritation, traumatic denudements, and burns may result from abnormalities of the receptors or the nerve filaments to them, and decreased sensation in callosities and scars may result from involvement of the end-organs and smaller filaments.

In focal peripheral neuropathies, the area of sensory abnormality corresponds to the distribution of the specific involved nerve. The areas of skin supplied by various nerves are shown in Figure 26.2. Within the involved area, all sensory modalities are affected. Sensory distributions

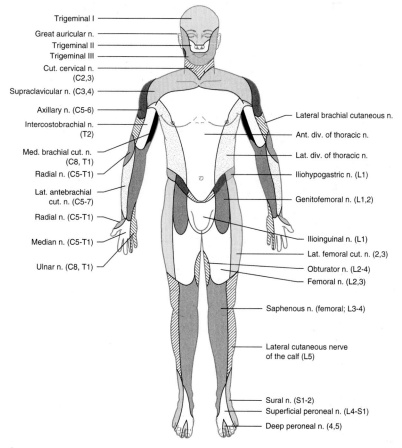

Trigeminal I
Great auricular n.
Trigeminal II
Trigeminal III
Cut. cervical n.
(C2,3)
Supraclavicular n. (C3,4)
Axillary n. (C5-6)
Intercostobrachial n. (T2)
Med. brachial cut. n. (C8, T1)
Radial n. (C5-T1)
Lat. antebrachial cut. n. (C5-7)
Radial n. (C5-T1)
Median n. (C5-T1)
Ulnar n. (C8, T1)

Lateral brachial cutaneous n.
Ant. div. of thoracic n.
Lat. div. of thoracic n.
Iliohypogastric n. (L1)
Genitofemoral n. (L1,2)
Ilioinguinal n. (L1)
Lat. femoral cut. n. (2,3)
Obturator n. (L2-4)
Femoral n. (L2,3)
Saphenous n. (femoral; L3-4)
Lateral cutaneous nerve of the calf (L5)
Sural n. (S1-2)
Superficial peroneal n. (L4-S1)
Deep peroneal n. (4,5)

**A**

*FIGURE 26.2* ● The cutaneous distribution of the peripheral nerves. **A.** On the anterior aspect of the body.

*(continued)*

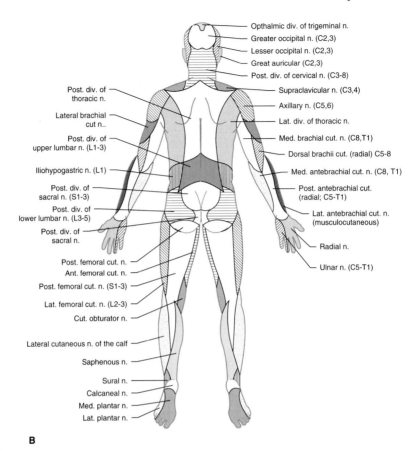

FIGURE 26.2  ●  (Continued) **B.** On the posterior aspect of the body.

may vary slightly from individual to individual, and the mapped area may not correspond precisely to a published text or atlas. An excellent source for a pictorial/graphic demonstration of peripheral nerve distributions is http://www.neuroguide.com/nerveindex.html.

The demonstrable area of pain and temperature loss is typically smaller than the area of light touch loss, and smaller than the published peripheral nerve or dermatome distributions. The deficit to light touch usually corresponds more closely to a nerve distribution than the pinprick loss. In a patient with a focal nerve or root lesion, it may be possible with careful testing to identify a dense zone of severe sensory loss, surrounded by areas of milder sensory loss. Occasionally, there is spread of sensory loss beyond the field of an injured nerve.

In generalized peripheral neuropathies, vibration is often the first modality affected, but in severe cases all exteroceptive, proprioceptive, and combined modalities are impaired. Most axonopathies are length dependent, and the distribution of sensory loss usually involves predominantly the distal segments, causing a stocking-glove distribution of blunted sensation. However, the margins of the involved area may be poorly demarcated, with no sharp border between the normal and hypesthetic areas. Some generalized neuropathies have a predilection to involve predominantly large or small fibers. Peripheral nerve disease may also cause paresthesias, or pain that is either constant or lancinating in character. The nerves themselves may be sensitive and tender to palpation, and there may be pain on brisk stretching of the affected nerves and increased susceptibility to ischemia. There sometimes is hyperalgesia or allodynia in the involved area, even though the sensory threshold is raised.

Disease of the dorsal root ganglia (DRG), or corresponding cranial nerve ganglia, is also associated with sensory changes. Although classically a remote effect of small cell carcinoma of the lung, sensory neuronopathy is associated with a number of other conditions, including pyridoxine intoxication, Sjögren syndrome, and lymphoma. In herpes zoster, there is severe, lancinating pain in the distribution of the affected ganglia.

Lesions of the nerve root, most often due to compression, are accompanied by diminution or loss of sensation, pain, or paresthesias, but the distribution is segmental and corresponds to the involved dermatome (Figure 26.3). As with focal neuropathy, in compressive radiculopathy the touch deficit is larger and often corresponds better to the published dermatome than the pinprick deficit. Pain may be either constant or intermittent, and is often sharp, stabbing, and lancinating. It is increased by movement, coughing, or straining. There may be either hypalgesia or hyperalgesia. Because of dermatome overlap, sensory changes may be difficult to demonstrate if only one root is involved.

With lesions of the spinal cord and brainstem, impairment of one or more modalities of sensation, or perversions of sensation in the form of either pain or paresthesias, may develop. The area of sensory involvement may involve all levels below the lesion, but occasionally the sensory level is well below the level of the lesion; a sensory level on the trunk has been reported in lesions of the lower brainstem. Sensory loss is usually dissociated, with impairment of certain modalities and sparing of others. Because of the redundancy of the touch pathways, pain and temperature testing may be more useful than tactile sensation in evaluating CNS disease. Testing for the ability to detect the direction of skin movement above and below the level of the lesion and searching for a vibratory level may be helpful.

Lesions high in the cervical spinal cord and in the medulla may impair kinesthetic sensation in the upper extremities more than in the lower. Patients with pontine, medullary, or spinal cord lesions occasionally experience "central" pain. Lhermitte sign, sudden electric-like or painful sensations spreading down the body or into the back or extremities on flexion of the neck due to involvement of the posterior columns, may occur with focal lesions of the cervical cord, multiple sclerosis, or other degenerative processes.

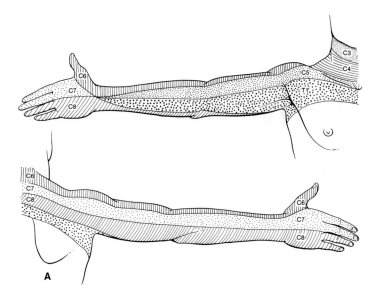

**FIGURE 26.3** • The segmental innervation. A. The upper extremity.

*(continued)*

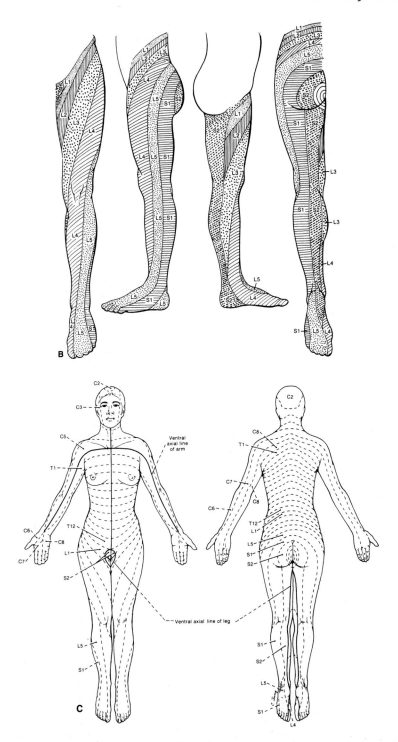

**FIGURE 26.3** ● *(Continued)* **B.** The lower extremity. **C.** The anterior and posterior aspects of the entire body. (Modified from Keegan JJ, Garrett FD. *Anat Rec* 102:409–437, 1943.)

The pattern of sensory return with recovering spinal lesions is variable; the impairment may recede downward in a segmental manner; the return may start in the sacral distribution and ascend, or there may be a gradual recovery of function over the entire affected area. Pressure sensation returns first and its recovery is usually the most complete, followed, in turn, by tactile, pain, cold, and heat sensibilities.

Sensory impulses that enter consciousness for interpretation by the parietal cortex must first pass through the thalamus. The thalamus is thought to be the end-station for pain, heat, cold, and heavy contact, where sensory impulses produce a crude, uncritical form of perception. Thalamic lesions usually cause impairment of all sensory modalities on the opposite side of the body. A severe and extensive lesion may cause gross impairment of all forms of sensation. Marked loss of appreciation of heavy contact, posture, passive movement, and deep pressure perception occurs, and the thresholds for light touch, pain, and temperature sensations are raised. Thalamic lesions are often associated with sensory perversions, such as paresthesias and hyperesthesias, or painful hyperpathias. In the thalamic pain (Dejerine-Roussy) syndrome, there is blunting, or raising of the threshold, of all forms of sensation on the opposite side of the body, without true anesthesia. Suprathreshold stimuli excite unpleasant sensations, and any stimulus, even the lightest, may evoke a disagreeable, often burning, pain. Slight hot and cold stimuli, or light cutaneous sensations, cause marked discomfort. The overreaction is termed hyperpathia. Impairment of sensation accompanied by intractable pain in the hypesthetic regions is called anesthesia dolorosa. In addition to the sensory changes, hemiparesis and hemianopia usually occur and, less frequently, hemiataxia, choreoathetosis, and unmotivated emotional responses. Pain of central origin is most often associated with thalamic lesions, but may occasionally result from involvement of other central pain pathways. Occasionally, pleasurable stimulation, such as application of a warm hand to the skin on the affected side, may be markedly accentuated. This overreaction is due to a thalamic lesion or to release of thalamic function from normal cortical control by damage to higher centers. Every stimulus acting on the thalamus produces an excessive effect on the abnormal half of the body, especially as far as the affective element—the pleasant or unpleasant character in its appreciation—is concerned.

Involvement of the sensory radiations in the posterior limb of the internal capsule causes variable, sometimes extensive, impairment of all types of sensation on the opposite side of the body. Because the sensory fibers are crowded closely together, the sensory loss is more severe than with isolated cortical lesions. The changes are similar to those that follow a thalamic lesion, but pain is rare.

Lesions of the parietal cortex rarely cause complete loss of sensation, but there is a raising of the threshold for both exteroceptive and proprioceptive sensations of the opposite side of the body. Sensation is often disturbed more in the upper than in the lower extremity, trunk, or face. The distal parts of the extremities are affected more than the proximal portions, with a gradual transition to more normal perception approaching the shoulder and hip. Parietal lesions primarily cause disturbances in discriminatory sensation. Detailed and critical examination of sensory functions may be necessary to detect parietal lobe lesions. The threshold for pain stimuli is raised very little in parietal lesions, although a prick may feel less sharp than on the normal side; with deeper lesions the threshold is more definitely raised. Qualitative appreciation of heat and cold are present, but there is loss of discrimination for slight variations in temperature, especially in the intermediate ranges. Light touch perception is little disturbed, but tactile discrimination and localization may be profoundly affected. There often is severe impairment of position sense resulting in sensory ataxia and pseudoathetosis, but vibratory sensation is only rarely affected (another instance where vibration and position sense loss are dissociated). Astereognosis is common, but both small and large objects may have to be used to detect the deficit; sometimes a delay in answering when objects are placed in the affected hand, with no delay with the other hand, may be a clue to minimal involvement. Bilateral simultaneous testing for stereognostic sense, placing identical objects in both hands, may be useful. Sensory inattention, or extinction, is often an early and important diagnostic finding in parietal lobe lesions. Other possible findings include baragnosis, agraphesthesia, impairment of two-point discrimination, autotopagnosia, anosognosia, or Gerstmann syndrome.

The ability to distinguish two cutaneous stimuli to the same side of the body but separated by a brief time interval is also impaired with parietal lobe lesions. Spontaneous discharges from the parietal cortex frequently cause contralateral paresthesias that may constitute a focal sensory seizure or the sensory aura preceding a jacksonian motor convulsion. Only rarely do spontaneous discharges from the parietal cortex cause pain.

## NONORGANIC SENSORY LOSS

Nonorganic sensory abnormalities are usually areas of decreased sensibility. Areas of hypesthesia, hypalgesia, anesthesia, and analgesia are commonly encountered that may be complete or partial, affect all modalities or be dissociated. Even normal individuals, or those with organic sensory loss, may be suggestible and have spurious sensory findings.

One of the obvious clues that sensory loss is nonorganic is failure to follow any sort of anatomical distribution. The demarcation between normal and abnormal often occurs at some strategic anatomical point that has no neurologic significance, such as a joint or skin crease, causing a finding such as numbness circumferentially below the elbow, wrist, shoulder, ankle, or knee. Nonorganic facial sensory loss often stops at the hairline and angle of the jaw, a nonanatomic distribution. A real spinal sensory level on the trunk slants downward from back to front; a functional level may be perfectly horizontal. The term stocking-glove sensory loss is used to describe both hysteria and peripheral neuropathy. The key to understanding this confusing usage is the type of stocking. When sensory loss due to length-dependent peripheral neuropathy extends to about the level of the knees it appears in the hands, causing loss in a glove-knee sock distribution; with hysteria the impairment may be distal to the wrists and ankles: a glove-ankle sock distribution. The border between normal and abnormal is usually abrupt and well demarcated, more discrete than in organic sensory loss, and may vary from examination to examination, or even from minute to minute. Sensation may be different on the ventral and dorsal surfaces. Responses are typically inconsistent. In spite of complete loss of cutaneous sensibility, the patient may have intact stereognosis and graphesthesia, or in spite of complete loss of position sense may be able to perform skilled movements and fine acts without difficulty, and have no Romberg sign. On finger-to-nose testing, the examiner may touch one finger of the "anesthetic" hand and ask the patient to touch her nose with it; a patient with organic exteroceptive sensory loss will not know which finger was touched, while those with organic proprioceptive loss can't find their nose. The hand wandering widely before eventually finding the nose suggests histrionic tendencies. In the search test, the patient holds the involved hand in the air and searches for it with the unaffected hand. In nonorganic loss there may be no difficulty, but with bona fide proprioceptive loss, performance is poor with either hand.

Clinical subterfuge is often used to establish that sensory loss is nonorganic. The author has seen all of these "tricks" fail (i.e., indicate the sensory loss is not real when it is), at one time or another, save one: the SHOT syndrome. In the SHOT syndrome, the patient claims to have no Sight in the eye, no Hearing in the ear, no Olfaction in the nose, and no Touch sensation on the body, all on the same side. This pattern is of course utterly impossible on an anatomic basis and its presence reliably indicates that hemi-body numbness is nonorganic. Another sometimes helpful technique to bring out nonorganic sensory loss is the "yes if you feel it/no if you don't" maneuver. After demonstrating the patient is unable to feel a given stimulus in a given distribution, instruct her to close her eyes and say "yes" every time she feels a stimulus and "no" when she does not; the gullible will respond with "no" every time the alleged anesthetic region is stimulated.

It is often possible to confuse the patient and confirm the absence of organic changes by checking sensation while the hands are in some bewildering position where it is difficult to tell which side is which, such as crossed behind the back or intricately entwined. A commonly used technique is to have the patient cross the hyperpronated forearms and hold the hands with little fingers up, palms together, and fingers interlocked. The hands are then rotated downward and inward, then upward, so that the little fingers are facing the chest. Anyone who has ever done this knows how difficult it is to tell which finger belongs to which hand. The patient responds as digits are stimulated randomly. It matters little whether eyes are open or closed, and in fact the test may work better with eyes open. The patient with nonorganic hemianalgesia may make errors, while the one with organic loss will not. The nonorganic patient may respond slowly, delay answering, or betray signs of the effort required. It is of course imperative that the examiner accurately keep track of which side is which. With practice, performance improves rapidly, so the test is most conclusive the first time it is done.

Nonorganic sensory loss is often in a hemi-body distribution, almost invariably on the left side. Sensory changes along the midline may provide useful clues. Because of the overlap along the midline of the trunk, organic sensory loss does not usually extend to the midline, and, when stimulating from the hypesthetic to the normal side, sensation begins to return slightly before the midline is reached. With nonorganic loss, the change may take place abruptly at the midline or even beyond it. This finding is not reliable on the face, where organic sensory loss does more accurately obey the midline. With nonorganic hemi-anesthesia, the midline change may include the penis, vagina, and rectum, a finding rare with organic lesions. There may even be midline splitting of vibration, so that the patient claims to perceive a difference in the intensity of vibration when the fork is placed just to right or left of the midline over the skull, sternum, or symphysis pubis, each a single bony structure, or comparing the medial ends of the clavicles or the medial incisor teeth. In all these locations, the vibration is transmitted to both sides, and patients with organic hemi-anesthesia do not perceive any difference in vibration along the midline. Somatosensory evoked potential studies may aid in differentiating organic from nonorganic sensory loss.

# The Reflexes

# CHAPTER 27

## Introduction to the Reflexes

The reflex examination is important for several reasons. Reflex changes may be the earliest and most subtle indication of a disturbance in neurologic function. The testing of reflexes is the most objective part of the neurologic examination. Reflexes are under voluntary control to a lesser extent than most other parts of the neurologic examination, and reflex abnormalities are difficult to simulate. They are not as dependent on the attention, cooperation, or intelligence of the patient, and can be evaluated in patients who cannot or will not cooperate with other parts of the examination. In such circumstances, the integrity of the motor and sensory systems can sometimes be appraised more adequately by the reflex examination than by other means. Although the reflex examination is an essential component, it is only one part of the neurologic examination, and must be evaluated in the context of the other findings.

A reflex is an involuntary response to a sensory stimulus. Afferent impulses arising in a sensory organ produce a response in an effector organ. There are segmental and suprasegmental components. The segmental component is a local reflex center in the spinal cord or brainstem and its afferent and efferent connections. The suprasegmental component is made up of the descending central pathways that control, modulate, and regulate the segmental activity. Disease of the suprasegmental pathways may increase the activity of some reflexes, decrease the activity of others, and cause reflexes to appear that are not normally seen. A reflex response may be motor, sensory, or autonomic.

The stimulus is received by the receptor, which may be a sensory ending in the skin, mucous membranes, muscle, tendon, or periosteum or, in special types of reflexes, in the retina, cochlea, vestibular apparatus, olfactory mucosa, gustatory bulbs, or viscera. Receptor stimulation initiates an impulse that travels along the afferent pathway to the central nervous system (CNS), where there is a synapse in a reflex center that activates the cell body of the efferent neuron. The efferent neuron transmits the impulse to the effector: the cell, muscle, gland, or blood vessel that then responds. A disturbance in function of part of the reflex arc—the receptor, afferent limb, reflex center, efferent limb, or effector apparatus—will disrupt the reflex arc, causing a decrease or loss of the reflex.

Most reflexes investigated clinically are more complex than the primitive reflex response just described. Complex reflexes involve connections between various segments on the same and opposite sides of the spinal cord, brainstem, and brain. The more complex the reflex, the greater the number of associated neurons and mechanisms involved. Stronger stimuli cause the excitation of a greater number of neurons: the phenomenon of irradiation.

Reflex activity is essential to normal functioning. Nociceptive reflexes help avoid injurious stimuli. Reflex activity is important in maintaining the body in its daily environment, in sustaining an upright position, in standing and walking, and in moving the extremities. It is an integral part of the response to visual, gustatory, auditory, and vestibular stimulation; and it is important in visceral functions.

Reflexes have been named in various ways: according to the site of elicitation, the body part stimulated, the muscles involved, the part of the body that responds, the ensuing movements, the joint acted on, or the nerve involved. Many carry the names of one or more individuals who are said to have first described them. Hundreds of reflexes have been identified. Since many are not clinically important and it is impractical to test all the reflexes routinely, only those more important for clinical diagnosis will be described. The majority of these are muscle responses. Reflex abnormalities due to disease involving the descending motor pathways are often clinically referred to as upper motor neuron, corticospinal or pyramidal signs, but the abnormalities likely result from dysfunction of related motor pathways rather than the corticospinal tract proper.

CHAPTER **28**

# The Deep Tendon
# or Muscle Stretch Reflexes

**W**hen a normal muscle is passively stretched, its fibers resist the stretch by contracting. Reflexes elicited by application of a stretch stimulus to either tendons or periosteum, or occasionally to bones, joints, fascia, or aponeurotic structures are usually referred to as muscle stretch or deep tendon reflexes. The reflex is caused by sudden muscle stretch, brought about by percussion of its tendon. Occasionally, the tendon is stretched by percussing a structure to which it is attached, as in the jaw jerk. Because of their critical roles in maintaining an erect posture, the extensor muscles of the legs, quadriceps and calf muscles, have better developed stretch reflexes than the flexors.

The term deep helps separate these reflexes from the superficial or cutaneous reflexes, which are quite different. The term deep tendon reflex (DTR) was introduced in 1875, and since at least 1885 some authorities have criticized it. The term DTR is in much wider use than muscle stretch reflex, and for both pragmatic and anti-pedantic reasons, the DTR abbreviation will be used in this text.

The primary problem areas in eliciting DTRs are poor tools and poor technique. These reflexes are best tested using a high-quality rubber percussion hammer. To properly obtain a reflex, a crisp blow must be delivered to quickly stretch the tendon. A heavy, high-quality reflex hammer is immensely helpful for this task. Proper technique is much more difficult to describe than to demonstrate. The hammer strike should be quick, direct, crisp, and forceful, but no greater than necessary. The most effective blow is delivered quickly with a flick of the wrist, holding the handle of the hammer near its end and letting it spin through loosely held fingertips. Putting the index finger on top of the handle and using primarily elbow motion, common faults, make it much harder to achieve adequate velocity at the hammer head. Another common mistake is "pecking": striking the tendon with a timid, decelerating blow, pulling back at the last instant.

The patient should be comfortable, relaxed, and properly positioned. It may help relaxation to divert the patient's attention with light conversation. Sometimes, as in the ankle reflex, positioning includes passively stretching the muscle slightly. An adequate stimulus must be delivered to the proper spot. Reinforcement methods are necessary if the reflex is not obtainable in the usual way. The part of the body to be tested should be in an optimal position for the response, usually about midway in the range of motion of the muscle to be tested. In order to compare the reflexes on the two sides of the body, the position of the extremities should be symmetric. During the reflex examination, the patient should keep the head straight, since looking to one side may alter reflex tone, especially in the arms (tonic neck reflex). The DTRs may be influenced to some degree by voluntary mental effort. Merely by concentrating some individuals are able to somehow alter reflex excitability. Mentally induced reflex asymmetry is possible and may be clinically relevant in some cases.

## TABLE 28.1

### The Commonly Elicited Deep Tendon (Muscle Stretch) Reflexes

| Reflex | Segmental Level | Peripheral Nerve |
| --- | --- | --- |
| Biceps | C5–C6 | Musculocutaneous |
| Triceps | C7–C8 | Radial |
| Brachioradialis | C5–C6 | Radial |
| Quadriceps | L3–L4 | Femoral |
| Achilles | S1 | Sciatic |

The examiner can feel as well as see the contraction. Placing one hand over the muscle is often useful, especially when responses are sluggish. A reflex quadriceps contraction can sometimes be felt even when insufficient to produce visible contraction or knee movement. The activity of a reflex is judged by the speed and vigor of the response, the range of movement, and the duration of the contraction. An absent reflex often makes a dull, thudding sound when the tendon is struck.

The DTRs usually examined include the biceps, triceps, brachioradialis, knee (quadriceps), and ankle (Achilles) tendon reflexes. Table 28.1 summarizes the reflex levels. Reflexes may be graded as absent, sluggish or diminished, normal, exaggerated, and markedly hyperactive. For the purposes of clinical note taking, most neurologists grade the DTRs numerically, as follows: 0 = absent; 1+ (or +) = present but diminished; 2+ (or ++) = normal; 3+ (or +++) = increased but not necessarily to a pathologic degree; and 4+ (or ++++) = markedly hyperactive, patho-logic, often with extra beats or accompanying sustained clonus. The "+" after the number is more traditional than informative, and is sometimes omitted. Signs are sometimes used to indicate subtle asymmetry, but generally a grade of 2 means the same as 2+. Another level, trace (or +/−), is frequently added to refer to a reflex, most often an ankle jerk, that appears absent to routine test-ing but can be elicited with reinforcement. Some add a grade of 5+ for the patient with extreme spasticity and clonus. In the 0 to 4 scale, level 1+ DTRs are still normal but somewhat sluggish and difficult to elicit, hypoactive but in the examiner's opinion not pathologic. Grade 3+ reflexes are "fast normal," quicker than 2+, sometimes very quick, but not accompanied by any other signs of upper motor neuron pathology such as increased tone, upgoing toes, or sustained clonus. Normality of the superficial reflexes, normal lower-extremity tone, and downgoing toes are reassuring evi-dence of fast normal rather than pathologically quick reflexes. Some use 3+ to indicate the presence of spread or unsustained clonus, with all other normal reflexes, even very fast ones, labeled as 2+. Grade 4+ reflexes are unequivocally pathological. The speed of the response is very fast, the threshold low, the reflexogenic zone wide, and there are accompanying signs of corticospinal tract dysfunction. Other scales are in use, but not widely. Reflexes may be charted in several ways, for example, as shown in Table 28.2, or as in Figure 28.1.

When reflexes are very active, responses may occur from muscles that have not been directly stretched, even in normal patients. The response may involve adjacent or even contralateral mus-cles, and the contraction of one muscle may be accompanied by contraction of other muscles. This is referred to as spread, or irradiation, of reflexes. It is normal for percussion of the brachioradialis tendon to also cause slight finger flexion. In the presence of spasticity and hyperreflexia, contrac-tion of the biceps or brachioradialis may be accompanied by pronounced flexion of the fingers and adduction of the thumb. Extension of the knee may be accompanied by adduction of the hip, or there may be bilateral knee extension. Judging how much spread is still within normal limits can be difficult. Under some circumstances, the expected response to percussion of a tendon is absent, but muscles innervated by adjacent spinal cord segments contract instead (e.g., inverted brachioradialis reflex). On other occasions, a reflex is absent and percussion of the tendon causes an inverted or

## TABLE 28.2

**Method of Recording the Commonly Tested Deep Tendon (Muscle Stretch) Reflexes**

|  | Right | Left |
|---|---|---|
| Biceps | 2+ | 2+ |
| Triceps | 2+ | 2+ |
| Brachioradialis | 2+ | 2+ |
| Patellar | 2+ | 2+ |
| Achilles | 2+ | 2+ |
| Plantar | Down | Down |

Grades 0 to 4+ (see text) used for all but plantar reflex, which is down (normal), absent (0), equivocal (+/−), or up (abnormal). Other reflexes may be added and charted as needed.

paradoxical contraction, e.g., elbow flexion on attempted elicitation of the triceps reflex (see Inverted and Perverted Reflexes further on).

In some patients, DTRs may be markedly diminished, or even apparently absent, although there is no other evidence of nervous system disease. Under such circumstances, reinforcement techniques are often useful. Reflex reinforcement probably involves supraspinal, fusimotor, and long-loop mechanisms. A reflex can be reinforced or brought out using several methods. In the Jendrassik maneuver, the patient attempts to pull the hands apart with the fingers flexed and hooked together, palms facing, as the tendon is percussed (Figure 28.2). The effect is very brief, lasting only 1 to 6 seconds, and is maximal for only 300 milliseconds. The Jendrassik maneuver is obviously only useful for lower-extremity reflexes. Other techniques include having the patient clench one or both fists, firmly grasp the arm of the chair, side of the bed, or the arm of the examiner. Reinforcement may also be carried out by having the patient look at the ceiling, grit the teeth, cough, squeeze the knees together, take a deep breath, count, read aloud, or repeat verses at the time

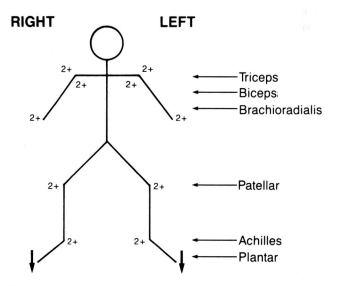

*FIGURE 28.1* ● Alternate method of recording the commonly tested muscle stretch reflexes. For grading, see text and Table 28.2.

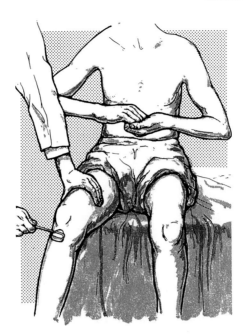

*FIGURE 28.2* ● Method of reinforcing the patellar reflex.

the reflex is being tested. A sudden loud noise, a painful stimulus elsewhere on the body—such as the pulling of a hair or a bright light flashed in the eyes—may also be a means of reinforcement.

Procedures other than distraction are also helpful in reflex reinforcement. A slight increase in tension of the muscle being tested may reinforce the reflex response. A simple and effective method to reinforce a knee or ankle jerk is to have the patient maintain a slight, steady contraction of the muscle whose tendon is being tested (e.g., slight plantar flexion by pushing the ball of the foot against the floor or the examiner's hand to reinforce the ankle jerk). The patient may tense the quadriceps by extending the knee slightly against resistance as the knee jerk is being elicited. Reinforcement may increase the amplitude of a sluggish reflex or bring out a latent reflex not otherwise obtainable. Reflexes that are normal on reinforcement, even though not present without reinforcement, may be considered normal. Slight muscle contraction due to inability to relax may be one reason for the slightly hyperactive reflexes often seen in patients who are tense or anxious.

The DTRs are instrumental in the evaluation of weakness. Under most circumstances, weakness accompanied by hyporeflexia is of lower motor neuron origin, and weakness accompanied by hyperreflexia of upper motor neuron origin. The presence of pathologic reflexes and abnormalities of associated movements are also helpful in the differential diagnosis (Table 28.3).

## THE UPPER-EXTREMITY REFLEXES

The biceps, triceps, brachioradialis, and finger flexor reflexes are the most important upper-extremity reflexes.

### The Biceps Reflex

With the arm relaxed and the forearm slightly pronated and midway between flexion and extension, the examiner places the palmar surface of her extended thumb or finger on the patient's biceps tendon, and then strikes the extensor surface with the reflex hammer (Figure 28.3). Pressure on the tendon should be light; too much pressure exerted with the thumb or finger against the tendon makes the reflex much harder to obtain. The hands may lie in the patient's lap, or the examiner

## TABLE 28.3

### Reflex Patterns with Different Neurologic Disorders

| Site of Type of Lesion | Muscle Stretch Reflexes | Superficial Reflexes | Pathologic Reflexes | Associated Movements |
|---|---|---|---|---|
| Neuromuscular junction | Normal or decreased | Normal | Absent | Normal |
| Muscle | Usually normal; may be decreased in proportion to weakness | Normal | Absent | Normal |
| Peripheral nerve | Decreased to absent | Normal, or decreased to absent in distribution of involved nerve(s) | Absent | Normal |
| Corticospinal tract (upper motor neuron syndrome) | Hyperactive (especially in speed of response) | Decreased to absent | Present | Pathologic associated movements present |
| Extrapyramidal system | Normal; occasionally slightly increased or decreased | Normal or slightly increased | Absent | Normal associated movements absent |
| Cerebellum | Pendular | Normal | Absent | Normal |
| Psychogenic | Normal or increased (especially in range of response) | Normal or increased | Absent | Normal or bizarre |

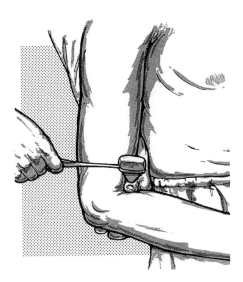

*FIGURE 28.3* ● Method of obtaining the biceps reflex.

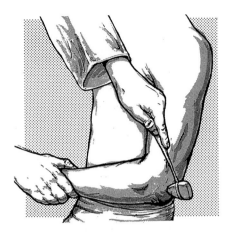

***FIGURE 28.4*** ● Method of obtaining the triceps reflex.

may hold the patient's arm with the elbow resting in her hand. The major response is a contraction of the biceps muscle with flexion of the elbow. Since the biceps is also a supinator, there is often a certain amount of supination. If the reflex is exaggerated, the reflexogenic zone is increased and the reflex may even be obtained by tapping the clavicle; there may be abnormal spread with accompanying flexion of the wrist and fingers and adduction of the thumb.

## The Triceps Reflex

This reflex is elicited by tapping the triceps tendon just above its insertion on the olecranon process of the ulna. The arm is placed midway between flexion and extension, and may be rested in the patient's lap, on her thigh or hip, or on the examiner's hand (Figure 28.4). The response is contraction of the triceps muscle with extension of the elbow. The most common error in eliciting the triceps jerk is simply too timorous a blow.

## The Brachioradialis (Radial Periosteal or Supinator) Reflex

Tapping just above the styloid process of the radius with the forearm in semiflexion and semi-pronation causes flexion of the elbow, with variable supination (Figure 28.5). The supination is

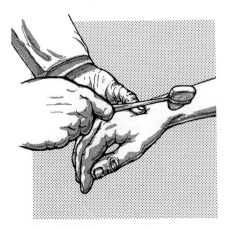

***FIGURE 28.5*** ● Method of obtaining the brachioradialis reflex.

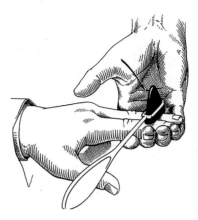

***FIGURE 28.6***  ●  Method of obtaining the finger flexor reflex.

more marked with the forearm extended and pronated, but there is less flexion. The principal muscle involved is the brachioradialis. The tendon can be percussed not only at its insertion on the lateral aspect of the base of the styloid process of the radius, but also at about the junction of the middle and distal thirds of the forearm or at its tendon of origin above the lateral epicondyle of the humerus. The most common error is hitting the muscle belly rather than the tendon. The muscle becomes tendinous at about midforearm. A local contraction can be elicited from any muscle by directly striking the muscle belly. The point in eliciting a DTR is to lengthen the muscle by stretching its tendon. An idiomuscular contraction can be obtained by striking the brachioradialis muscle belly in the proximal third of the forearm; this is not a DTR. If the reflex is exaggerated, there is associated flexion of the wrist and fingers, with adduction of the forearm. When the afferent limb of the reflex is impaired, there may be a twitch of the flexors of the hand and fingers without flexion and supination of the elbow; this is termed inversion of the reflex.

### The Finger Flexor Reflex (Wartenberg Sign)

To elicit the finger flexor reflex, the patient's hand is in supination, resting on a table or a solid surface, with the fingers slightly flexed. The examiner places her fingers against the patient's fingers, and taps the backs of her own fingers lightly with the reflex hammer (Figure 28.6). The response is flexion of the patient's fingers and the distal phalanx of the thumb. The reflex may be reinforced by having the patient flex her fingers slightly as the blow is delivered. An alternate technique is for the patient to hold the hand in the air, palm down, the examiner touching fingers with palm up, with the blow delivered in an upward direction from below.

## MUSCLE STRETCH REFLEXES OF THE LOWER EXTREMITIES

### The Patellar Reflex (Quadriceps Reflex, Knee Jerk)

The patellar reflex is contraction of the quadriceps femoris muscle, with resulting extension of the knee, in response to percussion of the patellar tendon. A firm tap on the tendon draws the patella down, stretching the quadriceps, provoking reflex contraction. If the reflex is brisk, the contraction is strong and the amplitude of the movement is large. If the examiner places one hand over the muscle, and with the other hand taps the patellar tendon just below the patella, she can palpate the contraction as well as observe the rapidity and range of response. Palpation helps in judging the latency between the time of the stimulus and the resulting response. The knee jerk can be elicited in various ways.

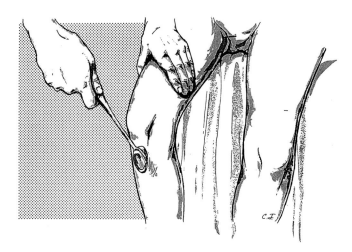

*FIGURE 28.7*  ●  Method of obtaining the patellar (quadriceps) reflex with the patient seated.

The patient may sit in a chair with the knees slightly extended and the heels resting on the floor, or sit on an examination table with the legs dangling (Figure 28.7). If the patient is lying in bed, the examiner should partially flex the knee by placing one hand beneath it and then tap the tendon (Figure 28.8).

If there is reflex spread, extension of the knee may be accompanied by adduction of the hip, which on occasion is bilateral, or there may be bilateral knee extension. If the reflex is exaggerated, the response may be obtained not only by tapping the tendon in the usual spot, but also just above the patella (suprapatellar or epipatellar reflex); the tendon can be tapped directly, or, with the patient recumbent, the examiner can place her index finger on the upper border of the patella and tap the finger to push down the patella. Contraction of the quadriceps causes a brisk upward movement of the tendon, together with extension of the leg (Figure 28.9). Marked exaggeration of the patellar reflex may be accompanied by patellar clonus.

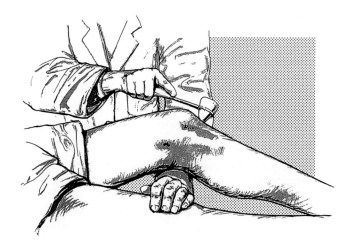

*FIGURE 28.8*  ●  Method of obtaining the patellar (quadriceps) reflex with the patient recumbent.

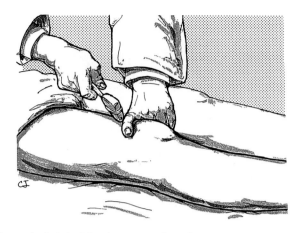

*FIGURE 28.9* ● Method of obtaining the suprapatellar reflex.

## The Achilles Reflex (Ankle Jerk, Triceps Surae Reflex)

The ankle jerk is obtained by striking the Achilles tendon just above its insertion on the calcaneus. The resulting contraction of the posterior crural muscles, the gastrocnemius, soleus, and plantaris, causes plantar flexion of the foot at the ankle. If the patient is seated or lying in bed, the thigh should be held in moderate abduction and external rotation and the knee flexed. If the patient is supine, access to the tendon requires placing the legs into a frog-leg position with the knees apart and the ankles close together. Some prefer to have the patient cross the leg to be examined atop the other shin or ankle ("figure four position," as the legs form a 4). The examiner should place one hand under the foot and pull upward slightly to passively dorsiflex the ankle to about a right angle (Figure 28.10). The Achilles reflex is mediated by the tibial nerve (S1).

The ankle jerk is by far the most difficult reflex to master. There are two critical variables: proper stretch and efficient striking. Of the two, proper stretch is the more difficult to learn. If the reflex is difficult to obtain, the patient may be asked to press her foot lightly against the examiner's hand in order to tense the muscle and reinforce the reflex. Using a driving analogy and asking the patient to imagine pressing on an accelerator enough to go "17 mph" communicates the need for

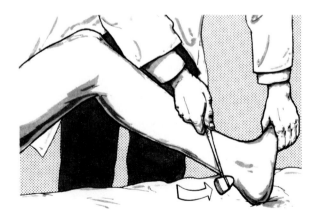

*FIGURE 28.10* ● Method of obtaining the Achilles (triceps surae) reflex with the patient recumbent.

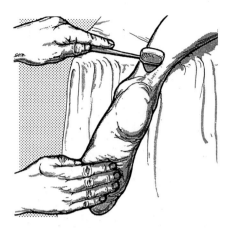

**FIGURE 28.11** ● Method of obtaining the Achilles (triceps surae) reflex with the patient kneeling.

a low-level but precisely graded contraction, which is then easy to adjust up or down to the proper level. The reflex may also be elicited by having the patient kneel on a chair or similar surface, with the feet projecting at right angles; the Achilles tendons are percussed while the patient is in this position (Figure 28.11). This method is particularly useful for comparing reflex activity on the two sides. Another method for supine examination is to strike the ball (sole) of the foot, or strike the examiner's hand placed flat against the sole. This plantar stretch reflex is considered equivalent to the ankle jerk for clinical purposes. Although the Achilles reflex, when carefully elicited, should be present in normal individuals, it tends to diminish with age and its bilateral absence in elderly individuals is not necessarily of clinical significance.

## INTERPRETATION OF THE DEEP TENDON (MUSCLE STRETCH) REFLEXES

The most valuable DTRs for clinical diagnosis are the biceps, triceps, brachioradialis, patellar, and Achilles (see Table 28.1); under most circumstances, and using good technique, these are elicitable in every normal person. One or more of these reflexes may be absent in occasional individuals with no other evidence of disease of the nervous system. They are present even in the majority of premature infants. The activity of a DTR is judged by the latency, speed, vigor, and duration of contraction, and the range of movement. Of these, the latent period between the time the stimulus is applied and the time the response occurs is most important for clinical evaluation of disease states.

## ABNORMALITIES OF THE DEEP TENDON (MUSCLE STRETCH) REFLEXES

Abnormal DTRs are either hypoactive or hyperactive. When hypoactive, the response varies from diminished or sluggish to complete absence of the reflex. Hyperactive reflexes are characterized by varying degrees of decreased latency, increased speed and vigor of response, increased range of movement, decrease in threshold, extension of the reflexogenic zone, and prolongation of the muscular contraction. Table 28.3 summarizes the patterns of reflex responses seen with lesions at various sites.

Reflexes are judged in both absolute and relative terms. Clearly hyperactive or hypoactive reflexes speak for themselves. But a reflex that is normal in absolute terms may be judged abnormal in comparison to the patient's other reflexes. The reflexes should be compared on the two sides of the body, the arms to the legs, and the knees to the ankles. The DTRs are normally symmetric, and reflexes otherwise normal may be abnormal if different from expected. For example, a 1+ biceps jerk in a patient with suspected cervical radiculopathy, while "normal," may be judged abnormal if the

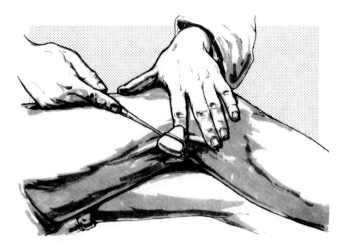

*FIGURE 28.12* ●  Method of obtaining the biceps femoris reflex.

opposite biceps jerk is 2+. The DTRs are usually comparable in the upper and lower extremities. Slight differences are permissible but a pronounced difference may be significant (e.g., in thoracic myelopathy the DTRs in the legs may be much brisker than in the arms, even though not clearly pathologic). A proximal to distal gradient may also be significant. Symmetric 1+ ankle jerks when all of the other reflexes are 2+ may signal mild peripheral neuropathy. When asymmetry is the main finding, it is sometimes difficult to tell whether one side is increased or the other side decreased.

## Hypoactive Reflexes

When a reflex is hypoactive, there is a sluggish response and/or a diminution in the range of response. An increase in stimulus intensity may be necessary to elicit the reflex, or repeated blows may be necessary, for a single stimulus may be subliminal. A DTR is absent if it is not obtained even with reinforcement. A depressed or absent reflex results from dysfunction of some component of the reflex arc. Interference with the afferent limb may be caused by lesions involving the sensory nerve, posterior root, dorsal root ganglion, or intramedullary pathways between the dorsal root entry zone and the anterior horn (e.g., syringomyelia). Abnormalities of the motor unit and final common pathway that make up the efferent limb of the reflex arc occur in many conditions, but particularly with radiculopathy and peripheral nerve lesions. In neurogenic processes, DTRs are lost out of proportion to atrophy and weakness. With a peripheral nerve lesion, a reflex may not return until much of the motor function has recovered. Sometimes there is persistent areflexia following lesions of the nerve root or peripheral nerve, even after complete return of both motor and sensory functions.

## Hyperactive Reflexes

Reflex hyperactivity is characterized by the following: a decrease in reflex threshold; a decrease in the latency, the time between tendon percussion and the reflex contraction; an exaggeration of the power and range of movement; prolongation of the reflex contraction; extension of the reflexogenic zone (or zone of provocation); and spread of the reflex response. When the reflex threshold is decreased, a minimal stimulus may evoke the reflex, and reflexes that are not normally obtained may be elicited with ease. Very hyperactive DTRs may sometimes be elicited with extremely slight percussion. Another manifestation of decreased reflex threshold may be a widening of the area from which the reflex may be elicited, and application of the stimulus to sites at some distance from the usual one may evoke the response; the patellar reflex may be elicited by tapping the tibia or dorsum of the foot, and the biceps and other arm reflexes by tapping the clavicle or scapula. There may also be abnormal spread of the response. One stimulus may provoke repetitive responses and sometimes elicit sustained clonus.

The DTRs become hyperactive with lesions of the corticospinal or pyramidal system. Spasticity and hyperreflexia are likely related to involvement of a variety of structures in the descending motor pathways at cortical, subcortical, midbrain, and brainstem levels. Hyperreflexia results from a lowering of the reflex threshold due to increased excitability of the lower motor neuron pool related to dysfunction of some or all of these structures. A lesion at any level of the corticospinal system or other related upper motor neuron components, from the motor cortex to just above the segment of origin of a reflex arc, will be accompanied by spasticity and hyperreflexia. The characteristic posture in hemiplegia is flexion of the upper extremities, with more marked weakness of the extensors; and extension of the lower extremities, with more marked weakness of the flexors. Consequently, the flexor reflexes are exaggerated to a greater degree in the upper extremities, and the extensor reflexes in the lower. The reflexes may be present in spinal cord lesions in spite of the absence of sensation.

Exaggeration of the DTRs may occur in psychogenic disorders, and in anxiety, fright, and agitation (Table 28.3). The reflexes vary in these conditions; they may be normal, or they may be decreased owing to voluntary or involuntary tension of the antagonistic muscle, but they are most frequently increased. Hyperactivity may be marked, but it is an exaggeration not in the speed of the response but in the excursion or range of response. The foot may be kicked far into the air and held extended for a time after the patellar tendon is tapped, but the contraction and relaxation takes place at a normal rate. There is often a bilateral response with extraneous and superfluous jerking of remote parts, including whole body jerks, when a reflex is tested. There is no increase in the reflexogenic zone in psychogenic lesions, and although there may be irregular repeated jerky movements (spurious clonus), no true clonus is present. Furthermore, there are no other signs of organic disease of the corticospinal system.

In lesions of the extrapyramidal system there are no consistent reflex changes (Table 28.3). In diseases of the cerebellum the reflexes may be diminished (Table 28.3) and pendular: Eliciting the patellar reflex while the foot is hanging free may elicit a series of to-and-fro pendular movements of the foot and leg before the limb finally comes to rest.

## Inverted and Perverted Reflexes

Occasionally, percussion of a tendon produces unexpected results. In the presence of hyperreflexia, there may be spread to other muscles, as in the crossed adductor response. Inverted or paradoxical reflexes are contractions the opposite of those expected. With an inverted triceps or patellar reflex there is elbow or knee flexion instead of extension. Under these circumstances, the segmental reflex is absent, but there is an underlying hyperreflexia lowering the threshold for activation of the antagonist muscle, perhaps because of transmitted vibration. Degenerative spine disease with radiculomyelopathy is the usual mechanism. An inverted brachioradialis (often referred to as an inverted radial periosteal) reflex does not result in true inversion (i.e., elbow extension), but instead produces a perverted response with finger flexion. When the brachioradialis reflex is present this finger flexion is simply referred to as spread; when the brachioradialis reflex is absent and the only response is finger flexion, the reflex is commonly said to be inverted.

# CHAPTER 29

# The Superficial
# (Cutaneous) Reflexes

Superficial reflexes are responses to stimulation of either the skin or mucous membrane. Cutaneous reflexes are elicited by a superficial skin stimulus, such as a light touch or scratch. The response occurs in the same general area where the stimulus is applied. Too painful a stimulus may call forth a defensive reaction rather than the desired reflex. Superficial reflexes are polysynaptic, in contrast to the stretch reflexes, which are monosynaptic. The superficial reflexes respond more slowly to the stimulus than do the stretch reflexes, their latency is longer, they fatigue more easily, and they are not as consistently present as tendon reflexes. The primary utility of superficial reflexes is that they are abolished by pyramidal tract lesions, which characteristically produce the combination of increased deep tendon reflexes and decreased or absent superficial reflexes. The superficial reflexes obtained most often are the abdominal and cremasteric. Unilateral absence of the superficial abdominal reflexes may be an early and sensitive indicator of a corticospinal tract lesion.

## THE SUPERFICIAL ABDOMINAL REFLEXES

The superficial abdominal reflexes consist of contraction of the abdominal muscles, elicited by a light stroke or scratch of the anterior abdominal wall, pulling the linea alba and umbilicus in the direction of the stimulus (Figure 29.1). The response can be divided into the upper abdominal and lower abdominal reflexes. The anterior abdominal wall can be divided into four quadrants by vertical and horizontal lines through the umbilicus. Light stroking or scratching in each quadrant elicits the response, pulling the umbilicus in the direction of the stimulus. The stimulus may be directed toward, away, or parallel to the umbilicus; stimuli directed toward the umbilicus seem more effective. The response is a quick, flicking contraction followed by immediate relaxation. The responses are typically brisk and active in young individuals with good anterior abdominal tone. They may be sluggish or absent in normal individuals with lax abdominal tone, in those who are obese, or in women who have borne children.

## THE SUPERFICIAL REFLEXES OF THE LOWER EXTREMITIES

### The Cremasteric Reflex

This reflex is elicited by stroking or lightly scratching or pinching the skin on the upper, inner aspect of the thigh. The response consists of a contraction of the cremasteric muscle with a quick elevation of the homolateral testicle. The innervation is through the ilioinguinal and genitofemoral nerves (L1-L2). The cremasteric reflex must not be confused with the scrotal, or dartos, reflex,

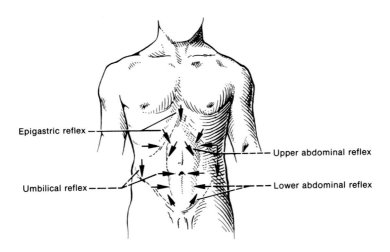

*FIGURE 29.1* ●   Sites of stimulation employed in eliciting the various superficial abdominal reflexes.

which produces a slow, writhing, vermicular contraction of the scrotal skin on stroking the perineum or thigh or applying a cold object to the scrotum. The cremasteric reflex may be absent in elderly males, in individuals who have a hydrocele or varicocele, and in those who have had orchitis or epididymitis. There is no female equivalent.

## The Plantar Reflex

Stroking the plantar surface of the foot from the heel forward is normally followed by plantar flexion of the foot and toes (Figure 29.2). The pathologic variation of the plantar reflex is the Babinski sign. In ticklish patients there may be voluntary withdrawal with flexion of the hip and knee, but in every normal individual there is a certain amount of plantar flexion of the toes on stimulation of the sole of the foot.

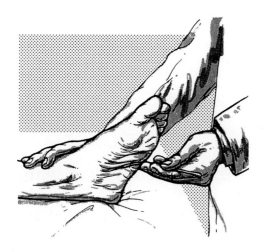

*FIGURE 29.2* ●   Method of obtaining the plantar reflex.

## The Superficial Anal Reflex

The cutaneous anal reflex (anal wink) consists of contraction of the external sphincter in response to stroking or pricking the skin or mucous membrane in the perianal region.

## Bulbocavernosus Reflex

The bulbocavernosus reflex (BCR) is related to the anal reflex in that both cause contraction of the anal sphincter, but in the BCR, the stimulus is delivered to the glans penis or clitoris. The response is best palpated with a gloved finger in the rectum. Some forewarning and preliminary explanation are necessary, but the stimulus should still come as a surprise. In the male, a grabbing, pinching, or tweaking of the glans evokes the response, felt as a tightening of the sphincter on the finger. The response is much more difficult to elicit in females and the significance of its absence more dubious. The BCR is primarily useful is assessing the integrity of the cauda equina, lower sacral roots, and conus medullaris.

## ABNORMALITIES OF THE SUPERFICIAL REFLEXES

The effect on the superficial reflexes of lesions at various sites is summarized in Table 28.3. The superficial reflexes are impaired or absent with a lesion that disturbs the continuity of the reflex arc. In addition, a lesion anywhere along the corticospinal pathway will usually cause either diminution or absence of the superficial reflexes. The reflex change is contralateral to a lesion above the pyramidal decussation, and ipsilateral to a lesion below the pyramidal decussation. Corticospinal tract disease causes dissociation of reflexes, absence of superficial reflexes, and exaggerated deep reflexes. So the superficial reflexes, especially the abdominal and cremasteric reflexes, have a special significance when their absence is associated with increased deep tendon reflexes or when they are absent when signs of corticospinal tract involvement are present. The abdominal and the cremasteric reflexes may occasionally be absent in persons without other evidence of neurologic disease.

The superficial reflexes may help distinguish physiologic from pathologic hyperreflexia. In physiologic hyperreflexia, seen most often in young individuals or patients with anxiety, the abdominal and cremasteric reflexes are usually present and active, but in pathologic hyperreflexia due to an upper motor neuron lesion they are usually absent.

# CHAPTER 30

# Pathologic Reflexes

**P**athologic reflexes are responses not generally found in the normal individual. Some are responses that are minimally present and elicited with difficulty in normals but become prominent and active in disease, while others are not seen in normals at all. Many are exaggerations and perversions of normal muscle stretch and superficial reflexes. Some are related to postural reflexes or primitive defense reflexes that are normally suppressed by cerebral inhibition but become enhanced when the lower motor neuron is separated from the influence of the higher centers. Others are responses normally seen in the immature nervous system of infancy, then disappear only to reemerge later in the presence of disease. A decrease in threshold or an extension of the reflexogenic zone plays a role in many pathologic reflexes.

Descending motor influences normally control and modulate the activity at the local, segmental spinal cord level to insure efficient muscle contraction and proper coordination of agonists, antagonists, and synergists. Disease of the descending motor pathways causes loss of this normal control so that activity spills from the motor neuron pool responsible for a certain movement to adjacent areas, resulting in the recruitment into the movement of muscles not normally involved. Some pathologic reflexes may also be classified as "associated movements," related to such spread of motor activity. Whether a certain abnormal response would be best classified as a reflex or an associated movement is not always clear. Responses that are more in the realm of an associated movement are sometimes referred to clinically as reflexes (e.g., the Wartenberg thumb adduction sign, an associated movement, is sometimes called a Wartenberg reflex).

Most pathologic reflexes are related to disease involving the corticospinal tract and associated pathways. They also occur with frontal lobe disease and occasionally with disorders of the extrapyramidal system. There is a great deal of confusion regarding names of reflexes and methods of elicitation, and in many cases there has been significant drift away from the original description. Many of the responses are merely variations in the method of eliciting the same responses, or modifications of the same reflex. The typical reflex pattern with lesions involving the corticospinal tract, the upper motor neuron syndrome, is exaggeration of deep tendon reflexes (DTRs), disappearance of superficial reflexes, and emergence of pathologic reflexes (Table 28.3).

Fontal release signs (FRS) are reflexes that are normally present in the developing nervous system, but disappear to a greater or lesser degree with maturation. While normal in infants and children, when present in an older individual they may be evidence of neurologic disease, although some may reappear in normal senescence. Many of these are exaggerations of normal reflex responses. Responses often included as FRS include the palmomental reflex (PMR), grasp, snout, suck, and others.

Frontal release signs occur most often in patients with severe dementias, diffuse encephalopathy (metabolic, toxic, postanoxic), after head injury, and other states in which the pathology is usually diffuse but involves particularly the frontal lobes or the frontal association areas. The significance and usefulness of some of these release signs or primitive reflexes has been questioned. The PMR is commonly seen in normal individuals. The Hoffman finger flexor reflex and its variants, which are sometimes classified as FRS and sometimes as corticospinal signs, are similarly present in a significant proportion of normal individuals. Clearly, these reflexes are a normal phenomenon in a significant proportion of the healthy population. They must be interpreted with caution and kept in clinical context. Even when such reflexes are briskly active in an appropriate clinical setting, the primitive reflexes do not have great localizing value, suggesting instead the presence of diffuse and widespread dysfunction of the hemispheres.

## PATHOLOGIC REFLEXES IN THE LOWER EXTREMITIES

Pathologic reflexes in the lower extremities are more constant, more easily elicited, more reliable, and more clinically relevant than those in the upper limbs. The most important of these responses may be classified as (a) those characterized in the main by dorsiflexion of the toes, and (b) those characterized by plantar flexion of the toes. The most important pathologic reflex by far is the Babinski sign, and a search for an upgoing toe is part of every neurologic examination. Searching for upper-extremity pathologic reflexes is much less productive and often omitted.

### Corticospinal Responses Characterized in the Main by Extension (Dorsiflexion) of the Toes

#### The Babinski Sign

In the normal individual, stimulation of the skin of the plantar surface of the foot is followed by plantar flexion of the toes (Figure 29.2). In the normal plantar reflex, the response is usually fairly rapid, the small toes flex more than the great toe, and the reaction is more marked when the stimulus is along the medial plantar surface. In disease of the corticospinal system there may be instead extension (dorsiflexion) of the toes, especially the great toe, with variable separation or fanning of the lateral four toes: the Babinski sign or extensor plantar response (Figure 30.1). The Babinski

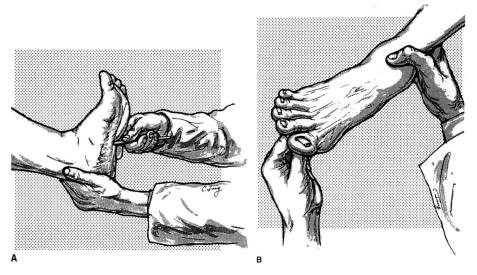

**A**                                                        **B**

*FIGURE 30.1* ● Method of eliciting the Babinski sign.

sign has been called the most important sign in clinical neurology. It is one of the most significant indications of disease of the corticospinal system at any level from the motor cortex through the descending pathways.

The Babinski sign is obtained by stimulating the plantar surface of the foot with a blunt point, such as an applicator stick, handle of a reflex hammer, a broken tongue blade, the thumbnail, or the tip of a key. Strength of stimulus is an important variable. It is not true that the stimulus must necessarily be deliberately "noxious," although most patients find it at least somewhat uncomfortable even if the examiner is trying to be considerate. When the response is strongly extensor only minimal stimulation is required. The stimulus should be firm enough to elicit a consistent response, but as light as will suffice. Some patients are very sensitive to plantar stimulation and only a slight stimulus will elicit a consistent response; stronger stimuli may produce confusing withdrawal. If the toe is briskly upgoing, merely a fingertip stimulus may elicit the response. If no response is obtained, progressively sharper objects and firmer applications are necessary. Although some patients require a very firm stimulus, it is not necessary to aggressively rake the sole as the opening gambit. Both tickling, which may cause voluntary withdrawal, and pain, which may bring about a reversal to flexion as a nociceptive response, should be avoided.

Plantar stimulation must be carried out far laterally, in the S1 root/sural nerve sensory distribution. More medial plantar stimulation may fail to elicit a positive response when one is present. Far medial stimulation may actually elicit a plantar grasp response causing the toes to flex strongly. The stimulus should begin near the heel and be carried up the side of the foot at a deliberate pace, not too quickly, usually stopping at the metatarsophalangeal joints. The response has usually occurred by the time the stimulus reaches the midportion of the foot. If the response is difficult to obtain, the stimulus should continue along the metatarsal pad from the little toe medially, but stopping short of the base of the great toe. The most common mistakes are insufficiently firm stimulation, placement of the stimulus too medially and moving the stimulus too quickly, so that the response does not have time to develop. The only movements of real significance are those of the great toe. Fanning of the lateral toes without an abnormal movement of the great toe is seldom of any clinical significance, and an absence of fanning does not negate the significance of great toe extension.

The patient should be relaxed and forewarned of the potential discomfort. The knee must be extended; an upgoing toe may be abolished by flexion of the knee. The best position is supine, with hips and knees in extension and heels resting on the bed. If the patient is seated, the knee should be extended, with the foot held either in the examiner's hand or on her knee. The response may sometimes be reinforced by rotating the patient's head to the opposite side.

Usually, the upward movement of the great toe is a quick, flicking motion sometimes mistaken for withdrawal by the inexperienced. The response may be a slow, tonic, sometimes clonic, dorsiflexion of the great toe and the small toes with fanning, or separation, of the toes. The slow great toe movement has been described as a "majestic rise." The nature of the stimulus may be related to the speed of the toe movement; primarily proprioceptive stimuli (e.g., Gonda, Stransky, Szapiro) are more apt to be followed by a slow, tonic response; exteroceptive stimuli by a brief, rapid extension. There may occasionally be initial extension, followed by flexion; less often brief flexion precedes extension. There may be extension of only the great toe, or extension of the great toe with flexion of the small toes.

The Babinski sign is a part of the primitive flexion reflex. The central nervous system is organized according to movement patterns, and one of the most basic patterns is avoidance or withdrawal from a noxious stimulus. In higher vertebrates, the flexion response includes flexion of the hip and knee, and dorsiflexion of the ankle and toes, all serving to remove the threatened part from danger. Descending motor systems normally suppress the primitive flexion response. When there is disease involving the corticospinal tract, the primitive flexion response may reappear, and the first clinical evidence of this is the Babinski sign. With more severe and extensive disease the entire flexion response emerges, so that stimulation of the sole causes dorsiflexion not only of the toe, but also the ankle, as well as flexion of the hip and knee (the "triple flexion" response). In addition, there is often contraction of the tensor fascia lata causing slight internal rotation at the hip and more rarely abduction of the hip.

There are many other corticospinal tract responses in the lower extremities characterized by dorsiflexion of the toes. With severe corticospinal tract disease, the threshold for eliciting an upgoing toe is lower, the reflexogenic zone wider, and more and more of the other components of the primitive flexion reflex appear as part of the response. This has led to a profusion of variations on the Babinski method of eliciting the extensor plantar response. The most useful variation is the Chaddock sign, and the Oppenheim is also often done.

The Chaddock sign is elicited by stimulating the lateral aspect of the foot, not the sole, beginning about under the lateral malleolus near the junction of the dorsal and plantar skin, drawing the stimulus from the heel forward to the small toe. The Chaddock is the only alternative toe sign that is truly useful. It may be more sensitive than the Babinski but is less specific. It produces less withdrawal than plantar stimulation. The two reflexes are complementary; each can occur without the other, but both are usually present. The Oppenheim sign is usually elicited by dragging the knuckles heavily down the anteromedial surface of the tibia from the infrapatellar region to the ankle. The response is slow and often occurs toward the end of stimulation. A common ploy is to combine the Oppenheim and the Babinski to make a suspicious toe declare itself, but this is more painful and less useful than the Chaddock.

When the response is very active and the reflexogenic zone wide, the toe may go up with such minor stimuli as pulling back the bed sheets or rapid removal of the sock or shoe. Occasionally there is a "spontaneous Babinski," occurring with no apparent manipulation of the foot. There may even be contralateral or bilateral responses. Sometimes the toes are held in a tonic position of dorsiflexion and fanning. A tonic extensor plantar response must be distinguished from a "striatal toe."

## Problems in Interpreting the Plantar Response

The extensor plantar response is one of the most reliable, dependable, and consistent signs in clinical neurology. But it is not perfect, and the response to plantar stimulation may at times be difficult to evaluate. The most common problem is distinguishing an upgoing toe from voluntary withdrawal. The Babinski sign is part of a withdrawal reflex, so flexion of the hip and knee are by no means reliable indicators that the withdrawal movement is voluntary. Voluntary withdrawal rarely causes dorsiflexion of the ankle, and there is usually plantar flexion of the toes. Voluntary withdrawal is more likely when the stimulus is too intense and uncomfortable. It helps if the patient understands the importance of holding still and receives some explanation of the relevance of this seemingly inane and cruel test. Some patients have ticklish feet and will pull away from even a light stimulus. If the patient is ticklish, it may help to simply hold the ankle firmly. Internal rotation of the leg during the "withdrawal" signals recruitment of the tensor fascia lata into the movement and makes it more likely the response is reflex and not voluntary.

The most important observation is the initial movement of the great toe. With repeated stimulation of the sole, the extensor movement may decrease and then disappear. So the crucial observation is the first toe movement on the first stimulation. Occasionally, withdrawal makes it impossible to be certain whether the toe was truly extensor or not; these are equivocal plantar responses. Some patients have no elicitable plantar response, in which case the plantars are said to be mute or silent. Asymmetry of the plantar responses may be significant; a toe that does not go down as crisply as its fellow may be suspect, even if it does not frankly go up. A toe is more likely to go up late in the day or when the patient is tired.

An extensor plantar response does not always signify structural disease; it may occur as a transient manifestation of physiologic dysfunction of the corticospinal pathways. A Babinski sign may sometimes be found in deep anesthesia and narcosis; drug and alcohol intoxication; metabolic coma such as hypoglycemia; deep sleep; post-ictally; and in other conditions of altered consciousness. The plantar response returns to normal with recovery of consciousness.

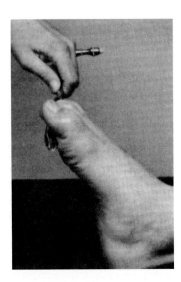

*FIGURE 30.2*  ●   Plantar grasp reflex. Brisk bending of toes to grasp reflex hammer handle. (Reprinted from Massey EW, Pleet AB, Scherokman BJ. *Diagnostic Tests in Neurology: A Photographic Guide to Bedside Techniques.* Chicago: Year Book Medical Publishers, Inc., 1985.)

## Corticospinal Tract Responses Characterized by Plantar Flexion of the Toes

In the newborn infant there is a grasp reflex in the foot as well as the hand, with flexion and adduction of the toes in response to a light pressure on the plantar surface of the foot, especially its distal and medial portions. The plantar grasp normally disappears by the end of the first year. A grasp reflex of the foot may reappear in adults, along with a grasp reflex of the hand, in disease of the opposite frontal lobe. The plantar grasp may be elicited by drawing the handle of a reflex hammer from the midsole toward the toes, causing the toes to flex and grip the hammer (Figure 30.2).

In addition to the superficial plantar reflex, there is a plantar muscle reflex consisting of contraction of the toe flexors following sudden stretching. This response is barely, if at all, perceptible normally, but becomes more obvious with reflex hyperactivity and, therefore, with corticospinal tract lesions. The best known of this group of reflexes is the Rossolimo sign (Figure 30.3). Tapping the ball of the foot or plantar surfaces of the toes causes a quick plantar flexion of the toes.

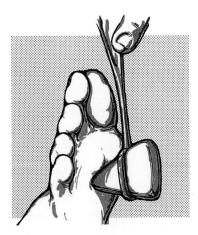

*FIGURE 30.3*  ●   Method of eliciting the Rossolimo sign.

# PATHOLOGIC REFLEXES IN THE UPPER EXTREMITIES

Abnormal reflex responses in the upper extremities are less constant, more difficult to elicit, and usually less significant diagnostically than those found in the lower extremities. A great deal of confusion exists concerning the nomenclature of these reflexes, with many variations and modifications of the same response. The upper-extremity pathologic reflexes primarily fall into two categories: frontal release signs (FRS) and exaggerations of or variations on the finger flexor reflex. The grasp and palmomental reflexes are usually classified as FRS. The finger flexor related responses are usually a manifestation of the spasticity and hyperreflexia that occur in lesions involving the corticospinal tract, so the Hoffman and Trömner signs are usually classified as corticospinal tract signs. These responses occur only with lesions above the C5 or C6 segment of the cervical spinal cord.

## The Grasp (Forced Grasping) Reflex

The grasp reflex is usually classified as an FRS. Forced grasping is an involuntary flexor response of the fingers and hand following stimulation of the skin of the palmar surface of the fingers or hand. The palmar grasp is normally present at birth and may be strong enough to suspend the infant by her own grasp. The response begins to diminish at the age of 2 to 4 months. It reappears primarily in association with extensive neoplastic or vascular lesions of the frontal lobes or with cerebral degenerative processes, usually contralaterally but occasionally ipsilaterally. Although the grasp reflex is usually classified as an FRS or primitive reflex, it may also occur as evidence of corticospinal tract dysfunction in spastic hemiplegia. The grasping responses are exaggerations of normal reactions and occur as release phenomena; the groping response is a more complicated reaction that is modified by visual and tactile integration at the cortical level.

## The Palmomental Reflex

The palmomental reflex (PMR), or palm-chin reflex, is contraction of the mentalis and orbicularis oris muscles causing wrinkling of the skin of the chin with slight retraction and sometimes elevation of the angle of the mouth in response to scratching or stroking the palm of the ipsilateral hand. The reflex is best elicited by stroking a blunt point over the thenar eminence, either from wrist toward thumb or vice versa, or by tapping this area. The PMR is so frequently present in normal persons that significance can only be attached to a marked exaggeration of the response or a conspicuous asymmetry between the two sides. If the response is marked, the reflexogenic zone may be wide, including the hypothenar area. The localizing value and clinical significance of these reflexes are limited. A unilateral PMR may occur with bilateral, contralateral, or ipsilateral lesions.

## The Hoffmann and Trömner Signs and the Flexor Reflexes of the Fingers and Hand

The finger flexor reflex (Wartenberg sign) is flexion of the patient's fingers and distal phalanx of the thumb in response to a stretch stimulus delivered with a reflex hammer (Figure 28.6). The Hoffmann and Trömner signs are alternative methods of delivering the stretch stimulus. They are prominent when the other upper-extremity DTRs are hyperactive, as in corticospinal tract lesions. These signs are not necessarily pathologic and are often present to some degree in normal individuals. As with the PMR, they are only of clinical significance when markedly active or very asymmetric. A very active, complete Hoffmann or Trömner sign, especially if unilateral or associated with other reflex abnormalities or a consistent history, is certainly suggestive if not diagnostic of corticospinal tract involvement.

To elicit the Hoffmann sign the patient's relaxed hand is held with the wrist dorsiflexed and fingers partially flexed. With one hand, the examiner holds the partially extended middle finger between her index finger and thumb or between her index and middle fingers. With a sharp, forcible flick of the other thumb, the examiner nips or snaps the nail of the patient's middle finger, forcing the distal finger into sharp, sudden flexion followed by sudden release (Figure 30.4). The rebound of the distal phalanx stretches the finger flexors. If the Hoffmann sign is present, this is followed by flexion and adduction of the thumb and flexion of the index finger, and sometimes

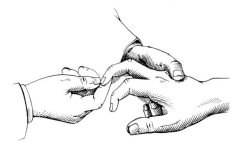

**FIGURE 30.4** ● Method of eliciting the Hoffmann sign.

flexion of the other fingers as well. If only the thumb or only the index finger responds the sign is "incomplete." In the Trömner sign, the examiner holds the patient's partially extended middle finger, letting the hand dangle, then, with the other hand, thumps or flicks the finger pad (Figure 30.5). The response is the same as that in the Hoffmann test. The two methods are equivalent and either manner of testing may be used; both are sometimes referred to as the Hoffmann test.

### Other Frontal Release Signs

The orbicularis oris (snout) reflex is puckering and protrusion of the lips, primarily the lower, often with depression of the lateral angles of the mouth, in response to pressing firmly backward on the philtrum of the upper lip, a minimal tap to the lips, or sweeping a tongue blade briskly across the lips. When exaggerated, the response may include not only puckering and protrusion of the lips, but also sucking and even tasting, chewing, and swallowing movements. The sucking reflex is normal in infants; stimulation of the perioral region is followed by sucking movements of the lips, tongue, and jaw. A rooting (searching) reflex is when the lips, mouth, and even head deviate toward a tactile stimulus delivered beside the mouth or on the cheek. The sucking reflex disappears after infancy, when sucking becomes a voluntary rather than reflex phenomenon. Like the other FRS, it may reappear in some patients with diffuse cerebral disease.

## Clonus

Clonus is a series of rhythmic involuntary muscular contractions induced by the sudden passive stretching of a muscle or tendon. It often accompanies the spasticity and hyperactive DTRs seen in corticospinal tract disease. Clonus occurs most frequently at the ankle, knee, and wrist, occasionally

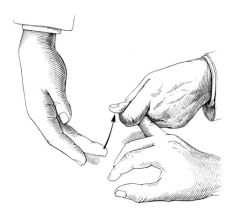

**FIGURE 30.5** ● Method of eliciting the Trömner sign.

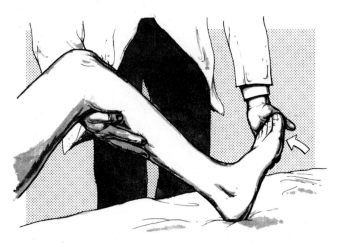

**FIGURE 30.6** ● Method of eliciting ankle clonus.

elsewhere. Ankle clonus consists of a series of rhythmic alternating flexions and extensions of the ankle. It is easiest to obtain if the examiner supports the leg, preferably with one hand under the knee or the calf, grasps the foot from below with the other hand, and quickly dorsiflexes the foot while maintaining slight pressure on the sole at the end of the movement (Figure 30.6). The leg and foot should be well relaxed, the knee and ankle in moderate flexion, and the foot slightly everted. The response is a series of alternating contractions. Unsustained clonus fades away after a few beats; sustained clonus persists as long as the examiner continues to hold slight dorsiflexion pressure on the foot. Unsustained (transient, exhaustible, or abortive) symmetric ankle clonus may occur in normal individuals with physiologically fast DTRs. Sustained clonus is never normal. In severe spasticity clonus may occur spontaneously or with the slightest stimulus. Slight plantar flexion pressure, as in stepping on the accelerator of a car, may cause violent, uncontrollable, repetitive jerking of the foot. A single tap on the tendon to elicit the ankle jerk will occasionally provoke clonus.

Patellar clonus consists of a series of rhythmic up-and-down movements of the patella. It may be elicited if the examiner grasps the patella between index finger and thumb and executes a sudden, sharp, downward thrust, holding downward pressure at the end of the movement. The leg should be extended and relaxed. Patellar clonus may appear when eliciting the patellar or suprapatellar reflex. Clonus of the wrist or of the fingers may be produced by a sudden passive extension of the wrist or fingers. Clonus of the jaw occurs occasionally. Nonorganic clonus occurs rarely. False clonus (pseudoclonus) in psychogenic disorders is poorly sustained and irregular in rate, rhythm, and excursion. At the ankle, true clonus can usually be stopped by sharp passive plantar flexion of the foot or the great toe; false clonus is not altered by such a maneuver.

## DECEREBRATE AND DECORTICATE RIGIDITY

Severe lesions of the brainstem often produce increased tone in the extensor, or antigravity, muscles of the limbs and the spine. This phenomenon is known as decerebrate rigidity. In patients with extreme decerebrate rigidity, there is opisthotonos, with all four limbs stiffly extended, the head back, and the jaws clenched. The arms are internally rotated at the shoulders, extended at the elbows, and hyperpronated, with the fingers extended at the metacarpophalangeal joints and flexed at the interphalangeal joints. The legs are extended at the hips, knees, and ankles, and the toes are plantar flexed. The position is an exaggeration or caricature of the normal standing position. The deep tendon reflexes are exaggerated, the tonic neck and labyrinthine reflexes are present, and the righting reflexes abolished.

Decerebrate rigidity may follow severe insults to the brainstem at any level between the superior colliculi or the decussation of the rubrospinal pathway and the rostral portion of the vestibular nuclei. The vestibular nuclei enhance extensor tone, and integrity of the vestibular nuclei is necessary for decrebrate rigidity to occur. These nuclei are intact, but isolated from the midbrain, specifically from the red nuclei and rubrospinal tracts. Activity in the reticular formation is also important, particularly the pontine reticular nuclei and the medial reticulospinal tract, which also facilitates extensor muscle tone. Experimentally, decerebrate rigidity is abolished by section of the vestibulospinal pathways. In patients, when the process extends to involve the medulla the decerebration disappears. The most common cause of decerebrate rigidity in humans is trauma, and the presence of extensor posturing is a poor prognostic indicator.

Decorticate rigidity is characterized by flexion of the elbows and wrists with extension of the legs and feet. The causative lesion is higher than that causing decerebrate rigidity, preserving the function of the rubrospinal tract, which enhances flexor tone in the upper extremities.

# CHAPTER 31

# Associated Movements

An associated movement (AM) is an unintentional, involuntary, spontaneous, automatic movement that accompanies some other voluntary (or involuntary) movement. The associated, or synkinetic, movement is often one that serves to fix a part of the body as another part is voluntarily activated. Associated movements often occur because of activation of the synergistic and fixation muscles involved in a particular motion, or spread of the activation to nearby motor neuron pools. This activity is normally suppressed by the descending motor pathways, but in the face of disease becomes clinically apparent. The corticospinal pathways are concerned primarily with fine, fractionated, discrete movements of the distal extremities. Disease in the corticospinal pathways may eliminate discrete distal movement but not affect mass movements of the proximal muscles. The mass movements usually play a secondary, supportive role, particularly in fixation of the part to be moved. However, when the distal movements are paralyzed, the primary movement left may be the associated mass movement. Associated movements are, to a certain extent, postural or righting reflexes that have a peculiarly widespread distribution. They may be clinical homologues of movements seen in decerebrate animals. Associated movements are more complex manifestations of motor function than the simple reflexes, but are more primitive than voluntary movements. They are probably initiated and largely controlled by the extrapyramidal system and its connections, although the corticospinal system also plays a role.

## PHYSIOLOGIC ASSOCIATED MOVEMENTS

Many AMs are present physiologically; in fact they play a part in all normal motor activity. The activity of the antagonists, synergists, and muscles of fixation in any motor response may be considered AMs. Generally, the term is used for more widespread responses. Common examples of normal AMs include the following: pendular swinging of the arms when walking; facial contortions or grimaces with violent exertion; movements of the head and neck with movements of the eyes; and normal extension of the wrist with flexion of the fingers. In some disease states, normal AMs may decrease or disappear. The normal AMs are lost in diseases of the extrapyramidal system, especially in the parkinsonian syndromes, where masking of facial expression and absence of arm swing when walking are prominent manifestations. In other conditions, normal AMs may be exaggerated, and abnormal AMs may be present. With lesions of the corticospinal system, a number of AMs may appear that are not present normally. Table 28.3 correlates the site of a lesion with the pattern of AMs. The AMs not usually present in the normal individual are discussed in the following paragraphs.

# PATHOLOGIC ASSOCIATED MOVEMENTS

Abnormal or pathologic AMs are usually activity in paretic muscle groups that are brought out by active movement of other groups, and seen predominantly in disease of the corticospinal pathways. They usually accompany vigorous voluntary movements of another part, and occur on the hemiplegic side. Associated movements are slow, forceful movements of the already spastic parts that lead to the adoption of new postures. The greater the spasticity, the greater the extent and duration of the AMs.

## Generalized Associated Movements

Generalized AMs occur in hemiplegia, where they tend to emphasize or enhance the characteristic hemiplegic posture. The AMs often occur with exertion. Straining and attempts to grip with the paretic hand may cause an increase in the spasticity, with increased flexion of the wrist, elbow, and shoulder; this is sometimes accompanied by associated facial movements on the involved side. The new posture may be maintained until the grip is relaxed. An involuntary, automatic movement such as a yawn may cause the affected arm to extend at the elbow, wrist, and fingers, remaining rigidly in this new attitude until the yawn passes off. Movements such as coughing or stretching may cause similar reactions. Tonic neck reflexes may also influence these generalized AMs. Turning the head toward the hemiplegic side may cause increased extensor tonus on that side, and turning it to the normal side may be followed by either increased flexor tonus on the paretic side or flexion of the arm and extension of the leg.

## Symmetric (Imitative or Contralateral) Associated Movements (Mirror Movements)

In the normal infant there is a tendency for movements of one limb to be accompanied by similar involuntary movements of the opposite limb; this disappears as coordination and muscle power are acquired. Mirror movements usually disappear or become inconspicuous at adolescence, their persistence to any marked degree should be considered pathologic. They may occur in patients with brain injuries, disturbances of cerebral development, and dysplasias of the upper portion of the spinal cord; under such circumstances there are usually associated abnormalities of motor function, tone, and reflexes. Occasionally, persisting mirror movements are familial, and not accompanied by other signs of neurologic disease.

In certain neurologic disorders, forceful voluntary movements of one limb may be accompanied by identical involuntary movements of the same limb on the other side. They are usually seen in the paretic limb when the opposite healthy one is forcefully moved, although occasionally such movements may appear in the healthy limb on extreme attempts to move the affected extremity (especially in extrapyramidal disease). They appear particularly during exertion to carry out a quick or strenuous movement. When squeezing the examiner's hand with the healthy hand, the paretic hand may flex. Any forceful movement on the normal side may be followed by a similar but slow tonic duplication of the movement on the paretic side. Imitation synkinesias by themselves have little localizing significance, occurring with lesions in various portions of the neuraxis. Their value in neurologic assessment is in conjunction with other findings. Mirror movements may occur on the unaffected or less affected side in early or mild asymmetric parkinsonism.

## Coordinated Associated Movements

Coordinated associated movements are involuntary movements of synergistic muscle groups that accompany a voluntary movement of a paretic limb. They are exaggerations or perversions of ordinary synergistic and cooperative movements, and may be classified into three groups: (a) movements, not present normally, which accompany movements of a paretic limb; (b) contralateral

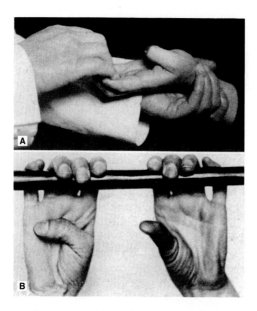

**FIGURE 31.1** ● Associated movement of thumb (Wartenberg sign). **A.** Patient bends his last four fingers against resistance of four hooked fingers of examiner. Thumb moves toward palm. Mild spastic paralysis of hand. **B.** With his fingers hooked over a horizontally fastened rod, patient is asked to pull it down. Right thumb performs an associated movement toward the palm. Right-sided spastic hemiplegia. (From Wartenberg R. *Diagnostic Tests in Neurology.* Chicago: Year Book Medical Publishers, 1953.)

coordinated associated movements; and (c) associated movements, normally present, which are abolished in cerebral hemiplegia. These responses may be useful in the differentiation between organic and nonorganic deficits.

## Coordinated Associated Movements in the Paretic Limb

Coordinated AMs that accompany voluntary motion of involved extremities in patients with hemiparesis are characterized by a spread of movement from one muscle or group of muscles to others. They alter the position of the part and lead to the adoption of new postures. They do not appear in the normal individual or in nonorganic weakness. The best known of these are the Wartenberg thumb adduction sign, the Babinski trunk-thigh sign, and the tibialis sign of Strumpell.

### Wartenberg Sign

Active flexion of the terminal phalanges of the four fingers of a paretic hand about a firm object, or against resistance offered by the examiner's fingers similarly flexed, is followed by adduction, flexion, and opposition of the thumb (Figure 31.1). In a normal extremity the thumb remains in abduction and extension. A variation is for patient and examiner to hook and pull with only the index fingers; the response is the same.

### The Trunk-Thigh Sign of Babinski, or Combined Flexion of the Trunk and Thigh

The patient, lying supine with legs abducted, attempts to sit up while holding the arms crossed on the chest. Normally, the legs remain motionless and the heels down. In corticospinal hemiparesis, the hip flexes as the trunk flexes and there is an involuntary elevation of the paretic limb off the bed

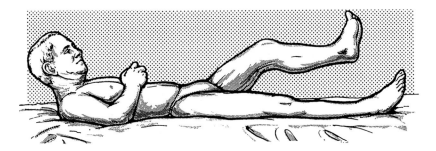

**FIGURE 31.2** ● Trunk-thigh sign in patient with left hemiparesis.

(Figure 31.2). The toes may spread out in a fanlike fashion. The normal limb remains on the bed or rises slightly, but not as high as the paretic one. In paraparesis, both legs rise equally. In nonorganic weakness, the normal leg rises and the paretic one does not, or neither leg rises. If the patient tries to sit up with the legs hanging over the edge of the bed, the hip flexes and the knee extends on the involved side. The same phenomenon occurs if the standing patient bends over (Figure 31.3).

### The Tibialis Sign of Strümpell

Normally, vigorous flexion of the hip and knee are accompanied by plantarflexion of the foot. In lower-extremity weakness due to a corticospinal tract lesion, voluntary flexion of the hip and knee is accompanied by involuntary dorsiflexion and inversion of the paretic foot; there may also be dorsiflexion of the great toe or of all the toes. The patient is unable to flex the hip and knee without

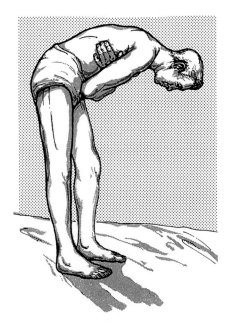

**FIGURE 31.3** ● Combined flexion of the thigh and leg in a patient with left hemiparesis.

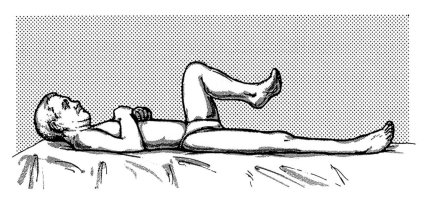

*FIGURE 31.4* ● Tibialis sign in a patient with left hemiparesis.

dorsiflexing the foot (Figure 31.4). The response is accentuated if the movement is carried out against resistance.

## Contralateral Coordinated Associated Movements

Coordinated AMs in which the response is contralateral are similar to the symmetric AMs, but the response is not always imitative and may involve muscles other than those used in the primary movement.

## Loss of Coordinated Associated Movements

Certain coordinated AMs normally present are abolished in pyramidal lesions. Normal associated and automatic movements, such as swinging of the arms in walking and synergistic movements used in rising and sitting down, are also lost in disorders of the extrapyramidal system, especially parkinsonian syndromes. In upper motor neuron facial weakness, the platysma may fail to contract as it normally does when the patient opens the mouth as widely as possible, grimaces, or touches the chin to the chest (platysma sign of Babinski).

# Coordination and Gait

# CHAPTER 32

# Cerebellar Function

The cerebellum is tasked with bringing finesse to the motor system. Although not primarily involved in the mechanisms for production of muscle power, it is necessary for normal control and regulation of muscle contraction. The major function of the cerebellum, from a clinical point of view, is the coordination of movement. The cerebellum is the portion of the brain through which the cerebral motor cortex achieves the synthesis and coordination of individual muscle contractions required for normal voluntary movements. Without it, movements are gross, uncoordinated, clumsy, and tremulous, and precise movements become impossible. Lesions of the cerebellum do not cause weakness, but rather loss of coordination and inability to gauge and regulate, as Gordon Holmes said, the "rate, range, and force" of movement. Although motor strength and power are preserved, active movements are severely compromised.

A major manifestation of cerebellar lesions is ataxia (Gr. a "without," taxis "order"); a rough translation is "not orderly." The essential feature in ataxia is that movements are not normally organized. Although the term is a general one, indicating chaotic and disorganized movement, it is used clinically primarily to refer to the motor control abnormalities—including incoordination, tremor, and impaired rapid alternating movements—that occur with cerebellar lesions. Ataxia is not specific for cerebellar disease, and lesions in other parts of the nervous system must be excluded before attributing ataxia to cerebellar disease. Impaired proprioception may cause sensory ataxia and lesions involving pathways that originate in the frontal lobe may cause frontal lobe ataxia. Other common manifestations of cerebellar disease include nystagmus, impaired balance, and difficulty walking.

## TABLE 32.1

Clinical Manifestations of Disorders of the Cerebellum (Related to the Different Zones of the Cerebellum)

| Zone of Cerebellum | Clinical Manifestation | Possible Disorder |
|---|---|---|
| Flocculonodular lobe (archicerebellum) | Nystagmus; extraocular movement abnormalities | Medulloblastoma |
| Vermis (paleocerebellum) | Gait ataxia | Alcoholic degeneration |
| Hemisphere (neocerebellum) | Appendicular ataxia | Tumor; stroke |
| Pancerebellar | All of the above | Paraneoplastic |

## CLINICAL MANIFESTATIONS OF CEREBELLAR DYSFUNCTION

Patients with cerebellar dysfunction suffer from various combinations of tremor, incoordination, difficulty walking, dysarthria, and nystagmus, depending on the parts of the cerebellum involved (Table 32.1). Cerebellar disease may also cause hypotonia, asthenia or slowness of movement, and deviation or drift of the outstretched limbs. Disease involving the cerebellar connections in the brainstem causes abnormalities indistinguishable from disease of the cerebellum itself. When cerebellar ataxia results from dysfunction of the cerebellar connections in the brainstem there are usually other brainstem signs.

### Dyssynergia

The essential disturbance in cerebellar disease is dyssynergia. Normally, there is harmonious, coordinated action between the various muscles involved in a movement so that they contract with the proper force, timing, and sequence of activation to carry out the movement smoothly and accurately. Cerebellar disease impairs the normal control mechanisms that organize and regulate the contractions of the different participating muscles and muscle groups to insure smooth, properly coordinated movement. There is a lack of speed and skill in performing movements that require the coordinated activity of several groups of muscles or of several movements. The cerebellum is instrumental in timing the activation of the different muscles involved in a movement. Lack of integration of the components of the act results in decomposition of movement—the act is broken down into its component parts and carried out in a jerky, erratic, awkward, disorganized manner. The cerebellum is particularly important in coordinating multi-joint movements.

### Dysmetria

Dysmetria refers to errors in judging distance and gauging the distance, speed, power, and direction of movement. Cerebellar dysfunction leads to loss of the normal collaboration between agonist and antagonist. When reaching for an object 50 cm away, the hand shoots out 55 cm, overshooting the target (hypermetria), or fails to reach the target (hypometria). Hypermetria is more common. The movement may be carried out too slowly or too rapidly with too much or too little force. The patient with dysmetria does not make a movement along a straight line between two points, but erratically deviates from the intended track.

### Agonist-Antagonist Coordination

A disturbance in reciprocal innervation results in a loss of the ability to stop the contraction of the agonists and rapidly contract the antagonists to control and regulate movement. Impairment of the ability to carry out successive movements and to stop one act and follow it immediately by its diametric opposite causes dysdiadochokinesia, loss of checking movements, and the rebound phenomenon. Dysdiadochokinesia (or adiadochokinesia) is a clumsy term (coined by Babinski) that means inability to make rapid repetitive or rapid alternating movements (RAMs). The patient with impaired RAMs has difficulty with such tests as patting the palm of one hand alternately with the palm and dorsum of the other hand, rapid tapping of the fingers, tapping out a complex rhythm, or tapping the foot in steady beat. Inability to rapidly reverse an action also causes impairment of the check response, producing the Holmes rebound phenomenon (see section on Impaired Check and the Rebound Phenomenon).

## Tremor

The most common type of cerebellar tremor is an intention (active, kinetic, or terminal) tremor that is not present at rest but becomes evident on purposeful movement. In the upper extremity, when the patient reaches to touch an object there are irregular, to-and-fro, jerky movements perpendicular to the path of movement that increase in amplitude as the hand approaches the target. A postural tremor of the outstretched limbs may also occur, without the patient reaching for a target. Cerebellar tremor often involves the proximal muscles. When severe, cerebellar tremor may involve not only the extremities, but also the head or even the entire body. Severe cerebellar tremor may at times take on an almost myoclonic character; some conditions cause both cerebellar ataxia and myoclonus. The tremors and other movements probably result from disease involving the cerebellar efferent pathways or their connections with the red nucleus and thalamus (dentorubral and dentothalamic pathways, or superior cerebellar peduncle), and are sometimes referred to as a cerebellar outflow tremor. A rubral tremor is present at rest but worsens with action, and probably results from a lesion involving the cerebellar outflow tracts.

## Hypotonia

Hypotonia, or muscle flaccidity, with a decrease in resistance to passive movement, is often seen in cerebellar disease. Cerebellar dysfunction results in a decrease in the tonic output of the cerebellar nuclei, causing loss of cerebellar facilitation to the motor cortex. The muscles are flabby and assume unnatural attitudes; the parts of the body can be moved passively into positions of extreme flexion or extension. The stretch reflexes are normal or diminished in disease limited to the cerebellum. Occasionally, the tendon reflexes are "pendular." Tapping the patellar tendon with the foot hanging free results in a series of to-and-fro movements of the foot and leg before the limb finally comes to rest. Pendular reflexes are caused by muscle hypotonicity and the lack of normal checking of the reflex response. The superficial reflexes are unaffected by cerebellar disease. Cerebellar disease may also cause a characteristic position of the extended hand, probably because of hypotonia. The wrist is flexed and arched dorsally, with the fingers hyperextended, and a tendency toward overpronation. The hand is similar to that seen in Sydenham chorea. A cerebellar lesion may cause a decrease in the normal pendular movement of the affected arm when walking. A decreased arm swing may also occur with extrapyramidal disorders and with mild hemiparesis. In the shoulder-shaking test, a cerebellar lesion causes an increase in the range and duration of swinging of the involved arm, although the movements may be irregular and nonrhythmic.

## Dysarthria

Cerebellar disease often affects speech. Articulation may be slow, ataxic, slurred, drawling, jerky, or explosive in type, because of dyssynergy of the muscles of phonation. A scanning type of dysarthria is particularly characteristic of cerebellar disease. The scanning speech of multiple sclerosis and the staccato speech of Friedreich ataxia are probably the result of cerebellar dysfunction.

## Nystagmus

Nystagmus and other disturbances of ocular motility may occur with lesions of the cerebellum. Nystagmus often indicates involvement of vestibulocerebellar pathways. The ocular abnormalities often result from involvement of the connections of the cerebellum with other centers rather than actual cerebellar dysfunction. Cerebellar disease may cause gaze paretic nystagmus. The patient is unable to sustain eccentric gaze and requires repeated saccades to gaze laterally. With a lesion of one hemisphere the eyes at rest may be deviated 10 degrees to 30 degrees toward the unaffected side. When the patient attempts to gaze elsewhere, the eyes saccade toward the point of fixation with slow return movements to the resting point. The movements are more marked and of greater amplitude when the patient looks toward the affected side. When a tumor of the cerebellopontine angle is present, the nystagmus is coarse on looking toward the side of the lesion and fine and rapid on gaze to the opposite side (Bruns nystagmus). Other ocular motility disturbances seen with cerebellar disease include skew deviation, ocular dysmetria, ocular flutter, opsoclonus, and saccadic intrusions. Rebound nystagmus is a type of nystagmus that may be unique to cerebellar disease; the fast component is in the direction of lateral gaze, but transiently reverses direction when the eyes come back to primary position.

## Other Abnormalities

Abnormalities of posture and gait with abnormal attitudes and spontaneous deviation of the head and parts of the body may be seen in cerebellar disease. In unilateral cerebellar disease there may be deviation of the head and body toward the affected side, with past pointing of the extremities toward the affected side. When standing, there is an inclination to fall, and when walking a tendency to deviate, toward the side of the lesion. The outstretched extremities deviate laterally, toward the affected side. There may be a decrease or absence of the normal pendular movement of the arm in walking. In midline, or vermis, lesions the patient may not be able to stand erect and may fall either backward or forward. The gait is staggering, reeling, or lurching in character, without laterality.

## EXAMINATION OF COORDINATION AND CEREBELLAR FUNCTION

Clinical tests for cerebellar dysfunction are basically designed to detect dyssynergia, decomposition of movement, and dysmetria. The combination of incoordination, awkwardness, errors in the speed, range, and force of movement, along with dysdiadochokinesia and intention tremor is referred to as cerebellar ataxia. Simple observation can be as informative as a detailed clinical examination. Watching as the patient is standing, walking, dressing and undressing, buttoning and unbuttoning clothing, and tying shoelaces may reveal tremor, incoordination, clumsiness, and disturbed postural fixation. The patient may be asked to write, use simple tools, drink from a glass, and trace lines with a lightweight pen while no support is given at the elbow. The examination of infants and children may be limited to simple observation, noting the child's ability to reach for and use toys and objects. Tests for coordination may be divided into those concerned with equilibratory and nonequilibratory functions.

### Equilibratory Coordination

Equilibratory coordination refers to the maintenance of balance and the coordination of the body as a whole. The examination of station and gait assesses equilibratory coordination; these are discussed further in Chapter 44.

### Nonequilibratory Coordination

Tests of nonequilibratory coordination assess the patient's ability to carry out discrete, oftentimes relatively fine, intentional movements with the extremities. Although these are primarily tests of coordination, other neural systems must be intact for normal performance. It is important to consider handedness in judging coordination, and to allow for the normal slight clumsiness of the non-dominant side. Patients who are fatigued or sedated may have incoordination that is not normal for the individual. Fine motor skills may also be assessed functionally by asking the patient to do such things as thread a needle, pick up a pin, string beads, pour water, or draw circles.

## The Finger-to-Nose (Finger-Nose-Finger) Test

There are several variations on the theme of having the patient touch his index finger to his nose, all of which will be included as the finger-to-nose (FTN) test. All may be carried out with the patient lying, seated, or standing. The patient extends the arm completely and then touches the tip of the index finger to the tip of the nose, slowly at first, then rapidly, with the eyes open and then closed. The examiner may place the outstretched extremity in various positions, and have the test carried out in different planes and from various angles. The patient may be asked to touch the tip of his index finger to his nose, then touch the tip of the examiner's finger, and then back to the tip of his nose. It is helpful to demonstrate the requested movement, lest the patient make some odd interpretation of the verbal request; an occasional patient will attempt to put his index finger on the examiner's finger without removing it from his own nose. The examiner's finger may be moved about during the test, and the patient asked to try to touch the moving target as the finger is placed in different locations at different distances, and to move both slowly and quickly. The examiner may pull his finger away and make the patient chase it; fully extending the arm in this way can bring out mild intention tremor.

During these movements note the smoothness and accuracy with which the act is executed, and look for oscillations, jerkiness, and tremor. An intention tremor becomes more marked, coarse, and irregular as the finger approaches the target. There may be little tremor during the midrange of the movement, but near the end the tremor erupts; when the finger contacts the target the tremor stops. In cerebellar ataxia, the difficulty may vary from slight incoordination, with a blundering type of movement, to wild oscillations causing complete inability to execute the act. A patient with severe appendicular ataxia may not be able to touch hand to head, much less finger to nose.

With dysmetria the patient may stop before he reaches his nose, pause and then complete the act slowly and unsteadily, or overshoot the mark and bring the finger to the nose with too much speed and force. With dyssynergy the act is not carried out smoothly and harmoniously; there may be irregular stops, accelerations, and deflections, or the movement may disintegrate into its component parts. Performing the FTN test against slight resistance may cause mild ataxia to become more obvious, or latent ataxia evident. The examiner may apply resistance by placing his fingers against the patient's forearm and exerting slight pressure as the patient moves his arm toward the nose, or by placing a long rubber band around the patient's wrist and pulling gently on it during the test. Another test is to have the patient draw a line, starting and then stopping at fixed points. He may have difficulty in starting at the correct point and may either stop short of the second point or overshoot the mark. This may also demonstrate tremor, with side-to-side oscillations along the intended tract. The patient with cerebellar disease may have macrographia, using large characters that become larger across the page, the opposite of the writing disturbance seen in Parkinson disease.

In the finger-to-finger (fingertips in the midline) test, the patient abducts the arms widely to the horizontal and then brings in the tips of the index or middle fingers through a wide arc to touch them exactly in the midline. This is done slowly and rapidly, with the eyes first open and then closed. With unilateral cerebellar disease the finger on the involved side may fail to reach the midline, and the finger on the normal side may cross the midline to reach it. Also, the arm on the affected side may sag or rise, causing the finger on that side to be below or above the one on the normal side.

In hysteria or malingering there may be bizarre responses of various types. The patient may act as if unable to touch the finger to the nose, or circle around it with widespread, wandering movements but eventually touch the very tip. Or the patient may repeatedly but precisely touch some other part of the face, implying there is no loss of sensation or coordination.

Similar tests may be used to evaluate the lower extremities. In the heel-to-shin (heel-knee-shin/toe) test, the patient is asked to place the heel of one foot on the opposite knee, tap it up and down on the knee several times, push the point of the heel (not the instep) along the shin in a straight line to the great toe, and then bring it back to the knee. The patient with cerebellar disease is likely to raise the foot too high, flex the knee too much, and place the heel down above the knee. The excursions along the shin are jerky and unsteady. With sensory ataxia, the patient may have difficulty locating the knee with the heel, groping around for it; there is difficulty keeping the heel on the shin, and it may slip off to either side while sliding down the shin. In the toe-to-finger test, the patient tries to touch his great toe, knee bent, to the examiner's finger. If there is dysmetria, he will undershoot or overshoot the mark; intention tremor and oscillations may also be evident. The patient may be asked to draw a circle or a figure eight with his foot, either in the air or on the floor; in ataxia the movement will be unsteady and the figure irregular.

## Rapid Alternating Movements

With dysdiadochokinesia, one act cannot be immediately followed by its diametric opposite; the contraction of one set of agonists and relaxation of the antagonists cannot be followed immediately by relaxation of the agonists and contraction of the antagonists. Patients with cerebellar ataxia may have great difficulty making these kinds of movements. A common test for dysdiadochokinesia is to have the patient alternately pronate and supinate his hands, as in patting alternately with the palm and dorsum of the hand on the thigh or on the palm or dorsum of the other hand, or imitating screwing in a lightbulb or turning a doorknob. The movements are performed repetitively and as rapidly as possible. Any movement involving reciprocal innervation and alternate action of agonists and antagonists can be used, such as: alternate opening and closing of the fists, quickly flexing and extending individual fingers, touching the tip of the index finger to the tip or extended interphalangeal joint of the thumb, or patting rapidly against a table top with hand or fingertips. A good test is to have the patient touch the tip of his thumb with the tip of each finger rapidly and in sequence—starting with the index finger and proceeding to the little finger, repeating with the little finger and going to the index finger, and so forth. Another good test is to have the patient tap out a simple rhythm with each hand (e.g., 1-2-3/pause in steady beat), and then a more complex but familiar rhythm (e.g., "Happy Birthday" song). Testing RAMs in the lower extremity is much more limited. The patient may be asked to pat the foot steadily, against the floor if standing, against the examiner's palm if recumbent, or to repetitively touch the heel up and down to the knee if supine. Rapid alternating movements of the tongue may be tested by having the patient move the tongue in and out or from side to side as rapidly as possible.

In all of these tests, note the rate, rhythm, accuracy, and smoothness of the movements. In patients with ataxia, the RAMs are either carried out slowly and hesitantly, with pauses during transition between the opposing motions, or unsteadily and irregularly, with loss of rhythm. There may be a rapid fatigability: The movements may be executed satisfactorily in the beginning, but after a few attempts they become awkward and clumsy. The two extremities are usually compared, but patients with bilateral abnormalities are common and the examiner must rely on experience or use another control. Demonstrating the movements to the patient provides an opportunity for the examiner to be the control. For some maneuvers, such as rapid, repetitive finger movements the two extremities can be examined simultaneously and one side compared with the other. Simultaneous testing may also cause accentuation of the abnormality on the affected side.

## Impaired Check and the Rebound Phenomenon

Checking movements involve contraction of the antagonists after a load is unexpectedly removed during strong contraction of the agonist. The agonists must immediately relax and the antagonists must contract to provide braking after the sudden release of resistance. Since cerebellar dysfunction causes impairment of the reciprocal relationship between agonist and antagonist, patients may have impairment of the checking response.

In the Holmes (Stewart-Holmes) rebound test, the patient holds the arm adducted at the shoulder and flexed at the elbow, with the forearm supinated and the fist firmly clenched. The elbow may rest on a table or be held unsupported close to the body. The examiner pulls on the wrist, and the patient strongly resists the examiner's attempt to extend the elbow. The examiner then suddenly releases his grip on the wrist. Normally, with the sudden unloading the contraction of the elbow flexors immediately ceases and is rapidly followed by contraction of the elbow extensors to arrest the sudden flexion movement and stop the patient from hitting himself. The normal patient is able to control the unexpected flexion movement of the elbow. In cerebellar disease, when the strongly flexed extremity is suddenly released the patient cannot stop the flexor contraction and engage the extensors to stop the elbow movement. Because of loss of the checking response, the fist flies up to the shoulder or mouth, often with considerable force. The examiner's free arm should be placed between the patient's fist and face to block the blow. The prevalent description of this as the Holmes rebound phenomenon is not precisely correct. Stewart and Holmes used rebound to refer to the jerk back in the opposite direction, the recoil, on release of the restraint. The rebound phenomenon is present normally and exaggerated in spastic limbs. It is the absence of rebound (usually accompanied by impaired checking) in limbs affected by cerebellar disease that is abnormal. The rebound test may be carried out in other ways. Elbow extension against resistance may be tested instead of flexion. With both arms outstretched in front of the patient, the examiner may press either down or up on them as the patient resists and then suddenly lets go. This allows comparison of the rebound phenomenon and loss of checking movements on the two sides. In the lower extremities, rebound can be tested by sudden release after the patient has been resisting either flexion or extension at the knee, hip, or ankle. Impaired checking and the rebound phenomenon are not invariably present in cerebellar disease, and may sometimes be present in normal limbs or even exaggerated in spastic limbs. An abnormal rebound test unilaterally is more significant than when present bilaterally. In the arm-stopping test, the patient holds both arms overhead or by his sides, the examiner holds his arms outstretched horizontally, and then the patient tries to quickly bring his arms up or down so that his fingertips are at the exact same level as the examiner's. With a unilateral hemispheric lesion, the good arm will stop on target, the affected arm often overshoots and then corrects in the opposite direction, oscillating around the target before eventually coming to rest.

## Deviation and Past Pointing

Patients with cerebellar disease often have difficulty maintaining normal alignment of the limbs or body when performing a task such as holding the arms outstretched or walking, especially with eyes closed. The patient may miss when trying to reach out to touch a target (past pointing), drift to one side when walking eyes closed, or have drift of the outstretched arm. Similar findings may occur with vestibular lesions.

To perform the traditional test for past pointing, the patient and examiner should be facing, either seated or standing, the outstretched upper extremity of each held horizontally with the index fingers in contact. The patient raises his arm to a vertical position, finger pointed directly upward, and then returns to horizontal to again touch the examiner's finger. The maneuver should be tried a few times with the eyes open and then executed with the eyes closed. The arms may be tested sequentially or simultaneously. The test is less commonly done with the patient raising the arm from below up to the horizontal. Normally, the patient will return to the starting position fairly accurately, without any drift or deviation. In labyrinthine disease or with a cerebellar hemispheric lesion, the arm will deviate to the involved side on the return track, more so with the eyes closed. This deviation is called past pointing. A simpler way to test for past pointing is to have the patient close his eyes while doing the finger-nose-finger test. With eyes open the pointing is accurate, but with eyes closed the patient points off to the side of the target. Repeating the test several times may produce greater deviation. With severe lesions, past pointing may occur even with eyes open. The pattern is different in vestibular as opposed to cerebellar past pointing. In vestibular disease, past pointing occurs with both upper extremities toward the involved side; in unilateral cerebellar disease past pointing occurs toward the side of the lesion, but only in the ipsilateral arm.

A cerebellar lesion may also cause drift of the outstretched upper extremities. Three types of drift may occur when the patient attempts to hold the arms outstretched with eyes closed: pyramidal drift, parietal drift, and cerebellar drift. In pronator drift (Barré sign) due to a pyramidal lesion, the arm sinks downward and there is accompanying pronation of the forearm. In parietal drift, the arm usually rises and strays outward (updrift). With cerebellar drift the arm drifts mainly outward, either at the same level, rising or less often sinking. Testing is done with arms outstretched and eyes closed. With disease involving one cerebellar hemisphere, the arm drifts toward the side of the lesion. The deviation may be accentuated by having the patient raise and lower the arms several times, or by tapping the patient's outstretched wrists. Tapping on the wrists may also create an up-and-down oscillation because of impaired checking, so that the arm swings up and down a few times, and gradually drifts laterally and often upward.

Position-holding can also be tested in the lower extremities. The patient, lying supine, raises the legs one at a time. When there is ataxia, the leg cannot be lifted steadily or in a straight line. There may be adduction, abduction, rotation, oscillations, or jerky movements from one position to another. When the limb is lowered, the patient may throw it down heavily and it may not return to its original position beside its mate but may be deviated across it or away from it. When the seated patient extends the legs without support and attempts to hold them steady, a unilateral cerebellar lesion may cause oscillations and lateral deviation of the ipsilateral extremity. The extended supported leg may show an increased range and duration of pendulousness when released or given a brisk push. If the prone patient bends the knees and tries to maintain the shins vertically, there may be marked oscillations and lateral deviation of the leg on the side of the lesion.

Deviation and drift may also occur when the patient tries to walk with eyes closed. As in vestibulopathy, the patient drifts to the side of the lesion. Walking back and forth with eyes closed may reveal a "compass" or "star" gait due to deviation toward the involved side. When walking around a chair, the patient shows a tendency to fall toward the affected side.

## DISEASE OF THE CEREBELLUM

Cerebellar disease may affect all or only a specific part of the cerebellum. There are two clearly defined cerebellar syndromes: a midline or vermis syndrome, and a lateral or hemispheric syndrome. With the vermis, or midline, syndrome the outstanding symptoms are abnormalities of station and gait, with abnormalities ranging from slight widening of the base on walking in mild disease (gait ataxia), to total inability to sit or walk in severe disease. Disease of the cerebellar hemispheres produces appendicular ataxia, disturbance in coordination of the ipsilateral extremities, the arm more than the leg. The primary clinical manifestations of dysfunction of the FN lobe or its connections are disturbances of equilibrium; nystagmus, often positional; and other abnormalities of extraocular movement. There is no limb ataxia. Table 32.1 summarizes the clinical manifestations of disease of these parts of the cerebellum.

The manifestations of cerebellar disease differ markedly in severity, depending upon the acuteness or chronicity of the process. The ability of the nervous system to compensate for a cerebellar lesion can be remarkable. If the lesion is acute, the symptoms are profound; if it is slowly progressive, they are much less severe. There may be considerable recovery from an acute lesion. If a lesion develops insidiously, there may be extensive involvement of the hemispheres without much in the way of clinical findings. The neural plasticity and compensation are such that some patients with little remaining cerebellar tissue can eventually function quite well. The symptoms of cerebellar disease are similar regardless of the etiology of the disease process, and whether the lesion is congenital or acquired.

## Midline Syndrome

The vermis is important in the control of axial structures, or those that are bilaterally innervated; vermian lesions primarily affect midline functions, such as walking and coordination of the head and trunk. A patient with mild vermian disease has gait ataxia. The base is widened, tandem gait is particularly difficult, and there may be decompensation on turning. The Romberg test is negative—the imbalance does not worsen significantly with eyes closed. With severe dysfunction of the vermis, there may be gross postural and locomotor disturbances of the entire body. There is no lateralization, and the tendency to fall may be either backward or forward. The gait is wide-based and characterized by swaying and staggering; the patient may reel in a drunken manner to either side. With truncal ataxia there is swaying and unsteadiness when standing, and the patient may be unable to maintain an upright position. There may be loss of the ability to remain erect when seated, or to hold the neck and head steady and upright; when severe, the standing and sitting balance disturbance leads to constant, to-and-fro swaying, nodding, and weaving movements of the head and trunk when the patient is upright known as titubation. The head movements in titubation are primarily anteroposterior (yes-yes) at 3 to 4 Hz. Vermis dysfunction causes little or no abnormality of the extremities, especially the upper extremities, although all coordinated movements may be poorly performed. Muscle tone and reflexes are normal. Nystagmus may be present, but is usually not marked. Ocular dysmetria, rebound nystagmus, and pursuit abnormalities may also occur. Lesions involving the vermis may cause upbeat nystagmus. Dysarthria is often present. There is sometimes an abnormal rotated or tilted head posture.

Common causes of a midline cerebellar syndrome are alcoholic cerebellar degeneration and medulloblastoma. Alcohol preferentially poisons the vermis, leading to a characteristic syndrome of gait ataxia with sparing of the limbs. Such patients may have no demonstrable lower-extremity ataxia while lying supine, yet be totally unable to walk. Unwary examiners may conclude such findings represent hysteria. Medulloblastomas occur most often in the cerebellar vermis.

## Hemispheric Syndrome

With a lesion involving one cerebellar hemisphere, the manifestations are appendicular rather than axial. Cerebellar hemispheric deficits are unilateral and ipsilateral to the lesion, as the pathways are uncrossed (or, more correctly, double crossed). There is a disturbance of skilled movements of the extremities, with ataxia, dysmetria, dyssynergy, dysdiadochokinesia, and hypotonicity affecting the arm and hand more than the leg and foot. Distal movements are affected more than proximal and fine movements more than gross ones. Movements are performed irregularly, and there may be intention tremor or other hyperkinesias if the dentate nucleus or its efferent pathways are involved.

Posture and gait are not impaired as severely as in the vermis syndrome, but abnormalities do occur. There may be swaying and falling toward the side of the lesion. The patient may be able to stand one-legged using the contralateral but not the ipsilateral foot. He may be unable to bend his body toward the involved side without falling. The abnormalities often resemble those of a unilateral vestibular lesion. On walking, there may be unsteadiness, with deviation or rotation toward the involved side. There may be drift and past pointing toward the involved side. Dysarthria may occur, although disturbances of articulation are not as severe as in vermis lesions. Nystagmus is a common finding, usually horizontal but sometimes rotatory. It is usually more prominent when looking toward the side of the lesion. Common causes of a cerebellar hemispheric syndrome include cerebellar astrocytoma, multiple sclerosis, and lateral medullary stroke.

## TABLE 32.2

**Associated Findings Helpful in Distinguishing Sensory from Cerebellar Ataxia**

| Sensory Ataxia | Cerebellar Ataxia |
| --- | --- |
| Sensory loss, especially for joint position and vibration | Nystagmus, ocular dysmetria, and other eye movement abnormalities |
| Steppage gait | Reeling, ataxic gait |
| Decreased reflexes | Other signs of cerebellar disease (dyssynergia, dysmetria, dysdiadochokinesia, hypotonia, rebound, impaired check response) |

## Diffuse Cerebellar Dysfunction

Some conditions affect the cerebellum diffusely, causing midline and bilateral hemispheric abnormalities. Patients may have nystagmus, gait and truncal ataxia, and appendicular incoordination. Etiologies include the hereditary spinocerebellar ataxia syndromes, drugs (especially phenytoin), toxins, and paraneoplastic cerebellar degeneration.

## Sensory Ataxia

Incoordination may also result from a lack of proprioceptive input from the limbs. Sensory ataxia results from peripheral nerve disease affecting primarily sensory fibers, pathology involving the dorsal root ganglia, dorsal roots or posterior columns of the spinal cord, interruption of the proprioceptive pathways in the brainstem, or disease of the parietal lobe. Incoordination due to sensory ataxia can closely mimic that of cerebellar ataxia (Table 32.2). With cerebellar ataxia, it makes little difference whether the patient's eyes are open or closed. In sensory ataxia, performance is not normal with eyes open, but worsens markedly with eyes closed. The different components of the abnormality may behave slightly differently when visual input is removed. Some of the tremor in sensory ataxia is due to visually guided voluntary corrections of deviations from the intended track. Because of loss of appreciation of limb position in space, with eyes closed the patient may be unable to find his nose or the examiner's finger, but the tremor may actually abate because the patient cannot see that a deviation is occurring and does not attempt to correct it. He may be wildly off target but move in a straighter line. The distinction between cerebellar and sensory ataxia is also made by the associated findings (Table 32.2).

## Other Abnormalities

There are many potential causes for a lack of coordination of movement. All of the levels of the motor system are involved in performing smooth and accurate movement. Weakness of any origin may interfere with skill and precision. Abnormalities of tone of any type may interfere with coordination. Diseases of the extrapyramidal system may impair motor control because of rigidity, akinesia or bradykinesia, lack of spontaneity, and loss of associated movements. A corticospinal tract lesion may cause jerkiness and clumsiness of movement, loss of motor control, and poor integration of skilled acts. Nonorganic illness may cause difficulty with coordination simulating true ataxia. Hyperkinetic movement disorders may cause irregularity in the timing and excursion of successive movements. Proprioceptive abnormalities may impair motor performance. To always attribute ataxia to cerebellar disease is an oversimplification, since many conditions can cause incoordination and clumsiness. Often the cause is multifactorial. A good general rule is to avoid drawing conclusions about the meaning of "cerebellar signs" in the face of any significant degree of weakness, spasticity, rigidity, or sensory loss. When the examination shows no other abnormalities, incoordination and awkwardness of movement are usually due to cerebellar disease.

Frontal lobe ataxia refers to disturbed coordination due to dysfunction of the contralateral frontal lobe; it may resemble the deficits due to abnormalities of the ipsilateral cerebellar hemisphere. Frontal lobe ataxia results from disease involving the frontopontocerebellar fibers en route to synapse in the pontine nuclei. Frontal lobe lesions may produce other abnormalities, such as hyperreflexia, increased tone, and pathologic reflexes; while purely cerebellar lesions typically cause hypotonia, diminished or pendular reflexes, and no pathologic reflex responses. Pressure on the brainstem by a cerebellar mass lesion may cause corticospinal tract findings that can confuse the picture. Bruns ataxia refers to a gait disturbance seen primarily in frontal lobe lesions.

# CHAPTER 33

# Gait and Station

$\mathbf{I}$t is possible to learn more about neurologic status from watching a patient walk than from any other single procedure, and observation of gait should always be part of a neurologic examination. Abnormalities of gait are a common clinical problem with numerous causes, both neurologic and non-neurologic. A careful general evaluation is always necessary to exclude a non-neurologic cause.

Station is the way a patient stands, gait the way she walks. Standing and walking are active processes that depend upon a number of factors and reflex responses. The mechanisms are complex, especially in the human, whose biped gait and erect position over a narrow base require more efficient maintenance and control of equilibrium than is necessary in quadrupeds. Gait and station may be affected by abnormalities of proprioception, abnormalities of muscle power or tone, abnormalities of vestibular function, and by dysfunction of the basal ganglia, the cerebellum, or their connections.

Neurologic causes of an abnormal gait include conditions as varied as foot drop due to peroneal nerve palsy, myopathy, hydrocephalus, and cerebellar degeneration. The various gait abnormalities have different findings on physical examination in regard to the gait itself, such as a steppage pattern as opposed to a pelvic waddle. The differential diagnosis of the gait abnormality is also very dependent on the history and the other clinical signs present. Some of the more common abnormal gait patterns are summarized in Table 33.1.

## EXAMINATION OF STATION

Station is the patient's attitude, posture, or manner of standing. The healthy individual stands erect with her head up, chest out, and abdomen in. Abnormality of station may be an important indicator of neurologic disease. Station is tested by having the patient stand, feet closely together, noting any unsteadiness or swaying. More rigorous testing includes having the patient stand eyes open and eyes closed, on one foot at a time, on toes and heels, and tandem with one heel in front of the toes of the other foot. She may be given a gentle push to see whether she falls to one side, forward, or backward.

Patients with unsteadiness standing often attempt to compensate by placing the feet wide apart in order to stand on a broader and steadier base. In cerebellar disease, the patient usually stands on a broad base and there is swaying, to more or less an equal degree, with eyes open and closed. With a lesion of the vermis, the patient may sway backward, forward, or to either side. With a

## TABLE 33.1

**Some of the More Common Neurologic Abnormalities of Gait**

| Gait Disorder | Gait Characteristics | Usual Associated Findings |
|---|---|---|
| Spastic | Stiff legged, scissoring (wooden soldier) | Hyperreflexia, extensor plantar responses |
| Cerebellar ataxia | Wide based, reeling, careening (drunken sailor) | Heel-to-shin ataxia, other cerebellar signs |
| Sensory ataxia | Wide based, steppage | Positive Romberg, impaired joint position sense |
| Hemiparetic | Involved leg spastic, circumduction, often with foot drop | Weakness, hyperreflexia, extensor plantar response |
| Parkinsonian | Small steps, flexed posture, shuffling, festination | Tremor, rigidity, bradykinesia |
| Marche à petits pas | Small steps, slow shuffling | Dementia, frontal lobe signs |
| Foot drop (unilateral or bilateral) | High steppage pattern to clear the toes from the floor, double tap with toe strike before heel strike | Foot dorsiflexion weakness |
| Myopathic | Exaggerated "sexy" hip motion, waddling, lumbar hyperlordosis | Hip girdle weakness |

lesion of one hemisphere she sways or falls toward the affected side. Unilateral vestibular disease also causes falling toward the affected side. In a unilateral, cerebellar hemispheric lesion, or in a unilateral vestibulopathy, the patient may tilt the head toward the involved side with the chin rotated toward the sound side, with the shoulder on the involved side somewhat higher than the other and slightly in front of it. If the patient is given a light push—first toward one side and then toward the other—with a cerebellar hemispheric lesion she will lose balance more easily when pushed toward the involved side. If asked to stand on one foot at a time, the patient with a cerebellar hemispheric lesion may be unable to maintain equilibrium standing on the ipsilateral foot, but may stand without difficulty on the contralateral foot.

### The Romberg Sign

When proprioception is disturbed, the patient may be able to stand with eyes open, but sways or falls with eyes closed (Romberg or Brauch-Romberg sign). The Romberg sign is often misunderstood and misinterpreted. The essential finding is a difference between standing balance with eyes open and closed. In order to test this function, the patient must have a stable stance eyes open and then demonstrate a decrease in balance with eyes closed, when visual input is eliminated and the patient must rely on proprioception to maintain balance.

The Romberg test can be difficult to interpret. There is some variability, even among expert examiners, in how the Romberg test is performed and interpreted. Many patients sway slightly with eyes closed, and minimal amounts of sway, especially in elderly patients, are seldom significant. Minor, normal swaying may stop if the patient is simply asked to stand perfectly still. Most clinicians discount sway at the hips, and insist on seeing sway at the ankles before calling the test positive; some require the patient take a corrective step to the side; and some that the patient nearly fall. Some require the patient be barefoot. The "sharpened" or tandem Romberg is done by having the patient stand in tandem position with eyes open and closed; the limits of normality for this variation are conjectural.

The Romberg sign is used primarily as a test of proprioceptive, not cerebellar, function. The pioneering nineteenth-century clinicians thought it was particularly useful in separating tabes dorsalis from cerebellar disease. In fact, patients with cerebellar disease, particularly disorders of the vestibulocerebellum or spinocerebellum, may have some increase in instability with eyes closed, but not usually to the degree seen with impaired proprioception. A patient with an acute unilateral vestibulopathy may fall toward the side of the lesion when standing with eyes closed. Patients with cerebellar disease, or those with severe weakness, may not have a stable base eyes open. It may help to have the patient widen stance to the point where they are stable eyes open, then close the eyes, and check for any difference. Only a marked worsening of balance with eyes closed qualifies as a positive Romberg sign. A patient who cannot maintain balance feet together and eyes open does not have a positive Romberg.

Some histrionic patients will sway with eyes closed in the absence of any organic neurologic impairment (false Romberg sign). The swaying is usually from the hips and may be exaggerated. If the patient takes a step, the eyes may remain closed, which never happens with a bona fide Romberg. The instability can often be eliminated by diverting the patient's attention. Effective distractors are to ask the patient to detect numbers the examiner writes with her finger on the forehead, wiggle the tongue, or to perform finger-to-nose testing. Having the shoes off and watching the toe movements may be very informative. The toes of the patient with histrionic sway are often extended; the patient with organic imbalance flexes the toes strongly and tries to grip the floor.

## PHYSIOLOGY OF GAIT

The brainstem and spinal cord in lower forms contain "central pattern generators," which are groups of interneurons that coordinate the activity in pools of motor neurons to produce patterned movements. Although the existence of such cell groups in humans is unproven, locomotion likely depends on activity in pattern generators. The pattern generators control the activity in lower motor neurons that execute the mechanics of walking. Higher centers in the subthalamus and midbrain, particularly the pedunculopontine nucleus, modulate the activity in the spinal cord pattern generators through the reticulospinal tracts.

## EXAMINATION OF GAIT

The first step in analyzing gait is to check the width of the base. The wider the base the worse the balance, and spreading the feet farther apart is the first compensatory effort in most gait disorders. Under normal circumstances the medial malleoli pass within about 2 in of each other during the stride phase, a narrow and well-compensated gait. Any spread more than this may signal some problem with gait or balance.

The forefoot on each side should clear the ground to about the same degree; asymmetry of toe lift may be the earliest evidence of foot drop. A shortened stride length may be early evidence of bifrontal or extrapyramidal disease. Excessive movement of the hips may occur with any process causing proximal muscle weakness. Note the reciprocal arm swing; a decreased swing on one side is sometimes an early indicator of hemiparesis or hemi-parkinsonism. Watch the hands for tremor or chorea.

Tandem walking stresses the gait and balance mechanisms even further. Elderly patients may have difficulty with tandem gait because of obesity or deconditioning. In relatively young patients with a low likelihood of neurologic disease, a quick and effective substitute for the Romberg is simply to have the patient close her eyes while walking tandem. This is a difficult maneuver and has high value as a screening test. Having the patient walk briskly and then stop abruptly on command, or make quick turns, first in one direction and then in the other, may bring out ataxia and incoordination not noticeable on straightaway walking. The patient may be asked to walk sideways and overstep, or cross one foot over the other. Having the patient walk on heels and toes may bring out weakness of dorsiflexion or plantar flexion. An excellent screening test is to have the patient hop on either foot.

This simultaneously assesses lower-extremity strength, especially of the gastrosoleus, plus balance functions. Individuals who can hop adroitly on either foot are unlikely to have significant neurologic disease. Note whether the patient has any obvious orthopedic limitations, such as a varus deformity of the knee, genu recurvatum, pelvic tilt, or any other abnormalities.

## ABNORMAL GAITS

### Cerebellar Ataxia

The gait of cerebellar disease is caused by involvement of the coordinating mechanisms in the cerebellum and its connecting systems. There is a clumsy, staggering, unsteady, irregular, lurching, titubating, wide-based gait, and the patient may sway to either side, back, or forward. Leg movements are erratic, and step length varies unpredictably. The patient is unable to walk tandem or follow a straight line on the floor. There may be tremors and oscillatory movements involving the entire body. With a lesion of the cerebellar vermis, the patient will exhibit a lurching, staggering gait, but without laterality, the ataxia will be as marked toward one side as the other. Cerebellar ataxia is present with eyes both open and closed; it may increase slightly with eyes closed, but not so markedly as in sensory ataxia. A gait resembling cerebellar ataxia is seen in acute alcohol intoxication. With a hemispheric lesion the patient will stagger and deviate toward the involved side. In disease localized to one cerebellar hemisphere or in unilateral vestibular disease, there is persistent swaying or deviation toward the abnormal side. As the patient attempts to walk a straight line or to walk tandem she deviates toward the side of the lesion. Walking a few steps backward and forward with eyes closed may bring out "compass deviation" or a "star-shaped gait." When attempting to walk a fixed circle around a chair, clockwise then counterclockwise, the patient will tend to fall toward the chair if it is on the side of the lesion, or to spiral out away from the chair if on the opposite side. Either unilateral cerebellar or vestibular disease may cause turning toward the side of the lesion on the Fukuda stepping test. For all the tests that bring out deviation in one direction, other findings must be used to differentiate between vestibulopathy and a cerebellar hemispheric lesion. Unilateral ataxia may be demonstrated by having the patient attempt to jump on one foot, with the eyes either open or closed. The patient with bilateral vestibular disease may seek to minimize head movement during walking, holding the head stiff and rigid; having the patient turn the head back and forth during walking may bring out ataxia.

### Sensory Ataxia

Sensory ataxia occurs when the nervous system is deprived of the sensory information, primarily proprioceptive, necessary to coordinate walking. Deafferentation may result from disease of the posterior columns (e.g., tabes dorsalis or subacute combined degeneration), or disease affecting the peripheral nerves (e.g., sensory peripheral neuropathy). The term spinal ataxia is sometimes used, but the pathology is not always in the spinal cord. The patient loses awareness of the position of the lower extremities in space, or even of the body as a whole, except as provided by the visual system. The patient is extremely dependent on visual input for coordination. When deprived of visual input, as with eyes closed or in the dark, the gait deteriorates markedly. The difference in walking ability with and without visual input is the key feature of sensory ataxia. If the condition is mild, locomotion may appear normal when the patient walks eyes open; more commonly it is wide based, and poorly coordinated.

The term "steppage gait" refers to a manner of walking in which the patient takes unusually high steps. Sensory ataxia is one of the causes of a steppage gait. The patient takes a high step, throws out her foot, and slams it down on the floor in order to increase the proprioceptive feedback. The heel may land before the toe, creating an audible "double tap." An additional sound effect may be the tapping of a cane, creating a "slam, slam, tap" cadence. The sound effects may be so characteristic that the trained observer can make the diagnosis by listening to the footfalls. The patient with sensory ataxia watches her feet and keeps her eyes on the floor while walking. With eyes closed, the feet seem to shoot out, the staggering and unsteadiness are increased, and the patient may be unable to walk. There is less reeling and lurching in sensory ataxia than with a comparable degree of cerebellar ataxia. The difficulty is even worse walking backward, since the patient cannot see where she is going. The patient with bilateral foot drops, however, also has a steppage gait and a double tapping sound. In all of these tests, sensory ataxia can be differentiated from predominantly cerebellar ataxia by accentuation of the difficulty with eyes closed; and unilateral cerebellar or vestibular disease from vermis involvement by laterality of unsteadiness.

## The Gait of Spastic Hemiparesis

The gait of spastic hemiparesis may be caused by a lesion interrupting the corticospinal pathways to one half of the body, most commonly stroke. The patient stands with a hemiparetic posture, arm flexed, adducted, and internally rotated, and leg extended (Figure 19.1). There is plantar flexion of the foot and toes, either due to foot dorsiflexion weakness or to heel cord shortening, rendering the lower extremity on the involved side functionally slightly longer than on the normal side, referred to as an equinus deformity. When walking, the patient holds the arm tightly to the side, rigid and flexed; she extends it with difficulty and does not swing it in a normal fashion. She holds the leg stiffly in extension and flexes it with difficulty. Consequently, the patient drags or shuffles the foot and scrapes the toes. With each step, she may tilt the pelvis upward on the involved side to aid in lifting the toe off the floor (hip hike) and may swing the entire extremity around in a semicircle from the hip (circumduction). The stance phase is shortened because of weakness, and the swing phase shortened because of spasticity and slowing of movement. The sound produced by the scraping of the toe, as well as the wear of the shoe at the toe, may be quite characteristic. The patient is able to turn toward the paralyzed side more easily than toward the normal side. Loss of normal arm swing and slight circumduction of the leg may be the only gait abnormalities in very mild hemiparesis.

## Scissoring

This gait pattern occurs in patients who have severe spasticity of the legs. It occurs in patients who have congenital spastic diplegia (Little disease, cerebral palsy) and related conditions, and in chronic myelopathies due to conditions such as multiple sclerosis and cervical spondylosis. There is characteristic tightness of the hip adductors causing adduction of the thighs, so that the knees may cross, one in front of the other, with each step (scissors gait). The patient walks on an abnormally narrow base, with a stiff shuffling gait, dragging both legs and scraping the toes. The steps are short and slow; the feet seem to stick to the floor. There may be a marked compensatory sway of the trunk away from the side of the advancing leg. Swaying and staggering may suggest an element of ataxia, but usually there is no true loss of coordination. The shuffling, scraping sound—together with worn areas at the toes of the shoes—are characteristic. The equinus position of the feet and heel cord shortening often cause the patient to walk on tiptoe.

## The Spastic-Ataxic Gait

Some neurologic disorders cause involvement of both the corticospinal and the proprioceptive pathways (e.g., combined system disease due to vitamin $B_{12}$ deficiency, or multiple sclerosis), resulting in a gait that has features of both spasticity and ataxia. The relative proportion of each abnormality depends on the particulars of the case. The ataxic component may be either cerebellar or sensory. In vitamin $B_{12}$ deficiency it is predominantly sensory; in multiple sclerosis, both components may be present. In amyotrophic lateral sclerosis there may be bilateral foot drops, as well as spasticity, resulting in an abnormality in walking that may suggest a spastic ataxic gait. The gait has been described as "jiggling" or "bobbing," with tremulous, bouncing, up-and-down body movements.

## The Parkinsonian Gait

The gait in most akinetic-rigid, parkinsonian syndromes is characterized by rigidity, bradykinesia, and loss of associated movements. The patient is stooped, with head and neck forward and knees flexed; the upper extremities are flexed at the shoulders, elbows, and wrists, but the fingers are usually extended (Figure 21.1). The gait is slow, stiff, and shuffling; the patient walks with small, mincing steps. Difficulty walking may be one of the earliest symptoms of the disease. The same gait disorder can occur with any condition causing parkinsonism, such as drug side effects.

## Marche à Petits Pas (Frontal Gait)

The marche à petits pas (walk of little steps) gait resembles that of parkinsonism, but lacks the rigidity and bradykinesia. Locomotion is slow, and the patient walks with very short, mincing, shuffling, and somewhat irregular footsteps. The length of the step may be less than the length of the foot. There is often a loss of associated movements. This type of gait may be seen in normal elderly persons, but also occurs in patients who have diffuse cerebral hemispheric dysfunction, particularly involving the frontal lobes. It may also occur as part of the syndrome of normal pressure hydrocephalus, and in other types of hydrocephalus. The same gait disturbance is typical of multi-infarct dementia or lacunar state. In some patients with marche à petits pas there are bizarre movements such as dancing or hopping. There may be generalized weakness of the lower extremities or of the entire body, with the patient fatiguing easily.

## Gait Apraxia

Apraxia of gait is the loss of the ability to use the legs properly in walking, without demonstrable sensory impairment, weakness, incoordination, or other apparent explanation. Gait apraxia is seen in patients with extensive cerebral lesions, especially of the frontal lobes. It is a common feature of normal pressure hydrocephalus, and may occur in frontal lobe neoplasms, Binswanger disease, Pick disease, and other conditions that cause diffuse frontal lobe dysfunction. The patient cannot carry out purposeful movements with the legs and feet, such as making a circle or kicking an imaginary ball. In rising, standing, and walking there is difficulty in initiating movement, and the automatic sequence of component movements is lost. The gait is slow and shuffling, with short steps. The patients may have the greatest difficulty initiating walking, making small, feeble, stepping movements with minimal forward progress. Eventually the patient may be essentially unable to lift the feet from the floor, as if they were stuck or glued down; or may raise them in place without advancing them (magnetic gait, gait ignition failure, start hesitation). After a few hesitant shuffles, the stride length may increase (slipping clutch gait). When trying to turn, the patient may freeze (turn hesitation). The patient may be able to imitate normal walking movements when sitting or lying down, but eventually even this ability is often lost. In addition, perseveration, hypokinesia, rigidity, and stiffness of the limb in response to contact (gegenhalten) are often seen.

## Frontal Gait Disorder

The abnormal gait that occurs in frontal lobe disease is difficult to describe and classify, and is in many ways similar to, perhaps identical to, gait apraxia. Many terms have been used, which refer to more or less the same phenomenon, including: gait apraxia, frontal disequilibrium, Bruns apraxia/ataxia, magnetic gait, and lower half/body parkinsonism. Lesions of the frontal lobe, or of the frontal lobe connections with the basal ganglia and cerebellum, may lead to a gait disorder characterized by a slightly flexed posture, short, shuffling steps, and an inability to integrate and coordinate lower-extremity movements to accomplish normal ambulation. The disorder has been attributed to involvement of the frontopontocerebellar fibers at their origin in the frontal lobe, but the explanation is probably more complex. The abnormality is very similar to gait apraxia.

## Steppage (Equine) Gait

A problem arises with the use of the term "steppage," which means that the patient is lifting one or both legs high during their respective stride phases, as though she were walking up steps though the surface is level. Patients with foot drop may do this in order to help the foot clear the floor and avoid tripping. Patients with sensory ataxia, classically tabes dorsalis, may also lift the feet up high and then slap them down smartly to improve proprioceptive feedback. Since both of these gaits are "high-stepping," both have been referred to as steppage gaits, but the causes and mechanisms are quite different.

A patient with foot drop has weakness of the dorsiflexors of the foot and toes. When mild, this may be manifest only as a decrease in the toe clearance during the stride phase. With more severe foot drop the patient is in danger of tripping, and may drag the toe when she walks, characteristically wearing out the toe of her shoe. When foot drop is severe, the foot dangles uncontrollably during the swing phase. To compensate, she lifts the foot as high as possible, hiking the hip and flexing the hip and knee. The foot is thrown out and falls to the floor, toe first. The touching of the toe, followed by the heel creates a "double tap" that has a different sound than the heel-first double tap of sensory ataxia. The patient is unable to stand on her heel, and when standing with her foot projecting over the edge of a step, the forefoot drops. The foot drops and steppage gait may be unilateral or bilateral. Common causes of unilateral foot drop and steppage gait include peroneal nerve palsy and L5 radiculopathy. Causes of bilateral foot drop and steppage gait include amyotrophic lateral sclerosis, Charcot-Marie-Tooth disease and other severe peripheral neuropathies, and certain forms of muscular dystrophy.

## The Myopathic (Waddling) Gait

Myopathic gaits occur when there is weakness of the hip girdle muscles, most often due to myopathy, and most characteristically due to muscular dystrophy. If the hip flexors are weak there may be a pronounced lordosis. The hip abductor muscles are vital in stabilizing the pelvis while walking. Trendelenburg sign is an abnormal drop of the pelvis on the side of the swing leg due to hip abductor weakness. When the weakness is bilateral, there is an exaggerated pelvic swing that results in a waddling gait. The patient walks with a broad base, with an exaggerated rotation of the pelvis, rolling or throwing the hips from side to side with every step to shift the weight of the body. In the extreme forms, this gait pattern has a bizarre appearance. The patient walks with a pronounced waddle, shoulders thrown back and pelvis thrust forward. This form of gait is particularly common in facioscapulohumeral muscular dystrophy. The myopathy patient has marked difficulty climbing stairs, often needing to pull herself up with the hand rail. Patients also have difficulty going from a lying to standing position without placing the hands on the knees and hips to push themselves up (Gowers sign, Fig. 20.3).

## Cautious ("Senile") Gait

A cautious gait is seen in older patients who have no neurologic disease but are uncertain of their balance and postural reflexes. The gait takes on the characteristics seen when a healthy person walks on an icy surface: velocity slows, steps shorten, and the base widens.

## Hyperkinetic Gait

In conditions such as Sydenham chorea, Huntington disease, other forms of transient or persistent chorea, athetosis, and dystonia the abnormal movements may become more marked while the patient is walking, and the manifestations of the disease more evident. Walking may accentuate not only the hyperkinesias, but also the abnormalities of power and tone that accompany them. In Huntington disease, the gait may be grotesque, dancing or prancing with abundant extraneous movement. It may look histrionic but is all too real. In athetosis, the distal movements, and in dystonia the proximal movements, may be marked during walking, and in both there are accompanying grimaces.

## Gaits Associated with Focal Weakness

In addition to the steppage gait that accompanies foot drop, weakness limited to other muscle groups may cause gait difficulties. With paralysis of the gastrocnemius and soleus muscles, the patient is unable to stand on the toes, and unable to push off to enter the swing phase with the affected leg. This may cause a shuffling gait that is devoid of spring. In weakness of the quadriceps muscle (e.g., femoral neuropathy), there is weakness of knee extension, and the patient can only accept weight on the affected extremity by bracing the knee. When walking the knee is held stiffly, and there is a tendency to fall if the knee bends. The patient has less difficulty walking backward than forward. Lumbosacral radiculopathy may cause either foot drop or a unilateral Trendelenberg gait, or both. In addition, the patient with acute radiculopathy may walk with a list or pelvic tilt, accompanied by flattening of the normal lumbar lordosis because of low back muscle spasm. The patient may walk with small steps; if the pain is severe, she may place only the toes on the floor, since dorsiflexion of the foot aggravates the pain. Patients commonly use a cane to avoid bearing weight on the involved leg.

## NON-NEUROLOGIC GAIT DISORDERS

Abnormalities of gait may occur for many other reasons and may be confused with neurologic disorders. An antalgic gait is one in which walking is disordered because of pain. Pain in a lower extremity, for whatever reason, causes a shortening of the stance phase on the involved limb as the patient seeks to avoid bearing weight. On more than one occasion, neurologic consultation has been requested in a patient who ultimately proved to have acute podagra or a hip fracture. Arthritis may cause difficulties with gait that are secondary to both pain and deformity. In pregnancy, ascites, and abdominal tumors there may be a lordosis that resembles that seen in the muscular dystrophies. With dislocation of the hips, there may be waddling suggestive of a myopathic gait. A waddling gait is also typical of advanced pregnancy. Patients with severe orthostatic hypotension may complain of difficulty walking rather than dizziness. Marked stooping in ankylosing spondylitis may resemble parkinsonism. A gait abnormality due to generalized weakness may occur after a period of bed rest, or in wasting and debilitating diseases. It is characterized mainly by unsteadiness and the wish for support. The patient staggers and sways from side to side with a suggestion of ataxia. She moves slowly and the knees may tremble. If the difficulty is marked, she may fall.

## NONORGANIC GAIT ABNORMALITIES

Derangements of station and gait on a nonorganic basis are common. Affected patients may be unable either to stand or walk, despite the absence of weakness or other objective neurologic abnormalities. Testing for strength, tone, and coordination is normal if carried out supine.

The gait abnormality in hysteria (astasia-abasia) is nondescript and bizarre, and may take any number of forms that do not conform to a specific organic disease pattern. The gait is irregular and variable, with a great deal of superfluous movement and often marked swaying from side to side. The patient may appear to be in great danger of falling, but rarely does so, often demonstrating superb balance during the contortions. If she does fall, it is in a theatrical manner without injury. The bizarre movements often require better than normal coordination. The patient may balance on the stance leg for a prolonged period of time, while bringing up the swing leg with a great show of effort. The gait may suggest the presence of a monoparesis, hemiparesis, or paraparesis, yet the limbs can be used in an emergency. The gait may show skating, hopping, dancing, or zigzag characteristics; the legs may be thrown out wildly, or there may be a tendency to kneel every few steps. Tremulousness of the extremities or tic-like or compulsive features may be present.

Although the patient cannot walk forward, she may be able to walk backward or to one side or to run without difficulty. The term astasia-abasia originated in an 1888 monograph by Blocq, and the condition is sometimes referred to as Blocq syndrome. Blocq described patients who were able to jump, or walk on all fours, but unable to stand upright (astasia) or to walk (abasia). Astasia-abasia is characterized by normal lower-extremity function when recumbent, yet an inability to walk. This same pattern can occur in lesions involving the cerebellar vermis, such as alcoholic cerebellar degeneration or medulloblastoma.

# The Autonomic Nervous System

# CHAPTER 34

## The Autonomic Nervous System

The autonomic nervous system (ANS) is the system that controls nonstriated muscles and glands. There are three divisions of the ANS: sympathetic (thoracolumbar), parasympathetic (craniosacral), and enteric. The sympathetic and parasympathetic divisions are characterized by a two-neuron chain with two anatomic elements: a preganglionic (first order) neuron within the central nervous system (CNS) that terminates in a ganglion outside the CNS, and a post-ganglionic (second order) neuron that carries impulses to a destination in the viscera. The enteric nervous system is located in the walls of the gastrointestinal tract. In addition, dorsal root ganglion neurons convey afferent visceral impulses that arise in both sympathetic and parasympathetic fibers. There are also autonomic neurons within the CNS at various levels from the cerebral cortex to the spinal cord. Autonomic functions are beyond voluntary control and for the most part beneath consciousness.

### EXAMINATION

The history in patients with autonomic insufficiency may reveal symptoms related to orthostatic hypotension, abnormalities of sweating, or dysfunction of the GI or genitourinary tracts. Symptoms of orthostasis include dizziness or lightheadedness, feelings of presyncope, syncope, palpitations, tremulousness, weakness, confusion, or slurred speech, all worse with standing. Occasional patients complain only of difficulty walking. The symptoms of orthostasis are often worse postprandially, after a hot bath or ingestion of alcohol, or following exercise. Sweating abnormalities may produce abnormal dryness of the skin, sometimes with excessive sweating in uninvolved regions. Other symptoms include constipation, dysphagia, early satiety, anorexia, diarrhea (particularly at night), weight loss, erectile dysfunction, ejaculatory failure, retrograde ejaculation, urinary retention, urinary urgency, recurrent urinary tract infections, and urinary or fecal incontinence.

The general physical and neurologic examinations may reveal a variety of abnormalities in patients with disorders of the autonomic nervous system. Acromegaly, dwarfism, signs of endocrine imbalance or sexual immaturity may indicate a hypothalamic abnormality. Abnormal dryness of the skin may be a sign of sudomotor failure and could occur in a localized distribution, as with a peripheral nerve injury, or be generalized, as in diffuse dysautonomia. Lack of normal moisture in the socks may indicate deficient sweating. A simple bedside test to demonstrate the distribution of abnormal skin dryness related to loss of sweating is to note the resistance to stroking of the skin with a finger or an object such as the barrel of a pen or a spoon. When a spoon is drawn over the skin, it pulls smoothly over dry (sympathectomized) skin but irregularly and unevenly over moist, perspiring skin. It is often possible to see the sweat droplets on the skin, especially on the papillary ridges of the fingers, using the +20 ophthalmoscope lens. Other cutaneous signs of autonomic dysregulation include changes in skin temperature or color, mottling, alopecia, hypertrichosis, thickening or fragility of the nails, absent piloerection, decreased hand wrinkling in water, and skin atrophy. Acral vasomotor dysregulation may lead to pallor, acrocyanosis, mottling, erythema, or livedo reticularis. Patients with dysautonomia associated with a regional pain syndrome may have allodynia and hyperalgesia in addition to the autonomic changes.

Assessment of orthostatic changes in blood pressure (BP) and heart rate (HR) are basic tests of cardiovascular autonomic function. At the bedside, BP and pulse are taken with the patient supine and after standing for variable periods, typically the BP is determined at 1, 3, and 5 minutes after standing. Tilt table testing is more precise. Normally, systolic blood pressure (SBP) on standing does not decrease by more than 20 mm Hg, and the diastolic blood pressure (DBP) by not more than 10 mm Hg. There are more stringent diagnostic criteria that permit a 30-point drop in SBP or a 15-point drop in DBP in normals. When BP measurement is done with a standard sphygmomanometer, the cuff should be kept at heart level to minimize hydrostatic influence on the measurement. When routine measurements are unrevealing, orthostatic blood pressure declines can sometimes be detected by having the patient perform 5 to 10 squats and then repeating the measurements.

The HR should not increase by more than 30 beats per minute above baseline on standing. In hypovolemia, the most common cause of orthostasis, a reflex tachycardia develops in response to the fall in standing blood pressure. When autonomic cardiovascular reflexes are impaired, the reflex tachycardia may not occur. Patients with the postural tachycardia syndrome will develop a brisk tachycardia without orthostatic hypotension (increased pulse rate more than 30 beats per minute above baseline or more than 120 beats per minute). The sustained hand grip, mental stress, and cold pressor tests all look for increases in DBP of at least 15 mm Hg or an increase in HR of >10 beats per minute in response to peripheral vasoconstriction induced respectively by isometric hand exercise, mental arithmetic, or immersion of the hand in cold water. The cold face test assesses the trigeminovagal (diving) reflex. Resting tachycardia may be a sign of parasympathetic dysfunction.

Clinical assessment of bladder function is done by looking for evidence of distension by palpation and percussion, and by checking the anal wink and bulbocavernous reflexes. The bulbocavernous and superficial anal reflexes are somatic motor reflexes; the internal anal and scrotal reflexes are autonomic reflexes. The internal anal sphincter reflex is contraction of the internal sphincter on insertion of a gloved finger into the anus. If the reflex is impaired there is decreased sphincter tone and the anus does not close immediately after withdrawal. Post void residual urine volume is determined by catheterization after voiding.

Tear production by the lacrimal glands can be evaluated in a number of ways by ophthalmologists. A convenient and simple bedside assessment can be obtained with the Schirmer test, done by placing a strip of sterile filter paper in the lower conjunctival sac and measuring the degree of wetting over 5 minutes. Additional eye findings include excessive dryness with redness and itching, and ptosis. When autonomic failure occurs as part of a neurologic illness (such as multisystem atrophy), there may be findings related to the underlying condition such as extrapyramidal or cerebellar signs, abnormal eye movements, weakness, sensory loss, or reflex abnormalities.

## Autonomic Function Testing

Many different procedures have been developed to test the sympathetic and parasympathetic nervous systems. Tests of cardiac vagal tone include assessment of heart rate variability to deep breathing, standing, and performing Valsalva. The beat-to-beat changes in heart rate in response to autonomic reflexes occur quickly, often too quickly for bedside assessment to be accurate. It is possible at the bedside to determine if heart rate variability with respiration or to Valsalva is present and obvious (probably normal), present but minimal (possibly abnormal), or absent (abnormal). More precise testing requires equipment, and may include an indwelling arterial catheter to follow BP changes. The respiratory variability in heart rate is exaggerated when a Valsalva maneuver is performed.

Tilt-table testing evaluates the integrity of autonomic reflexes. Autonomic laboratories use different degrees of tilt, but usually in the range of 60 degrees to 80 degrees and for different durations. In neurocardiogenic (vasovagal, vasodepressor) syncope, or fainting, hypotension is accompanied by bradycardia, rather than the tachycardia that should occur. It occurs in response to emotional upsets such as fear, stress, or the sight of blood, occasionally in relation to micturition (micturition syncope) or coughing (cough syncope), and sometimes without identifiable provocation. Tilt-table testing has shown that a neurocardiogenic mechanism is responsible for a large proportion of the patients with recurrent, unexplained syncope. There are laboratory procedures available to assess thermoregulatory and sudomotor function.

## DISORDERS OF THE AUTONOMIC NERVOUS SYSTEM

Autonomic disorders can be divided into those that affect the central autonomic elements and are typically associated with other evidence of CNS disease, and those that affect the peripheral autonomic nervous system. Multiple system atrophy (MSA) is a degenerative neurologic disorder, which is usually accompanied by prominent dysautononia. The autonomic failure in MSA results from involvement of preganglionic neurons in the brainstem and spinal cord in the degenerative process. Autonomic dysfunction may also occur in patients with Parkinson disease, but usually late in the illness and not to the degree typical of MSA. Autonomic disturbances may accompany seizures, including cardiovascular changes, flushing, pallor, sweating, shivering, piloerection, vomiting, and respiratory abnormalities. Seizure-induced cardiovascular abnormalities include sinus tachycardia, bradyarrhythmia, sinus arrest, and ventricular tachyarrhythmias, including ventricular fibrillation.

Hypothalamic disorders may cause many abnormalities of autonomic function, including deficiencies in osmoregulation and thermoregulation, as well as abnormalities of appetite, and body weight; sleep disturbances; changes in carbohydrate, fat, and water metabolism; and respiratory abnormalities; together with, in many instances, behavioral abnormalities and personality changes. Hypothalamic lesions may cause either hyperthermia or hypothermia. Hyperthermia generally results from involvement of the tuberal region, especially the supraoptic nuclei or the rostral portion of the anterior hypothalamus. It is a common manifestation of third ventricular tumors, and may occur after head trauma or cranial surgery; terminal hyperthermia is a frequent manifestation of neurologic disease (central fever). Hypothermia tends to occur with involvement of the posterior hypothalamic area and mammillary bodies. Disorders of the anterior hypothalamus tend to cause loss of the ability to regulate against heat, and of the posterior hypothalamus with loss of the ability to regulate against cold.

The hypothalamus is closely related anatomically and physiologically to the pituitary gland. Since the hypothalamus controls the release of many of the anterior pituitary hormones, abnormalities of hypothalamic function may have a close relationship to some endocrine disorders. Lesions of the supraoptic nuclei or the supraopticohypophyseal tract cause diabetes insipidus. Diabetes insipidus is a common manifestation of tumors in the parasellar region, encephalitis, and meningitis, and it may develop after intracranial surgery or head injury.

Abnormalities of respiration may be caused by hypothalamic dysfunction. These include hyperpnea, apnea, Cheyne-Stokes respirations, and Biot breathing. Disturbances of the sleep cycle may occur with hypothalamic lesions, especially those involving its posterior portions, including the mammillary bodies. There may be hypersomnolence, inversion of the sleep cycle, or insomnia. Neurons in the lateral hypothalamus synthesize hypocretin, a chemical involved in the pathogenesis of narcolepsy. Disturbances of sexual function and sexual development occur with hypothalamic lesions, including precocious puberty and sexual infantilism.

The hypothalamus is involved with emotions. It is the center that coordinates the neural and humoral mechanisms of emotional expression. Hypothalamic lesions in animals may cause "sham rage," with pupillary dilatation, increased pulse rate and blood pressure, piloerection, and other signs of sympathetic overactivity. These physical manifestations suggest an intense emotional reaction is taking place, but there is no change in affect.

Brainstem disorders commonly cause autonomic dysfunction, including paroxysmal hypertension, profound bradycardia, intractable vomiting, central hypoventilation, neurogenic pulmonary edema, and Horner syndrome. The automatic and the voluntary breathing pathways are separated in the brainstem and upper spinal cord. Selective damage of the pathways subserving automatic breathing may cause respiratory insufficiency during sleep, with preserved respiration during wakefulness (Ondine curse). Myelopathy, particularly spinal cord injury, is often associated with severe dysautonomia. The Cushing reflex, or Cushing triad, is bradycardia, hypertension, and slow, irregular respirations due to brainstem compromise, and has ominous prognostic implications.

Peripheral autonomic failure results from disorders that involve the autonomic ganglia or postganglionic nerve fibers. The syndrome of pure autonomic failure is a slowly progressive, degenerative disorder of the ANS in which dysautonomia occurs in isolation, without other evidence of neurologic disease. Dysautonomia occurs commonly in some peripheral nerve disorders. The most common cause of autonomic neuropathy is diabetes mellitus. Patients typically develop orthostatic hypotension, impotence, gastroparesis, constipation alternating with diarrhea, nocturnal diarrhea, and difficulty voiding.

Dysautonomia may accompany disorders of neuromuscular transmission, particularly Lambert-Eaton syndrome and botulism, in which the defect is presynaptic and acetylcholine release is impaired at autonomic synapses as well as at neuromuscular junctions. Some autonomic disorders occur in a restricted distribution or involve a particular organ system. Autonomic disorders of the pupil include Argyll Robertson and Adie pupils, Horner syndrome, and third cranial nerve palsy. Dysautonomia primarily involving the vascular system may cause Raynaud phenomenon, acrocyanosis, erythromelalgia (Weir Mitchell syndrome), and livedo reticularis. Autonomic dysfunction of the genitalia causing erectile dysfunction and other abnormalities is common, especially in diabetes mellitus. Abnormalities of sweating occur frequently and are sometimes the only manifestation of the autonomic disturbance. Autonomic dysregulation is a common component of complex regional pain syndromes (reflex sympathetic dystrophy) and occurs in the same distribution as the pain.

## The Bladder

Bladder function involves both the autonomic and the voluntary nervous systems, and disorders of bladder function may follow lesions of the paracentral lobule, hypothalamus, descending pathways in the spinal cord, pre- or postganglionic parasympathetic nerves, or pudendal nerve. The detrusor muscle of the bladder is innervated by parasympathetic neurons located in the S2–S4 intermediolateral column. Onuf's nucleus consists of additional motor neurons located in the nearby anterior horn at the same levels. The axons from Onuf's nucleus innervate the external urethral sphincter. There is a curious preservation of the Onuf's nucleus neurons in amyotrophic lateral sclerosis. The internal urethral sphincter at the neck of the bladder receives its innervation from the intermediolateral column at the T12–L1 level, via the sympathetic prevertebral plexus and the hypogastric nerve.

Micturition is a spino-bulbo-spinal reflex. Normal micturition requires intact autonomic and spinal pathways, and cerebral inhibition and control of the external sphincter must be normal. Forebrain lesions may cause loss of voluntary bladder control, but do not affect the spino-bulbo-spinal reflex mechanisms. Disruption of the bulbospinal pathway from the pontine micturition center to the sacral cord, and lesions affecting the afferent and efferent connections between the bladder and the conus medullaris may cause severe disturbances in bladder function.

The term neurogenic bladder refers to bladder dysfunction caused by disease of the nervous system. Symptoms of bladder dysfunction are often among the earliest manifestations of nervous system disease. Frequency, urgency, precipitate micturition, massive or dribbling incontinence, difficulty in initiating urination, urinary retention, and loss of bladder sensation may occur.

## Sexual Function

Disturbed sexual function is common in dysautonomia. In the genital (sex, ejaculatory, coital) reflex, arousal causes penile erection and sometimes ejaculation. Erection is a parasympathetic function mediated through S2–S4; ejaculation is a largely sympathetic function mediated by the lumbar nerves. Autonomic insufficiency usually causes impotence, but pathologic exaggeration of the sexual reflex may occur as part of the mass reflex, a spinal defense reflex seen in severe myelopathy, and may produce priapism and occasionally ejaculation after minimal stimulation. In autonomic neuropathy, especially from diabetes, retrograde ejaculation may precede the development of impotence. Because the internal vesical sphincter does not close, semen goes into the bladder rather than externally through the urethra. The patient with retrograde ejaculation may notice milky-appearing urine.

# Special Methods of Examination

# CHAPTER 35

## The Examination in Coma

**W**orkup of the patient with coma or altered mental status is often complex and always urgent. The neurologic examination is only one of several diagnostic methods that can be brought to bear in coma; and imaging, cerebrospinal fluid (CSF), and laboratory investigations play a vital role. However, the findings on examination often determine the early management, and the urgency with which imaging and CSF studies are obtained. Coma is a complicated topic, and this discussion will focus on what can be learned from the examination.

Consciousness has two dimensions: arousal and cognition. Arousal is a primitive function sustained by deep brainstem and medial thalamic structures. Cognitive functions require an intact cerebral cortex and major subcortical nuclei. In coma, stupor, and hypersomnia there is a lowering of consciousness; in confusion and delirium there is a clouding of consciousness.

### THE ANATOMY OF CONSCIOUSNESS

The ascending reticular activating system (RAS) is a system of fibers which arises from the reticular formation of the brainstem, primarily the paramedian tegmentum of the upper pons and midbrain, and projects to the paramedian, parafascicular, centromedian, and intralaminar nuclei of the thalamus. Neurons in the reticular formation also receive collaterals from the ascending spinothalamic pathways and send projections diffusely to the entire cerebral cortex, so that sensory stimuli are involved not only with sensory perception but—through their connections with the RAS—with the maintenance of consciousness. The fibers in the RAS are cholinergic, adrenergic, dopaminergic, serotonergic, and histaminergic. Experimentally, stimulation of the RAS produces arousal, and destruction of the RAS produces coma. The hypothalamus is also important for consciousness; arousal can be produced by stimulation of the posterior hypothalamic region.

Processes producing coma can be characterized as either structural or metabolic. Although restricted, focal lesions of the RAS can produce profound alterations in consciousness; hemispheric lesions cause coma only when extensive and bilateral, such as with head injury, meningitis, encephalitis, or bilateral cerebral infarction. The degree of alteration in consciousness is roughly proportional to the volume of brain tissue involved in the process. Focal lesions restricted to either hemisphere rarely produce significant alterations of consciousness. Metabolic processes produce coma by diffusely affecting the cerebral hemispheres or depressing the activity in the RAS, or both.

## INITIAL MANAGEMENT OF COMA

Because of the dire consequences to the brain of lack of substrate, the initial management of coma, unless the cause is immediately apparent, is directed toward correction of possible deficiencies in glucose, oxygenation, and blood pressure; these emergency measures are necessary, even before a detailed history and examination. After initial determination of vital signs, attention should first be directed toward ensuring an adequate airway and oxygenation, blood pressure, and intravenous access. After obtaining emergency blood samples, 50 cc of 50% glucose should be given, followed quickly by 100 mg of thiamine IV in case the patient is alcoholic (Wernicke encephalopathy can be precipitated by IV glucose in such patients). Naloxone and flumazenil are often given empirically in case there has been an opiate or benzodiazepine overdose. A "coma cocktail," consisting of dextrose, flumazenil, naloxone, and thiamine is sometimes used in the initial management of the comatose patient. Because the rapid reagent test strips used for glucose determination are not infallible, studies favor empirical administration of dextrose and thiamine to patients with altered consciousness, but naloxone should probably be reserved for patients with signs and symptoms of opioid intoxication, and flumazenil best left for reversal of therapeutic conscious sedation and rare select cases of benzodiazepine overdose. Preparations for intubation, respiratory support, and use of pressor agents must be made, should they become necessary. Always assume a cervical spine injury may be present, and immobilize the neck until a fracture can be ruled out.

## DIAGNOSTIC ASSESSMENT

After ensuring adequate oxygenation and substrate for the central nervous system (CNS), a rapid neurologic examination should be performed to search for obvious signs, such as a dilated pupil, that may require urgent imaging and neurosurgical intervention. Otherwise, the initial emergent management should be followed by a history and general physical and neurologic examinations.

### History

Though often difficult and sometimes impossible to obtain, historical information is extremely important and well worth pursuing vigorously. In the absence of family, a phone call to the neighbor, landlord, or companion may yield valuable details about the sequence of events leading to coma, the patient's past health and illnesses, and current medications. A history of known seizure disorder, diabetes mellitus, hypertension, substance abuse, depression, or suicide attempts may emerge. Check the wallet or purse for medication lists, a doctor's card or phone number, medical alert card, or other pertinent information. Talk with police or ambulance drivers if they are involved.

## General Physical Examination

Findings on the general physical examination may be extremely helpful in elucidating the cause of altered consciousness (Table 35.1). The patient should always be examined carefully for bruises and hematomas, lacerations, fractures, and other signs of injury, especially about the head. It is essential to remember that two conditions may occur together (e.g., trauma and alcoholic intoxication). Simple vital signs may provide important clues. An elevated temperature suggests infection or serious intracranial disease. Extremely elevated blood pressure suggests hypertensive encephalopathy or subarachnoid hemorrhage. Hypotension suggests impaired CNS perfusion due to some systemic process, such as hemorrhage or myocardial disease. Hypotension rarely occurs because of primary CNS disease, except in the terminal phase. Either tachycardia or bradycardia may impair CNS perfusion. The combination of hypertension and bradycardia suggests brainstem dysfunction, often because of increased intracranial pressure (Cushing reflex).

Abnormalities of respiration are important in the evaluation of patients with depressed consciousness. Abnormal respiratory patterns due to neurologic disease include Cheyne-Stokes respirations (CSR), central neurogenic hyperventilation, ataxic breathing, and apneustic breathing. In CSR, periods of hyperpnea alternate with periods of hypopnea. Respirations increase in depth and volume up to a peak, and then decline until there is a period of apnea, after which the cycle repeats. In posthyperventilation apnea, a brief period of hyperventilation is followed by apnea lasting 15 to 30 seconds or longer. The mechanisms underlying CSR and posthyperventilation apnea are likely similar. Cheyne-Stokes respirations may be due to bilateral hemisphere lesions, as well as to increased intracranial pressure and cardiopulmonary dysfunction. In respiratory ataxia, the pattern of breathing is irregular, with erratic shallow and deep respiratory movements. Ataxic breathing occurs with dysfunction of the medullary respiratory centers, and may signify impending agonal respirations and apnea. Central neurogenic hyperventilation refers to sustained, rapid, and regular hyperpnea. It is primarily associated with disease affecting the paramedian reticular formation in the low midbrain and upper pons, but it may also occur with lesions in other brainstem locations, either intra-axial or extra-axial. Apneustic breathing, which is rare, causes a prolonged inspiratory phase, and occurs in pontine lesions just rostral to the trigeminal motor nuclei, or cervicomedullary compression. Abnormal respiratory patterns may occur because of systemic disease, such as diabetic ketoacidosis (Table 35.1). Slow, regular respirations are noted with a variety of substance or drug intoxications and in severe myxedema.

Note the patient's appearance and behavior, apparent age, grooming, and signs of acute or chronic illnesses such as fever, cyanosis, jaundice, pallor, and signs of dehydration and loss of weight. Assess responses to noises, verbal commands, visual stimuli, threats, and tactile and painful stimulation, and whether there has been incontinence. Note whether the patient, even in coma, appears to be comfortable and natural or assumes unnatural positions. Carefully observe spontaneous movements, and the reaction to various stimuli. Note general activity (immobile, underactive, restless, or hyperkinetic), tone (limp, relaxed, rigid, or tense), and the presence of abnormal movements (tremors, twitches, tics, grimaces, and spasms). Motor unrest and excessive activity are seen in both organic and psychogenic states. If there is seizure activity, note the distribution and pattern of spread of the convulsive movements, and any associated manifestations such as the degree of impairment of consciousness, frothing at the mouth, tongue biting, and incontinence.

The behavior of the patient should be observed closely and as often as necessary until the diagnosis is established. Note the patient's reactions to physicians, nurses, and relatives. Do the eyes follow people? Is there some awareness of what is happening in the immediate environment? The conduct may be constant or may vary from time to time. For instance, the patient may appear to be completely unconscious and fail to respond to any type of stimulation while the observer is in the room, yet when not aware of being watched, may open the eyes, make furtive glances, and move around.

## TABLE 35.1

**Findings on General Physical Examination that May Provide a Clue to the Etiology of Coma or Altered Mental Status**

| System | Finding | Possible Implications |
|---|---|---|
| Blood pressure | Hypotension | Hypovolemia, MI, intoxication (especially ETOH and barbiturates), Wernicke encephalopathy, sepsis |
| | Hypertension | Stroke, intracranial hemorrhage, increased ICP, hypertensive encephalopathy, renal disease |
| Heart rate | Bradycardia | Heart disease, intoxication, increased ICP |
| | Tachycardia | Hypovolemia, cocaine overdose, infection |
| Respiration | Breath odor | Acetone (DKA), ETOH (intoxication), fetor hepaticus, uriniferous (uremia), garlic odor (arsenic poisoning), household gas (carbon monoxide) |
| | Hyperventilation | Hypoxia, hypercapnia, acidosis, fever, liver disease, sepsis, pulmonary emboli, toxins or drugs producing metabolic acidosis, central neurogenic hyperventilation, salicylism |
| | Hypoventilation | Overdose, myxedema |
| | Cheyne-Stokes | Bilateral cerebral disease, impending transtentorial herniation, upper brainstem lesions, metabolic encephalopathy, CHF |
| | Cluster breathing | Increased ICP, posterior fossa lesion |
| | Apneustic breathing | Pontine lesion, transtentorial herniation, metabolic coma |
| | Ataxic breathing | Medullary lesion |
| | Ondine's curse | Medullary lesion |
| Temperature | Fever | Infection, inflammation, neoplasms (rare), anticholinergics, SAH, hypothalamic lesion, heatstroke, thyroid storm, malignant hyperthermia |
| | Hypothermia | Exposure, sepsis, shock, myxedema coma, Wernicke encephalopathy, drug intoxication (especially barbiturates), hypothalamic lesion, hypoglycemia |
| Head and neck | Scalp laceration or edema, Battle sign, raccoon eyes | Trauma |
| | Stiff neck | Meningitis, SAH, cerebellar tonsillar herniation |
| | Unilateral, fixed dilated pupil | Uncal herniation, aneurysm |
| | Small, reactive pupils | Metabolic coma, early transtentorial herniation |
| | Bilateral, large, fixed pupils | Midbrain or pretectal lesion (tectal pupils) |

## TABLE 35.1 *(Continued)*

### Findings on General Physical Examination that May Provide a Clue to the Etiology of Coma or Altered Mental Status

| System | Finding | Possible Implications |
|---|---|---|
| | Midposition, fixed pupils | Midbrain stage of transtentorial herniation |
| | Pinpoint pupils | Pontine hemorrhage or infarct, opiate overdose |
| | Fundus exam | Papilledema (increased ICP), hypertensive or diabetic retinopathy, subhyaloid hemorrhages, Roth spots |
| Skin | Needle tracks | Drug overdose |
| | Cyanosis | Hypoxia, cardiac disease, cyanide |
| | Cherry red | Carbon monoxide intoxication |
| | Jaundice | Hepatic encephalopathy, hemolysis |
| | Pallor | Anemia, hemorrhage, shock, vasomotor syncope |
| | Petechiae | DIC, TTP, meningococcemia, drugs, fat embolism |
| | Purpuric rash | Meningococcemia, RMSF, and others |
| | Maculopapular rash | Toxic shock syndrome, SBE, SLE, and others |
| | Bruises | Trauma, coagulopathy |
| | Bullous lesions | Drug overdose, especially barbiturates |
| | Sweating | Fever, hypoglycemia |
| | Flushing, erythema | Polycythemia, fever, alcohol intoxication |
| Heart | Arrhythmia | Cerebral embolism |
| | Murmur | SBE, embolism |
| Lungs | Pulmonary edema | Neurogenic pulmonary edema, CHF, anoxic encephalopathy |
| GI | Fecal incontinence | Seizure with post-ictal coma |
| | + stool blood | Hepatic encephalopathy, GI hemorrhage |
| GU | Urinary incontinence | Seizure with post-ictal coma |
| | Hematuria | Cerebral embolism |
| Extremities | Subtle twitching | Subclinical status epilepticus |

CHF, congestive heart failure; DIC, disseminated intravascular coagulation; DKA, diabetic ketoacidosis; ETOH, ethanol; GI, gastrointestinal; GU, genitourinary; ICP, intracranial pressure; MI, myocardial infarction; RMSF, Rocky Mountain spotted fever; SAH, subarachnoid hemorrhage; SBE, subacute bacterial endocarditis; SLE, systemic lupus erythematosus; TTP, thrombotic thrombocytopenic purpura.

After the general physical exam, a focused neurologic exam may help characterize the pathologic process. Specific attention should be paid to the level of responsiveness, pupils, eye movements, and motor responses.

## Neurologic Examination

The details of the neurologic examination in the various states of disordered consciousness necessarily vary with the degree of impairment and depth of coma. As a minimum, the following must be assessed: level of consciousness, pupils, eye movements (including reflex movements), fundoscopic, motor status, reflexes, and meningeal signs. Other portions of the examination then follow as necessary. Coma is most often due to a metabolic process. With rare exception, metabolic

SECTION J ● Special Methods of Examination

encephalopathies are characterized by reactive pupils and a symmetric neurologic examination. Any asymmetry in motor or sensory responses and any pupillary or eye movement abnormality should prompt an immediate, vigorous search for structural disease.

## Level of Responsiveness

Coma is a state of complete loss of consciousness from which the patient cannot be aroused by ordinary stimuli. There is complete unresponsiveness to self and the environment. The patient in coma has no awareness of herself, makes no voluntary movements, and has no sleep-wake cycles. Stupor is a state of partial or relative loss of response to the environment in which the patient's consciousness may be impaired to varying degrees. The patient is difficult to arouse, and although brief stimulation may be possible, responses are slow and inadequate. The patient is otherwise oblivious to what is happening in the environment, and promptly falls back into the stuporous state. The lethargic patient can usually be aroused or awakened and may then appear to be in complete possession of her senses, but promptly falls asleep when left alone. In a confusional state patients may be alert, but are confused and disoriented. Patients with delirium are confused, disoriented, and often agitated; the best example is delirium tremens. Terminologic description of the differences between various states of impaired altered consciousness is at best ambiguous. Because of imprecision and inconsistency in usage, such terms as semi-coma and semi-stupor, all describing changes across a spectrum of altered awareness, are best avoided. It is preferable to describe the patient's state of responsiveness, or use an objective and well-defined scheme, such as the Glasgow coma scale (GCS), which has gained wide acceptance in the evaluation of patients with impaired consciousness, particularly in head injury. In the GCS, scores are obtained for ocular, verbal, and motor functions (Table 35.2). An alert person with normal eye and motor responses would score 15 points; a patient in profound coma would score 3 points. Other coma scales are available. Coma must be distinguished from the persistent vegetative state, locked-in syndrome, and mutism.

## TABLE 35.2

### The Glasgow Coma Scale

| Eye opening | |
|---|---|
| Open spontaneously | 4 |
| Open only to verbal stimuli | 3 |
| Only to pain | 2 |
| Never open | 1 |
| Best verbal response | |
| Oriented and converses | 5 |
| Converses, but disoriented, confused | 4 |
| Uses inappropriate words | 3 |
| Makes incomprehensible sounds | 2 |
| No verbal response | 1 |
| Best motor response | |
| Obeys commands | 6 |
| Localizes pain | 5 |
| Exhibits flexion withdrawal | 4 |
| Decorticate rigidity | 3 |
| Decerebrate rigidity | 2 |
| No motor response | 1 |

The term altered mental status (AMS) is often used to describe a variety of abnormalities of cerebral function. It is used haphazardly to describe patients who have impaired alertness, impaired cognition, or a deficit of higher cortical function. Strictly speaking, the term AMS should imply a change in the level of consciousness, somewhere on a continuum between confusion and coma. It should not be used to describe patients who have impaired cognition with a clear sensorium—those patients have dementia; patients who have focal deficits of higher cortical function, such as aphasia; or used to describe patients who have psychiatric disorders, such as psychosis or mania. Neurologically naive clinicians may lump all these conditions together under the rubric AMS. They are in fact distinctly different conditions, with different etiologies and treatments, and especially with different prognostic implications. Patients with Wernicke aphasia are often thought to have AMS or an acute confusional state.

It is necessary to make reasonable attempts to arouse the patient, and this usually includes assessing the response to a painful stimulus. Commonly used painful stimuli are supraorbital pressure, sternal rub, and nailbed pressure. The stimulus must be adequate but remain humane and considerate. Avoid leaving bruises or other marks on the patient; the reason for these may be misinterpreted by family members and ancillary personnel. An effective and stealthy painful stimulus is to forcibly twist a key or the handle of a reflex hammer between two fingers or toes squeezed tightly together.

## Cranial Nerves

Although cranial nerve examination cannot be carried out in any detail in a patient with altered consciousness, examination of the pupils and extraocular movements are critical in evaluation of the comatose patient. The pupils are critical in the evaluation of altered consciousness. The size, shape, position, equality, and reactivity are all important. Bilateral pinpoint pupils occur with opiate toxicity and other lesions of the pons, such as pontine hemorrhage or thrombosis of the basilar artery. The bilateral miosis seen in large pontine lesions is probably due to dysfunction of the descending sympathetic pathways bilaterally. The light reaction is preserved with lesions involving the descending sympathetic system, but may be very difficult to see without magnification when the pupils are extremely small. Focusing on a tiny pupil with the ophthalmoscope, and turning the light off, then back on, may reveal the residual light reactivity. Hypothermia can cause small, unreactive pupils. Bilateral large pupils in coma are usually an ominous sign, especially when unreactive to light. They occur as a terminal condition in many patients. Bilateral mydriasis may also occur in botulism or anticholinergic intoxication. Midposition (3 mm to 6 mm) unreactive pupils result from lesions affecting both sympathetic and parasympathetic pathways. They occur commonly as a feature of central transtentorial herniation.

Pupillary asymmetry usually indicates structural disease. A unilaterally dilated pupil, especially if unreactive to light, is most often a sign of third nerve palsy, and in the setting of coma usually indicates uncal herniation. Because of the peripheral location of the pupillary fibers in the third nerve, they are especially susceptible to pressure, and pupillary dilation often occurs prior to any eye movement abnormality. Coma with a unilaterally dilated pupil could also result from subarachnoid hemorrhage due to a posterior communicating artery aneurysm. Lateral medullary syndrome may cause anisocoria due to Horner syndrome, along with evidence of brainstem dysfunction, but rarely causes coma. Horner syndrome may also occur with lesions involving the hypothalamus or thalamus (particularly hemorrhage). Ipsilateral Horner syndrome may occur because of carotid artery disease, especially occlusion, but is likely due to hypothalamic ischemia rather than dysfunction of the pericarotid sympathetic plexus. Rarely, seizures may cause transient anisocoria.

Pupillary reactivity is a key sign in distinguishing structural from metabolic coma. Normally reactive pupils in the setting of coma suggest metabolic encephalopathy, which typically affects consciousness and respiration earlier than pupillary function. Loss of pupillary reactivity is more consistent with structural disease or anoxia. Structural lesions of the brainstem usually cause abnormal pupillary responses, and in brain death pupillary responses are absent. Pupillary reactivity is usually preserved in drug-induced coma, except when extremely severe. A notable exception to the rule is that posterior fossa mass effect exerted primarily on the mid and lower brainstem, such as cerebellar infarction or hemorrhage, may initially spare the pupils. Pupillary light reaction is a key prognostic sign. Loss of reactivity portends a poor outcome. Brain injury patients, even those with a GCS of 3, if the pupils remain reactive, may survive. The ciliospinal reflex is another test of pupil reactivity, but it involves pathways caudal to the foramen magnum.

Eye movements and the oculocephalic and oculovestibular reflexes should be examined carefully. Note the position of the eyes at rest, whether there is any nystagmus, and whether the range of ocular movement is full in both directions to passive head movement or oculovestibular stimulation. If there is any possibility of trauma, a cervical spine series should precede neck manipulation for eye movement examination. Roving eye movements indicate that brainstem function is intact. Conjugate eye deviation away from the paralyzed extremities is seen in destructive frontal lobe lesions; conjugate deviation in the direction of the paralyzed extremities indicates a brainstem lesion. Conjugate gaze deviation, sometimes with accompanying nystagmoid jerking, may also occur because of seizure activity in the frontal eye fields on the side the patient is looking away from. Thalamic hemorrhage can cause "wrong-way eyes," with gaze deviation toward the hemiparesis. Vertical gaze deviations suggest brainstem disease; the most common is sustained downgaze with an upgaze deficit due to a lesion involving the upper midbrain or caudal thalamus. Hepatic encephalopathy can cause down-gaze deviation.

Reflex movements elicited by turning the head from side to side (doll's eye movements, oculocephalic reflex) or by the injection of ice water into the external auditory canal (caloric test, oculovestibular reflex) may reveal isolated weakness of particular extraocular muscles, gaze paresis, or other eye movement abnormalities (Figure 35.1). Supratentorial lesions and metabolic processes usually do not affect the oculocephalic reflex. Caloric testing assesses the same brainstem reflexes as the doll's eye maneuver, and is used if the oculocephalic reflex is not intact. After ensuring the external auditory canal is clear, the head is flexed to a 30-degree angle above horizontal and 10 cc to 20 cc of ice water is instilled into the canal. If no response is obtained, larger volumes are used.

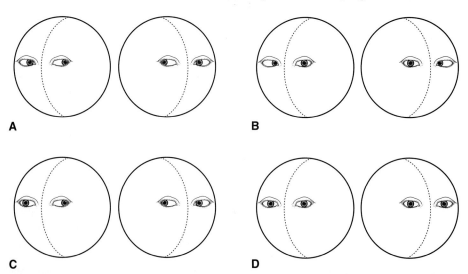

**FIGURE 35.1** ● Examples of oculocephalic responses that may be seen in comatose patients. When the brainstem is intact, the eyes move in the opposite direction from head rotation. **A.** Normal response, the usual response in a patient with metabolic encephalopathy. **B.** Bilateral sixth nerve palsies. **C.** Right third nerve palsy or internuclear ophthalmoplegia. **D.** Absent response, seen when the reflex pathways are impaired.

After 15 to 60 seconds, eye deviation begins and may last several minutes. The expected response in coma is tonic deviation of the eyes toward the side of the irrigated ear. Warm water causes the opposite response. Testing of the other side may be done after about 5 minutes. Brainstem lesions affecting the pathways and nuclei subserving the reflex may cause an abnormal response. In coma, absence of a response to cold calorics suggests sedative hypnotic drug intoxication, a structural lesion of the brainstem, or brain death, unless there is evidence of a vestibular disorder or exposure to vestibular-suppressant drugs. When the response is present, the eye movements may be dysconjugate. Some drugs, particularly sedative–hypnotic agents, tricyclics, and anticonvulsants, may affect eye movements in a comatose patient. Unusual spontaneous eye movements may occur in coma (e.g., ocular bobbing, ping-pong gaze), and the particular pattern often has localizing significance. If the patient is responsive enough, testing for optokinetic nystagmus may give important diagnostic information.

Note whether the eyes are open or closed, and the width of the palpebral fissures on the two sides. When the eyelids are closed in a comatose patient, the lower pons is still functioning. Asymmetry of the palpebral fissures may indicate either upper facial weakness on the side of the wider fissure, or ptosis on the side of the narrower. If the eyes are partially or completely closed, the examiner may try to open them by gently raising the upper lids, and then noting the speed with which the eyes close again. Unilateral orbicularis weakness may produce more leisurely closure on the affected side. In deep coma, the eyes may be open and a glassy stare evident. In profound illness, the patient often lies with the eyes only partially closed, even in sleep, so that a narrow portion of the cornea is visible between the upper and lower lids. In psychogenic unresponsiveness (hysterical coma), the patient may keep the eyes tightly closed and resist attempts to open them, yet open the eyes and glance around when unaware that someone is observing the action. Note whether there is any blinking, flickering, or tremor of the eyelids at rest or in response to a bright light or sudden noise. The corneal reflexes may be absent in coma; any asymmetry of the response may be significant.

In some patients it is possible to obtain facial movement by painful stimulation, such as supraorbital pressure, sternal rub, or pinprick stimulation of the face. The area of the upper nasolabial fold at the junction with the nose is particularly sensitive and a response to pinprick in this region can sometimes be obtained when there is no response over other parts of the face. It is important when examining facial sensation not to traumatize the face and leave pinprick marks, particularly in elderly patients with thin, fragile skin. Firm manual pressure over the supraorbital notch, at the point of emergence of the supraorbital nerve, will often produce facial grimacing. When facial movement does occur, compare the two sides for symmetry of the response. Elicitation of a blink response to loud noise provides a crude assessment of auditory function. The mouth may be either open or closed. In nonorganic unresponsiveness the patient may resist attempts to passively open the mouth. A gag reflex may or may not be present. If present, the palate should rise in the midline.

No neurologic evaluation of coma, stupor, or disordered consciousness is complete without an ophthalmoscopic examination. The presence of papilledema is, of course, indicative of some process causing increased intracranial pressure. Papilledema takes a period of time to develop, and may be absent in acute conditions. Normal spontaneous venous pulsations are a strong indicator of normal intracranial pressure, but absence of venous pulsations does not prove intracranial pressure is increased. Subarachnoid hemorrhage may produce subhyaloid hemorrhages in the retina. The ophthalmoscopic examination is also important in detecting systemic diseases responsible for altered consciousness (e.g., diabetes, hypertension, or endocarditis). It is not possible to test either visual acuity or the visual fields reliably if significant impairment of consciousness is present. If the patient is responsive enough it may be possible to determine if the patient follows objects, or blinks to threat.

## Examination of Motor Status

The motor examination in disorders of consciousness requires skilled observation. It may be difficult to recognize the presence of a hemiplegia in a comatose patient. If the hemiplegia has been of sudden onset, the paralyzed side of the body is usually flaccid. The width of the palpebral fissure is increased, the nasolabial fold is shallow, and the angle of the mouth droops on that side. There may be drooling of saliva and puffing out and retraction of the cheek on expiration and inspiration. If both arms are lifted, or placed with the elbows resting on the bed and the forearms at right angles to the arms, then released by the examiner, the affected extremity falls more rapidly and in a flail-like manner, while the normal arm drops slowly, or may even remain upright for a brief period before falling. If the lower extremities are lifted from the bed and then released, the affected extremity falls rapidly, while the normal limb drops more gradually to the bed. If the lower extremities are passively flexed with heels resting on the bed and then released, the paretic limb rapidly falls to an extended position with the hip in external rotation, while the unaffected limb maintains the posture for a few moments and then gradually returns to its original position. If the depression of consciousness is not too deep, there may be some response to painful stimulation. Pinching the skin on the normal side is followed by withdrawal of the part stimulated. In contrast, a painful stimulus on the paralyzed side causes no local movement, although grimacing or movements of the opposite side of the body may indicate that some sensation is retained. Other tests of motor function, such as evaluation of coordination and active movement, cannot be performed on unresponsive patients. It is important to appraise muscle tone, or resistance to passive movement, and to observe carefully for any abnormal movements. Occasionally, spasticity instead of flaccidity develops after acute cerebral lesions. A previous spastic hemiplegia or extrapyramidal syndrome may have caused an alteration in tone that persists even in coma, and arthropathies and skeletal abnormalities may also interfere with joint movements. In catatonia there may be a waxy resistance resembling that of extrapyramidal disease. Patients with AMS may have asterixis.

The motor responses to stimuli are probably the most important factor in gauging the depth of coma and prognosis. The highest level response is when the patient obeys simple commands (GCS 6). If there is no response to verbal commands, a painful stimulus is delivered. There are five possible outcomes. The patient may localize the painful stimulus and make appropriate movements to attempt to remove it (GCS 5). She may exhibit flexion withdrawal without localizing the stimulus (GCS 4). There may be abnormal flexor responses (decorticate rigidity, GCS 3), or, as the lowest level of response, an extensor response (decerebrate rigidity, GCS 2). The worst possible outcome is no response whatsoever (GCS 1).

Abnormal flexor and extensor responses are referred to as posturing. Abnormal posturing may occur spontaneously, as well as in response to stimuli. It is not uncommon for posturing to be different on the two sides of the body. When there is difficulty distinguishing purposeful withdrawal from decorticate posturing, a painful stimulus to the inner arm is useful. Abduction of the arm away from the stimulus is a high-level avoidance response; adduction into the stimulus is a low-level reflex response. Posturing usually indicates structural disease of the nervous system, and is particularly common after head injury. Posturing can also occur with severe metabolic encephalopathy, particularly sedative-hypnotic drug intoxication.

## Sensory Examination

Depending on the level of coma, the patient may not perceive even the most painful stimulus, or may respond to painful stimuli by wincing and withdrawing the part of the body stimulated. Often, the examination must be limited to comparing responses to painful stimulation on the two sides of the body. Sensory stimuli may be delivered by pinching the skin, pricking with a sharp object, pressing over the supraorbital notch, and squeezing the muscle masses and tendons, particularly the Achilles tendon.

## Reflexes

At a minimum, the principal tendon reflexes and the plantar responses should be tested. Frontal release signs (forced grasping, palmomental, and suck or snout responses) and paratonic rigidity may be present with AMS of either structural or metabolic origin. Asymmetry of responses may have some localizing value. Similarly, extensor plantar responses may occur with either structural or metabolic coma.

## Meningeal Signs

The examiner should attempt to elicit signs of meningeal involvement by flexing the neck passively and rotating it from side to side in order to detect nuchal rigidity. The Kernig, Brudzinski, and related signs may be absent in some cases of deep coma despite the presence of meningeal irritation. In subarachnoid hemorrhage, it requires some hours for meningeal signs to develop, and they may be absent at the time of presentation.

## DIFFERENTIAL DIAGNOSIS OF COMA

There are three possible etiologies for acute coma: (a) primary CNS disease, (b) depression of the CNS by a systemic metabolic process or drug intoxication, and (c) psychogenic unresponsiveness. Statistically, the most likely etiology is involvement of the CNS by a systemic metabolic process or drug intoxication. Patients with metabolic encephalopathy characteristically have a symmetrical examination, devoid of lateralizing or focal abnormalities, intact reflex eye movements, and reactive pupils.

## Structural Lesions

There are three mechanisms whereby structural lesions may cause coma: (a) a lateralized hemispheric mass lesion causes increased intracranial pressure, herniation, and compression or hemorrhage into the upper midbrain with secondary impairment of the RAS; (b) a brainstem lesion, such as hemorrhage or infarction, damages the RAS directly; and (c) a disease process affects both cerebral hemispheres, or both hemispheres and the RAS. The findings with a hemispheric mass lesion depend upon the stage of evolution of the process. In the early stages, there are usually lateralizing findings and asymmetries on examination consistent with a focal process. These include hemiparesis, focal seizures, aphasia, hemianopia, apraxia, and other signs of hemispheric dysfunction. As the lesion expands and intracranial pressure increases, the other hemisphere becomes involved, herniation develops, and the focal nature of the process becomes complicated by findings due to herniation. Asymmetric motor responses and abnormal eye movements usually persist until the terminal stages. Herniation syndromes are due to shifting of brain structures caused by increased intracranial pressure. They are evidence of severe disease, and are life-threatening. A number of different herniation syndromes have been recognized. The more common and important are central transtentorial, lateral transtentorial (uncal), and tonsillar (foramen magnum) herniation (Figure 35.2, Table 35.3).

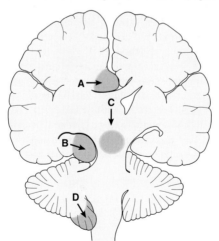

*FIGURE 35.2* ● Patterns of brain herniation. **A.** Herniation of the cingulate gyrus under the falx cerebri. **B.** Uncal (lateral transtentorial) herniation. **C.** Central transtentorial herniation. **D.** Herniation of the cerebellar tonsils through the foramen magnum. (Reprinted with permission from Wilkins RH, Rengachary SS. *Neurosurgery.* New York: McGraw-Hill, 1985.)

## TABLE 35.3

**Clinical Manifestations of Common Herniation Syndromes**

| Herniation Syndrome | Clinical Manifestations |
| --- | --- |
| Central transtentorial | Impaired consciousness, abnormal respirations, symmetric small or midposition fixed or minimally reactive pupils, decorticate evolving to decerebrate posturing, rostrocaudal deterioration |
| Lateral transtentorial (uncal) | Impaired consciousness, abnormal respirations, third nerve palsy (unilaterally dilated pupil), hemiparesis (may be false localizing), rostrocaudal deterioration |
| Cerebellar tonsillar (foramen magnum) | Impaired consciousness, neck rigidity, opisthotonos, decerebrate rigidity, vomiting, irregular respirations, apnea, bradycardia |
| Upward | Prominent brainstem signs, downward gaze deviation, upgaze palsy, decerebrate posturing (usually due to a cerebellar mass lesion) |

Central transtentorial herniation is due to symmetric downward displacement of the hemispheres causing impaction of the diencephalon and midbrain into the tentorial notch. Pressure effects on the diencephalon and midbrain often cause small hemorrhages in the upper midbrain (Duret hemorrhages). Uncal herniation occurs when the temporal lobe and uncus shift medially into the tentorial notch, causing compression of the third cranial nerve and adjacent midbrain. Tentorial herniation, unless reversed, evolves into an orderly progression of neurologic dysfunction referred to as rostrocaudal deterioration.

During rostrocaudal deterioration, neurologic dysfunction becomes progressively more dramatic. Clinical stages occur as if the brain had been transversely sectioned at a particular level (diencephalon, midbrain, pons, or medulla). Respirations become progressively more abnormal, evolving from a Cheyne-Stokes pattern early, to ataxic respirations to eventual apnea. Pupils become progressively more abnormal and eventually become fixed and unreactive. Reflex eye movements are eventually lost. Motor responses evolve from localizing to nonlocalizing to decorticate to decerebrate to flaccid. The end result of unchecked rostrocaudal deterioration is death.

Herniation of the cerebellar tonsils downward into the foramen magnum compresses the medulla and upper spinal cord, and can result in rapid failure of vital functions. A dreaded complication of lumbar puncture is herniation, especially cerebellar tonsillar herniation, due to removal of spinal fluid.

A primary lesion involving the brainstem (e.g., pontine hemorrhage or infarction) produces coma that is abrupt in onset, and causes focal or multifocal abnormalities, abnormal eye movements, pupillary abnormalities, pathologic reflexes, abnormal posturing, and other objective neurologic signs.

Disorders that cause bilateral hemispheric dysfunction or produce diffuse CNS involvement include bilateral subdural hematomas, bilateral cerebral infarction due to emboli, and other processes that may cause multifocal lesions. In addition, some processes affect the CNS in a more diffuse or widespread manner and cause coma by dysfunction of the cerebral hemispheres bilaterally or the cerebral hemispheres as well as the RAS. Such conditions include meningitis, encephalitis, and subarachnoid hemorrhage. These cause variable focality on examination, depending on the specifics of the process, and occasionally cause very little in the way of focal or lateralizing signs. There typically are objective neurologic signs in the form of reflex abnormality, pathologic reflexes, evidence of meningeal irritation, and abnormalities on fundoscopic examination. In addition, there may be fever or other evidence of systemic disease.

Metabolic encephalopathies are conditions that typically produce no focal or lateralizing signs on neurologic examination, preserved pupil reactivity, and usually do not affect eye movements or cause other signs of brainstem dysfunction. Metabolic encephalopathy often begins with a period of confusion or delirium, which gradually evolves into stupor, then coma. There are three common etiologies: (a) intoxication, (b) severe systemic metabolic disturbance, and (c) systemic infection. Intoxication is usually due to alcohol, opiates, or sedative-hypnotic drugs. These conditions sometimes produce other abnormalities on physical examination that may be a clue as to etiology, such as pinpoint pupils, respiratory depression, or skin lesions.

The most common systemic metabolic disturbance to cause coma is the hypoxic-ischemic encephalopathy that follows cardiac arrest. Other examples include hypoglycemia, diabetic ketoacidosis, nonketotic hyperosmolar state, hyperammonemia, hypercalcemia, and hypercarbia. Many of these conditions occur under obvious clinical circumstances, such as known diabetes, end-stage alcoholism with cirrhosis, or severe pulmonary disease with hypercarbia, and the etiology is often revealed by routine blood chemistries. Severe infections and septicemia occasionally cause altered mental status (septic encephalopathy).

Although metabolic encephalopathies in general produce a uniform clinical picture of a symmetric examination with reactive pupils and intact brainstem eye movement reflexes, in some conditions there may be deviations from this scheme. Occasionally, certain clinical features may provide clues as to etiology. In hypoglycemia there may be lateralized deficits, extensor posturing, hypothermia, and seizures. In hepatic encephalopathy there may be clinical evidence of alcoholism and end-stage liver disease, including ascites, jaundice, spider angiomas, palmar erythema, and gynecomastia. It is usually preceded by asterixis and confusion. There may be focal deficits, as well as abnormal posturing, and occasionally unusual eye findings, including ocular bobbing and gaze deviations. The encephalopathy of uremia is often associated with tremor, asterixis, myoclonus, seizures, and occasionally evidence of tetany. There may be mild focal deficits, but brainstem functions remain intact. Distinguishing features of the encephalopathy of hypercarbia include papilledema, asterixis, tremor, and myoclonus. Focal signs occur occasionally in hyponatremia, hypernatremia, and hyperosmolar coma. Sedative-hypnotic drug intoxication often affects eye movements, while pupillary light reactions remain unaffected. Abnormal posturing may also occur. This unusual combination of reactive pupils in the face of abnormal reflex eye movements and posturing is characteristic of sedative-hypnotic drug effects, but can also occur with posterior fossa mass lesions causing pressure on the lower and mid-brainstem with relative preservation of the midbrain. This picture can also occur with upward transtentorial herniation.

## Seizure Disorders

A seizure is a transient episode of uncontrollable motor activity, focal or generalized, usually accompanied by clouding or loss of consciousness. In addition to alteration of consciousness during the ictus, seizure disorders may also cause AMS due to postictal unresponsiveness, absence status, psychomotor status, and subclinical status epilepticus. In the postictal period there is often depression of consciousness, a desire to sleep, confusion, and disorientation. Coma or stupor may be a sequel of a recent seizure, although it may not be possible to obtain a history of either a recent convulsion or previous attacks. The patient may show evidence of tongue-biting, frothing at the mouth, bloody sputum, incontinence, and lacerations or other injuries to the body. Old scars may be found on the tongue. The postictal stupor is usually brief, but may be followed by either profound sleep or confusion and irrational behavior. A prolonged postictal encephalopathy may last many hours, rarely days. Postictal stupor occurs most commonly with generalized tonic clonic seizures, but may follow other seizure types. In the absence of a history of seizure disorder, it may be difficult to differentiate between the postictal state and cerebral trauma.

In status epilepticus there is prolonged seizure activity, or repeated convulsions with failure to regain consciousness between them. Status epilepticus may cause a state of altered consciousness that may be confused with AMS or coma. In absence (petit mal) status there is lowering and clouding of consciousness and the patient may appear to be in a trancelike stupor suggesting drug abuse or a psychiatric disorder. Patients in complex partial status epilepticus are commonly confused or lethargic. Subclinical status epilepticus, or seizures with subtle motor manifestations, may cause a coma-like state. Subclinical status may continue in patients when the motor manifestations have been suppressed with antiepileptic drugs. Patients with pseudoperiodic lateralized epileptiform discharges (PLEDs) are often comatose because of a hemispheric process, such as large infarction or subdural hematoma; and the electroencephalogram demonstrates characteristic discharges. The presence of myoclonus usually indicates that coma is of metabolic origin. Spontaneous, multifocal myoclonic jerking is common, particularly in uremia and hypercarbia. Massive generalized myoclonic jerks often occur as an aftermath of cardiac arrest and cerebral anoxia, and are an extremely poor prognostic sign.

## Locked-in Syndrome

In the locked-in syndrome, ventral brainstem destruction sparing the RAS renders the patient mute and quadriplegic but not comatose. There is complete paralysis of all four extremities and the lower cranial nerves but no associated impairment of consciousness. Patients with locked-in syndrome have quadriplegia and anarthria, but variable preservation of consciousness and intellect. The patient is awake but speechless and motionless, with little response to stimuli. The lesion usually involves the midpons and results in paralysis of facial movement and horizontal gaze. If the supranuclear vertical gaze pathways, which pass rostral to the other corticobulbar and corticospinal pathways, are spared there is preservation of vertical eye movements and the patient may be able to blink. With effort, communication may be established using eye movement or blink signals. Sensory pathways, hearing, and vision are largely spared, and the patient is effectively "de-efferented." Other findings vary with the particulars of the lesion. A fulminant neuropathy, such as Guillain-Barré syndrome, can result in a clinical state resembling brain death through diffuse de-efferentation. Jean-Dominique Bauby (deceased) bequeathed an eloquent and poignant description of the locked-in state from the victim's point of view in *The Diving Bell and the Butterfly: A Memoir of Life in Death* (Vintage Books, 1998). Bauby dictated his book by blinking one eyelid. The principal cause of locked-in syndrome is brainstem stroke (86%), but it may also occur after trauma (14%). The locked-in state is frequently mistaken for coma. Appreciation that the patient is not comatose or vegetative but locked-in does not usually occur for 2 to 3 months (mean 79 days), and the average survival locked-in is 71 months.

## Persistent Vegetative State

The pathology in patients with the persistent vegetative state (PVS) invariably entails massive bilateral hemispheric damage with a spared and intact brainstem. Preservation of the RAS permits behavioral arousal and sleep wake cycles, but existence is devoid of cognition. Positron emission tomography has demonstrated cerebral metabolic rates for glucose far too low to sustain consciousness. The PVS may develop as a sequel to acute insults, typically following a temporary period of coma, or as the end stage of a progressive neurologic illness, such as Alzheimer disease.

In PVS, patients are awake but unaware. Despite a seemingly alert demeanor, they display no speech, comprehension, or purposeful movement. Reflex eye movements and orientation to noise—brainstem level functions—may persist. Yawning, sneezing, bruxism, and occasional meaningless smiles may occur. Impaired motor function with spasticity, posturing, or contractures is common. Painful stimuli evoke nonspecific erratic reactions without discrete motor responses or localization. All patients are incontinent of stool and urine. In PVS, patients exist in eyes-open permanent unconsciousness, with intact sleep-wake cycles but no awareness of self or environment, and without voluntary action or behavior of any kind. Though seemingly awake, they display no interactive behavior and no ability to express emotion or engage another person on any level. Extended observation forms the primary and most important basis for the diagnosis of PVS. Such patients show no behavioral responses whatsoever over a prolonged period of time. Persistent vegetative state must be differentiated from catatonia and from the locked-in syndrome.

A number of other terms have been used to describe states of altered awareness that are similar, if not identical, to PVS (e.g., akinetic mutism, abulia, apallic state, coma vigil, and pseudocoma). Much of the nomenclature is outdated and perplexing, the distinctions vague and of marginal clinical utility.

## Psychogenic Unresponsiveness (Hysterical Coma)

In psychogenic unresponsiveness, usually due to either hysteria or malingering, the loss of consciousness is typically not deep, but the condition may occasionally simulate real coma. The patient often responds to painful stimuli, unless there is associated nonorganic sensory loss, and the reflexes are normal, with no pathologic responses. The temperature, pulse, respirations, and blood pressure are normal. The eyelids may flutter or the eyes may be closed tightly with the patient resisting attempts to open them. The vigorous eye closure may interfere with testing the corneal and pupillary reflexes, which are normal. When the eyelids are opened and then released by the examiner, they close gradually in the patient with real coma but quickly in the patient with factitious coma. The patient may resist other procedures, and glance around when unaware she is being watched. When a hand is raised and allowed to drop toward the face, the patient with psychogenic unresponsiveness will usually avoid hitting herself, but this rule is not infallible. In true coma, the hand will hit the face. Caloric testing produces nystagmus, which never occurs in real coma.

An episode of psychogenic unresponsiveness is usually precipitated by emotional stress, and the onset is often dramatic. The patient may appear to be in a trance, or coma may alternate with weeping and thrashing movements. The performance is appropriately staged, and occurs when observers are in the vicinity. Movements, if present, are not stereotyped, but appear to be coordinated and purposive. The patient may struggle, clutch at objects or parts of the body, or attempt to tear off clothes. Although the patient appears to be unconscious, some response to external stimuli may be evident. If there is muscle hypertonicity, it is usually of a rigid type, and there may be opisthotonos with the arc de cercle. If the patient can be persuaded to talk, the responses may be of the type seen in Ganser syndrome, with evasiveness and approximate but consistently inaccurate replies.

In psychotic states, there is rarely complete loss of consciousness. Severe depression, schizophrenia, and organic psychoses may cause mutism, in which the patient is either completely withdrawn from the environment or refuses to speak. Negativism, either passive or active, may be a symptom of various psychoses, but especially of schizophrenia. In severe depression the patient may show psychomotor retardation that may simulate AMS. In catatonic stupor there is apathy, mutism, and negativism, often with waxy rigidity of the extremities causing the patient to hold her limbs or entire body in bizarre and seemingly uncomfortable positions for long periods of time. Food may be held in the mouth.

## Brain Death

To meet clinical criteria for brain death, a high degree of certainty regarding the etiology of the brain death picture is imperative. Common causes include cerebral anoxia, cerebral hemorrhage, aneurysmal subarachnoid hemorrhage, and head injury. The patient must have no evidence of cerebral or brainstem activity, although segmental reflex activity mediated at the spinal cord level may persist. Preserved spinal cord reflex activity may lead to dramatic movements, such as the "Lazarus reflex." There may even be respiratory-like movements, with shoulder elevation and adduction, back arching, and intercostal expansion, but without significant tidal volumes. Deep tendon reflexes, superficial reflexes, and the Babinski sign may be present and do not countermand a diagnosis of brain death. Except for segmental reflexes, motor responses are absent. The pupils

## TABLE 35.4

### Summary of the Diagnostic Criteria for the Clinical Diagnosis of Brain Death from the American Academy of Neurology

A. Prerequisites. Brain death is the absence of clinical brain function when the proximate cause is known and demonstrably irreversible.
1. Clinical or neuroimaging evidence of an acute CNS catastrophe that is compatible with the clinical diagnosis of brain death
2. Exclusion of complicating medical conditions that may confound clinical assessment (no severe electrolyte, acid-base, or endocrine disturbance)
3. No drug intoxication or poisoning
4. Core temperature $>32°C$ ($90°F$)

B. The three cardinal findings in brain death are coma or unresponsiveness, absence of brainstem reflexes, and apnea.
1. Coma or unresponsiveness—no cerebral motor response to pain in all extremities (nail-bed pressure and supraorbital pressure)
2. Absence of brainstem reflexes
   a. Pupils
      i. No response to bright light
      ii. Size: midposition (4 mm) to dilated (9 mm)
   b. Ocular movement
      i. No oculocephalic reflex (testing only when no fracture or instability of the cervical spine is apparent)
      ii. No deviation of the eyes to irrigation in each ear with 50 mL of cold water (allow 1 minute after injection and at least 5 minutes between testing on each side)
   c. Facial sensation and facial motor response
      i. No corneal reflex to touch with a throat swab
      ii. No jaw reflex
      iii. No grimacing to deep pressure on a nail bed, supraorbital ridge, or temporomandibular joint
   d. Pharyngeal and tracheal reflexes
      i. No response after stimulation of the posterior pharynx with tongue blade
      ii. No cough response to bronchial suctioning
3. Apnea—testing performed as follows:
   a. Prerequisites
      i. Core temperature $>36.5°C$ or $97°F$
      ii. Systolic blood pressure $>90$ mm Hg
      iii. Euvolemia. Option: positive fluid balance in the previous 6 hours
      iv. Normal $PCO_2$. Option: arterial $PCO_2 <40$ mm Hg
      v. Normal $PO_2$ Option: preoxygenation to obtain arterial $PO_2 >200$ mm Hg
   b. Connect a pulse oximeter and disconnect the ventilator.
   c. Deliver 100% $O_2$, 6 L/min, into the trachea. Option: Place a cannula at the level of the carina.
   d. Look closely for respiratory movements (abdominal or chest excursions that produce adequate tidal volumes).
   e. Measure arterial $PO_2$, $PCO_2$, and pH after approximately 8 minutes and reconnect the ventilator.
   f. If respiratory movements are absent and arterial $PCO_2$ is $>60$ mm Hg (option: 20 mm Hg increase in $PCO_2$ over a baseline normal $PCO_2$), the apnea test result is positive (i.e., it supports the diagnosis of brain death).
   g. If respiratory movements are observed, the apnea test result is negative (i.e., it does not support the clinical diagnosis of brain death), and the test should be repeated.
   h. Connect the ventilator if, during testing, the systolic blood pressure becomes $<90$ mm Hg or the pulse oximeter indicates significant oxygen desaturation and cardiac arrhythmias are present; immediately draw an arterial blood sample and analyze arterial blood gas. If $PCO_2$ is $>60$ mm Hg or $PCO_2$ increase is $>20$ mm Hg over baseline normal $PCO_2$, the apnea test result is positive (it supports the clinical diagnosis of brain death); if $PCO_2$ is $<60$ mm Hg or $PCO_2$ increase is $<20$ mm Hg over baseline normal $PCO_2$, the result is indeterminate, and an additional confirmatory test can be considered.

(From Neurology 1995;1012–1014.)

are fixed, and oculocephalic and oculovestibular reflexes are absent, even with large volume ice water caloric testing. There must be no evidence of sedative drug effects or any systemic metabolic abnormality severe enough to produce the clinical picture of brain death. There must be no significant hypothermia, as hypothermia can mimic brain death. The presence of neuromuscular blocking agents obviously precludes evaluation of motor status. If the patient meets these clinical criteria, an apnea test is performed, and if there is no respiratory effort with an arterial $PCO_2$ of 60 mm Hg or more, the diagnosis of brain death can be made. The apnea test is not without danger. Dramatic spontaneous movements are most likely to occur during the apnea test when the patient becomes hypoxic. These clinical conditions should persist for some time, the exact interval depending on the specific circumstances. A repetition of the evaluation is often done to confirm the findings; there is no decreed interval, but 6 hours is reasonable. These criteria apply to adults and may have to be modified for children, especially neonates.

Table 35.4 summarizes the practice parameter on determining brain death in adults prepared by the Quality Standards Subcommittee of the American Academy of Neurology.

# CHAPTER 36

# Miscellaneous Neurologic Signs

**M**iscellaneous neurologic signs—some of them reflexes, some closely related to the defense and postural reflex mechanisms, and others more varied in nature—are elicited in certain diseases of the nervous system.

## SIGNS OF MENINGEAL IRRITATION

Meningeal signs are elicited most frequently when the meninges are inflamed—from infection (e.g., bacterial meningitis) or from the presence of a foreign material (e.g., blood in the subarachnoid space). Meningismus is a term that refers to the presence of nuchal rigidity and other clinical signs of meningeal inflammation. Meningism is sometimes used synonymously with meningismus, but it is also used to refer to a syndrome characterized by neck stiffness without meningeal inflammation, seen in patients with systemic infections, particularly young children.

The clinical manifestations of meningeal irritation are varied and depend on the severity of the process. Accompaniments depend on etiology but commonly include headache, pain and stiffness of the neck; irritability; photophobia; nausea and vomiting; and other manifestations of infection, such as fever and chills. The various maneuvers used to elicit meningeal signs produce tension on inflamed and hypersensitive spinal nerve roots, and the resulting signs are postures, protective muscle contractions, or other movements that minimize the stretch and distortion of the meninges and roots.

### Nuchal (Cervical) Rigidity

Nuchal rigidity is the most widely recognized and frequently encountered sign of meningeal irritation, and the diagnosis of meningitis is rarely made in its absence. It is characterized by stiffness and spasm of the neck muscles, with pain on attempted voluntary movement as well as resistance to passive movement. The degree of rigidity varies. There may be only slight resistance to passive flexion, or marked spasm of all the neck muscles. Nuchal rigidity primarily affects the extensor muscles, and the most prominent early finding in meningeal irritation is resistance to passive neck flexion. The physician is unable to place the patient's chin on his chest, but the neck can be hyperextended without difficulty; rotatory and lateral movements may also be preserved. With more severe nuchal rigidity there may be resistance to extension and rotatory movements as well. Extreme rigidity causes retraction of the neck into a position of opisthotonos, the body assuming a wrestler's bridge or arc de cercle position, with the head thrust back and the trunk arched forward. Rigidity may be absent in meningitis when the disease is fulminating or terminal, when the patient is in coma, or in infants.

Stiffness and rigidity of the neck may occur in other conditions. A common problem is to distinguish restricted neck motion due to cervical spondylosis or osteoarthritis from nuchal rigidity. Patients with osteoarthritis typically have difficulty with rotation and lateral bending of the neck; these motions are usually preserved in patients who have meningismus, unless the meningeal irritation is extremely severe. Restricted neck motion may also occur with retropharyngeal abscess, cervical lymphadenopathy, neck trauma, and as a nonspecific manifestation in severe systemic infections. Extrapyramidal disorders, particularly progressive supranuclear palsy, may also cause diffuse rigidity of the neck muscles. Meningeal signs may occur with increased spinal fluid pressure, and nuchal rigidity may be a manifestation of cerebellar tonsillar (foramen magnum) herniation. Meningeal irritation may also cause resistance to movement of the legs and back, with the patient lying with his legs drawn up and resisting passive extension.

## Kernig Sign

There is some variability in the descriptions of how to elicit a Kernig sign. Kernig described an involuntary flexion at the knee when the examiner attempted to flex the hip with the knee extended. The more common method is to flex the hip and knee to right angles, and then attempt to passively extend the knee. This movement produces pain, resistance, and inability to fully extend the knee; another definition of Kernig sign is inability to extend the knee to over 135 degrees while the hip is flexed (Figure 36.1). There is some overlap between Kernig sign and the Lasègue (straight leg raising) sign. The technique is similar, but Lasègue sign is used to check for root irritation in lumbosacral radiculopathy. Both Kernig sign and straight leg raising are positive in meningitis because of diffuse inflammation of the nerve roots and meninges, and positive with acute lumbosacral radiculopathy because of focal inflammation of the affected root. In radiculopathy the signs are usually unilateral, but in meningitis they are bilateral.

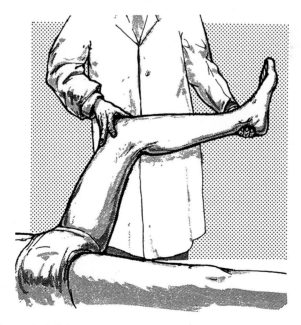

*FIGURE 36.1* ● Method of eliciting Kernig sign.

## Brudzinski Neck Sign

Placing one hand under the patient's head and flexing the neck while holding down the chest with the other hand causes flexion of the hips and knees bilaterally. With severe meningismus, it may not be possible to hold the chest down, and the patient may be pulled into a sitting position with only the examiner's hand behind the head. Occasionally there may be extension of the hallux and fanning of the toes, and sometimes arm flexion. The leg may fail to flex on one side when meningeal irritation and hemiplegia coexist.

## Other Meningeal Signs

To avoid spinal flexion, the patient with meningitis may sit in bed with the hands placed far behind, the head thrown back, the hips and knees flexed, and the back arched (Amoss, Hoyne, or tripod sign).

## SIGNS OF TETANY

The clinical manifestations of tetany include spasm and tonic contractions of the skeletal muscles, principally the distal muscles of the extremities. There may be carpopedal spasm, with tonic contraction of the muscles of the wrists, hands, fingers, feet, and toes. There is hyperexcitability of the entire peripheral nervous system, as well as the musculature, to even minimal stimuli. Sensory nerve involvement may cause paresthesias in the hands, feet, and perioral region. Tetany is related to a disturbance of calcium metabolism or alkalosis, causing a decrease in the ionized calcium level. Certain neurologic signs may be present that aid in making a diagnosis on the basis of the clinical examination alone. They are more easily obtained if the patient first hyperventilates for a few minutes (latent tetany). Severe tetany may cause seizures, laryngospasm, stridor, and respiratory arrest.

## Chvostek Sign

Tapping over the facial nerve causes spasm or a tetanic, cramplike contraction of some or all of the facial muscles. Two points of stimulation have been described: just below the zygomatic process of the temporal bone, in front of the ear (Chvostek sign) and midway between the zygomatic arch and the angle of the mouth. Sometimes the response may be elicited merely by stroking the skin in front of the ear. The sign is minimal if only a slight twitch of the upper lip or the angle of the mouth results; moderate if there is movement of the ala nasi and the entire corner of the mouth; maximal if the muscles of the forehead, eyelid, and cheek also contract. When the response is marked, even muscles supplied by the trigeminal nerve may respond. Chvostek sign is the result of a hyperexcitability of the motor nerves, in this instance the facial nerve, to mechanical stimulation. It is an important sign in tetany, but may occur in other conditions in which there is hyperreflexia, such as in lesions of the corticospinal tract. It is present in a majority of neonates and disappears during childhood.

## Trousseau Sign

Ischemia of the peripheral nerve trunks increases nerve excitability and causes spontaneous discharges. Compression of the arm by manual pressure, a tourniquet, or a sphygmomanometer cuff is followed first by distal paresthesias that progress centripetally, then twitching of the fingers, and finally by cramping and contraction of the muscles of the fingers and hand with the thumb strongly adducted and the fingers stiffened, slightly flexed at the metacarpophalangeal joints, and forming a cone clustered about the thumb (obstetrician's or accoucheur's hand, main d'accoucheur). There may be a latent period of 30 sec to 4 minutes. Similar pressure around the leg or thigh will cause pedal spasm. A modification is to keep a moderately inflated sphygmomanometer cuff on one arm for about 10 minutes, and then remove it and have the patient hyperventilate; typical tetanic spasm occurs earlier in the previously ischemic arm.

## SIGNS OF CERVICAL RADICULOPATHY

The history, especially patterns of pain radiation and paresthesias, can provide localizing information in suspected CR. Radiating pain on coughing, sneezing, or straining at stool (Dejerine sign) is significant but seldom elicited. Increased pain on shoulder motion suggests nonradicular pathology. Relief of pain by resting the hand atop the head (hand on head sign) is reportedly characteristic of CR, but the author has seen this phenomenon with a Pancoast tumor. Hand paresthesias at night suggest carpal tunnel syndrome, but carpal tunnel syndrome can occur in association with CR ("double crush syndrome"), so nocturnal acroparesthesias do not exclude coexistent radiculopathy.

Physical examination in patients with suspected CR should include an assessment of the range of motion of the neck and arm, a search for root compression signs, detailed examination of strength and reflexes, a screening sensory examination, and probing for areas of muscle spasm or trigger points. Patients with either weakness or reduced reflexes on physical examination are up to five times more likely to have an abnormal electrodiagnostic study. A normal physical examination by no means excludes CR (negative predictive value 52%).

The cervical spine range of motion is highly informative. Patients should be asked to put chin to chest and to either shoulder, each ear to shoulder and to hold the head in full extension; these maneuvers all affect the size of the intervertebral foramen. Pain produced by movements that narrow the foramen suggest CR. Pain on the symptomatic side on putting the ipsilateral ear to the shoulder suggests radiculopathy, but increased pain on leaning or turning away from the symptomatic side suggests a myofascial origin. Radiating pain or paresthesias with the head in extension and tilted slightly to the symptomatic side is highly suggestive of CR (Spurling sign or maneuver, foraminal compression test); brief breath holding or gentle Valsalva in this position will sometimes elicit the pain if positioning alone is not provocative. The addition of axial compression by pressing down on the crown of the head does not seem to add much. The Spurling test is specific, but not very sensitive. Light digital compression of the jugular veins until the face is flushed and the patient is uncomfortable will sometimes elicit radicular symptoms: unilateral shoulder, arm, pectoral or scapular pain, or radiating paresthesias into the arm or hand (Viets sign). A slight cough while the face is suffused may increase the sensitivity. In the past, clinicians sometimes went so far as to put a blood pressure cuff around the patient's neck to occlude the jugular veins (Naffziger sign). The two eponyms are often used interchangeably, and more often Naffziger sign is used for both techniques. Jugular compression is thought to engorge epidural veins or the cerebrospinal fluid (CSF) reservoirs, which in the normal individual is harmless. But when some element of foraminal narrowing and nerve root pressure exists, the additional compression causes the acute development of symptoms. The same mechanism likely underlies the exacerbation of root pain by coughing, sneezing, and straining. Like the Spurling test, the Viets/Naffziger sign is specific but insensitive. It is less useful in lumbosacral than in cervical radiculopathy. An occasional CR patient has relief of pain with manual upward neck traction, particularly with the neck in slight flexion (cervical distraction test). Some patients have a decrease in pain with shoulder abduction (shoulder abduction relief test); this sign is more likely to be present with soft disc herniation. The mechanism is uncertain but probably related to the hand on the head sign. Flexion of the neck may cause Lhermitte sign in patients with cervical spondylosis or large disc herniations. Pain or limitation of motion of any upper-extremity joint should signal the possibility of nonradicular pathology. The differentiation of CR from primary shoulder disease (e.g., bursitis, capsulitis, tendinitis, rotator cuff disease, or impingement syndrome) can be particularly difficult.

## SIGNS OF LUMBOSACRAL RADICULOPATHY

The utility, or lack thereof, of various physical examination findings has been studied. The straight leg raising (SLR, Lasègue) test remains the mainstay in detecting radicular compression. The test is performed by slowly raising the symptomatic leg with the knee extended (Figure 36.2). Pain

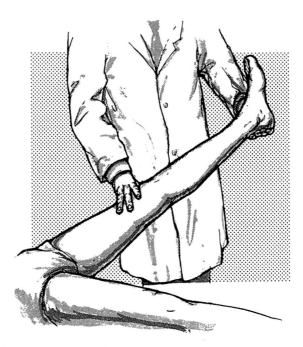

**FIGURE 36.2** ●  Method of eliciting the Lasègue sign.

caused by flexing the hip with the knee bent is suggestive of hip disease. During SLR tension is transmitted to the nerve roots between about 30 degrees and 70 degrees, and pain increases. Pain at less than 30 degrees raises the question of nonorganicity, and some discomfort and tightness beyond 70 degrees is routine and insignificant. There are various degrees or levels of positivity. Ipsilateral leg tightness is the lowest level, pain in the back more significant, and radiating pain in the leg highly significant. When raising the good leg produces pain in the symptomatic leg (crossed straight leg raising, Fajersztajn sign), the likelihood of a root lesion is very high. Rarely, SLR may even cause numbness and paresthesias in the distribution of the affected nerve root. The buckling sign is knee flexion during SLR to avoid sciatic nerve tension. Kernig sign is an alternate way of stretching the root. Various SLR modifications may provide additional information; all of these variations are referred to as root stretch signs. The pain may be more severe, or elicited sooner, if the test is carried out with the thigh and leg in a position of adduction and internal rotation (Bonnet phenomenon). The SLR can be enhanced by passively dorsiflexing the patient's foot (Bragard sign) or great toe (Sicard sign) just at the elevation angle at which the increased root tension begins to produce pain (Figure 36.3). The term Spurling sign is also used for either of these. A quick snap to the sciatic nerve in the popliteal fossa just as stretch begins to cause pain (bowstring sign, or popliteal compression test) accomplishes the same end, and may cause pain in the lumbar region, in the affected buttock, or along the course of the sciatic nerve. In severe cases, pain may be elicited merely by dorsiflexion of the foot or great toe as the patient lies supine with legs extended. A similar modification may be carried out by flexing the thigh to an angle just short of that necessary to cause pain, and then flexing the neck; this may produce the same exacerbation of pain that would be brought about by further flexion of the hip (Brudzinski, Lidner, or Hyndman sign). Occasionally, the pain may be brought on merely by passive flexion of the neck when the patient is recumbent with legs extended. The pain with SLR should be the same with the patient supine or seated. Failure of a patient with a positive supine SLR to complain or lean backward when the

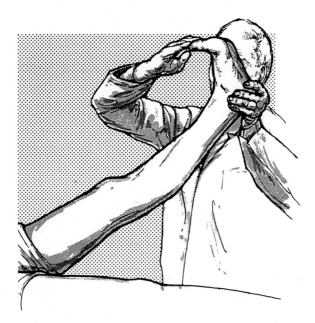

**FIGURE 36.3** ● Accentuation of the Lasègue sign by dorsiflexion of either the foot or the great toe.

extended leg is brought up while in the seated position (e.g., under the guise of doing the planter response) suggests nonorganicity. In the sitting position, the patient may be able to extend each leg alone, but extending both together causes radicular pain (Bechterew test).

The reverse SLR (femoral stretch or Ely test) is a way of eliciting root stretch in the evaluation of high lumbar radiculopathy. The patient lies prone, and the knee is pulled into maximum flexion; or the examiner pulls upward on the extended knee to passively extend the hip. In the bent knee pulling test the patient's knee is flexed and the examiner pulls upward on the ankle while pushing the buttock forward (in the same way as for eliciting the psoas sign used in the diagnosis of appendicitis). In all these variations, the normal individual should complain only of quadriceps tightness. With disc disease there is pain in the back or in the femoral nerve distribution on the side of the lesion.

The examiner should also look for abnormalities of posture, deformities, tenderness, and muscle spasm. With radiculopathy, there may be loss of the normal lumbar lordosis because of involuntary spasm of the paravertebral muscles. In addition, there is often a lumbar scoliosis, with a compensatory thoracic scoliosis. Most commonly, the list of the body is away from the painful side, and the pelvis is tilted so that the affected hip is elevated. The patient attempts to bear weight mostly on the sound leg. The list and scoliosis may sometimes be toward the painful side, and the patient's body may be bent forward and toward that side to avoid stretching the involved root. With very severe sciatic pain, the patient will avoid complete extension at the knee, and may place only the toes on the floor, since dorsiflexion of the foot aggravates the pain by stretching the nerve. The patient may walk with small steps and keep the leg semi-flexed at the knee. In bending forward, she flexes the knee to avoid stretching the nerve (Neri sign). When sitting, she keeps the affected leg flexed at the knee and rests her weight on the opposite buttock. She may rise from a seated position by supporting herself on the unaffected side, bending forward, and placing one hand on the affected side of the back (Minor sign). There may be areas of tenderness in the lumbosacral region, and manipulation or percussion over the spinous processes, or pressure just lateral to them, may reproduce or exacerbate the pain. A sharp blow with a percussion hammer, on or just lateral to the spinous processes, while the patient is bending forward, may bring out the pain. There may be not only spasm of the paravertebral muscles, but also the hamstrings and calf muscles. Flexion, extension, and lateral deviation of the spine are limited; the pain is usually accentuated with passive extension of the lumbar spine toward the affected side while the patient is standing erect. There may be localized tenderness at the sciatic notch and along the course of the sciatic nerve. Pelvic and rectal examination may be necessary in some instances.

The neurologic examination should include assessment of power in the major lower-extremity muscle groups, but especially the dorsiflexors of the foot and toes, and the evertors and invertors of the foot. Plantar flexion of the foot is so powerful that manual testing rarely suffices. Having the patient do 10 toe raises with either foot is a better test. As the patient is standing on one leg, look for the Trendelenburg sign. Normally the pelvis slants upward toward the unsupported leg. With a positive Trendelenburg the hip moves up and the shoulder moves down on the weight-bearing side, and the pelvis sags toward the unsupported leg. The Trendelenburg sign may occur when there is weakness of the hip abductors, as in L5 radiculopathy, but it may also occur with musculoskeletal disease, such as hip dislocation, fracture of the femoral head, or coxa vara. In addition to assessing power, it is important to look for atrophy and fasciculations. Sensation should be tested in the signature zones of the major roots. The status of knee and ankle reflexes reflects the integrity of the L3-L4 and S1 roots, respectively. There is no good reflex for the L5 root, but the hamstring reflexes are sometimes useful. An occasional L5 radiculopathy produces a clear selective diminution of the medial hamstring reflex.

Tests for nonorganicity are very useful in the evaluation of LBP. Pain during simulated spinal rotation, pinning the patient's hands to the sides while rotating the hips (no spine rotation occurs as shoulders and hips remain in a constant relationship) suggests nonorganicity. Also useful are a discrepancy between the positivity of the SLR between the supine and seated position, pain in the back on pressing down on top of the head, widespread and excessive "tenderness" (touch-me-not or Waddell sign), general overreaction during testing, and nondermatomal/nonmyotomal neurologic signs. The presence of three of these signs suggests, if not nonorganicity, at least embellishment.

# Index

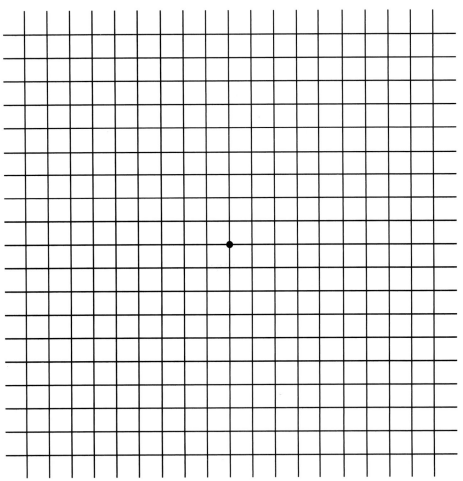

**FIGURE A-1** ● The Amsler grid for testing the central visual fields. *(1)* Test vision with one eye at a time, and use normal glasses for reading. *(2)* Hold chart at normal reading distance. *(3)* Stare at central dot and look for distortion or blind spots in the grid.

# Appendix A-2

**TABLE A-2**

### The Glasgow Coma Scale

| | |
|---|---|
| Eye opening | |
| Open spontaneously | 4 |
| Open only to verbal stimuli | 3 |
| Only to pain | 2 |
| Never open | 1 |
| Best verbal response | |
| Oriented and converses | 5 |
| Converses, but disoriented, confused | 4 |
| Uses inappropriate words | 3 |
| Makes incomprehensible sounds | 2 |
| No verbal response | 1 |
| Best motor response | |
| Obeys commands | 6 |
| Localizes pain | 5 |
| Exhibits flexion withdrawal | 4 |
| Decorticate rigidity | 3 |
| Decerebrate rigidity | 2 |
| No motor response | 1 |

# Appendix A-3

## Short Orientation-Memory-Concentration Test for Cognitive Impairment

Ask the patient to:

1. Name the month
2. Name the year
3. State the time of day
4. Remember the following memory phrase: "John Brown, 42 Market Street, Chicago"
5. Count backward from 20 to 1
6. Name the months of the year in reverse
7. Recall the memory phrase

See Katzman R, Brown T, Fuld P, et al. Validation of a short orientation-memory-concentration test of cognitive impairment. *Am J Psychiat* 1983;140:734, for expected scores in various age groups.

## HUNT & HESS SCALE

Patient Name: _____

Rater Name: _____

Date: _____

**For non-traumatic sub-arachnoid hemorrhage patients.**

**(Choose single most appropriate grade.)**

| Description | Grade |
|---|---|
| Asymptomatic, mild headache, slight nuchal rigidity | 1 |
| Moderate to severe headache, nuchal rigidity, no neurologic deficit other than cranial nerve palsy | 2 |
| Drowsiness/confusion, mild focal neurologic deficit | 3 |
| Stupor, moderate-severe hemiparesis | 4 |
| Coma, decerebrate posturing | 5 |

**GRADE (1–5):** _____

## References

Hunt WE, Hess RM. "Surgical risk as related to time of intervention in the repair of intracranial aneurysms." *Journal of Neurosurgery* 1968 Jan;28(1):14–20.

Hunt WE, Meagher JN, Hess RM. "Intracranial aneurysm. A nine-year study." *Ohio State Medical Journal* 1966 Nov;62(11):1168–71.

*FIGURE A-4* ● Hunt & Hess Scale

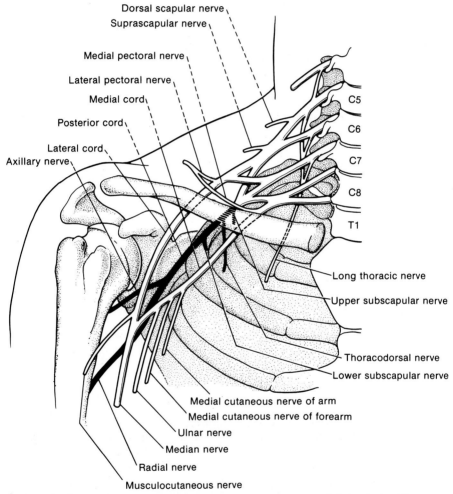

Dorsal scapular nerve
Suprascapular nerve

Medial pectoral nerve

Lateral pectoral nerve

Medial cord

Posterior cord

Lateral cord
Axillary nerve

C5

C6

C7

C8

T1

Long thoracic nerve

Upper subscapular nerve

Thoracodorsal nerve

Lower subscapular nerve

Medial cutaneous nerve of arm
Medial cutaneous nerve of forearm
Ulnar nerve
Median nerve
Radial nerve
Musculocutaneous nerve

*FIGURE A-5* ● Brachial plexus showing its various constituents and their relationship to structures in the region of the upper chest, axilla, and shoulder.

| | | Point | Jaeger | Distance equivalent |
|---|---|---|---|---|
| **95** | | | | $\frac{20}{800}$ |
| **874** | | | | $\frac{20}{400}$ |
| **2843** | | 26 | 16 | $\frac{20}{200}$ |
| 638 ᗑ Ш ᗐ XOO | | 14 | 10 | $\frac{20}{100}$ |
| 8745 ᗐ ᙢ Ш O X O | | 10 | 7 | $\frac{20}{70}$ |
| 63925 ᙢ ᗑ ᗐ X O X | | 8 | 5 | $\frac{20}{50}$ |
| 428365 Ш ᗑ ᙢ o x o | | 6 | 3 | $\frac{20}{40}$ |
| 374258 ᗐ Ш ᗐ x x o | | 5 | 2 | $\frac{20}{30}$ |
| 937826 Ш ᙢ ᗑ x x o | | 4 | 1 | $\frac{20}{25}$ |
| 428739 ᗑ Ш ᙢ o o x | | 3 | 1+ | $\frac{20}{20}$ |

Card is held in good light 14 inches from eye. Record vision for each eye separately with and without glasses. Presbyopic patients should read through bifocal segment. Check myopes with glasses only.

**PUPIL GAUGE (mm.)**

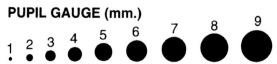

*FIGURE A-6* ● Pocket vision screener. (Courtesy of J.G. Rosenbaum, MD.)

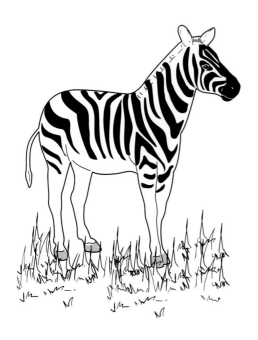

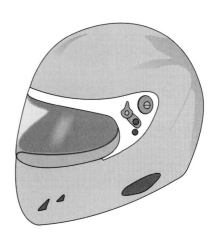

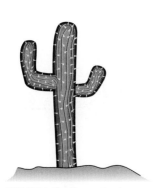

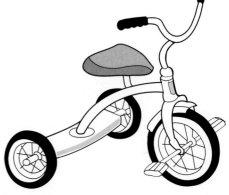

*FIGURE A-7* ● Difficult naming items for testing for anomia.

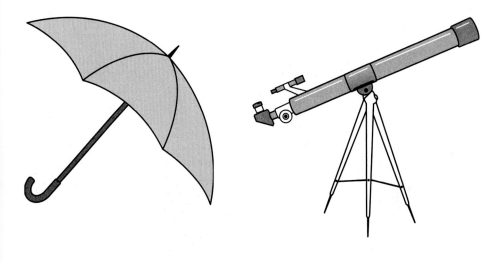

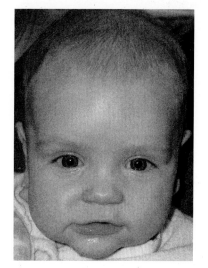

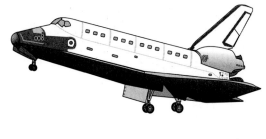

***FIGURE A-7*** ● ***(Continued)*** Difficult naming items for testing for anomia.

# Appendix A-8

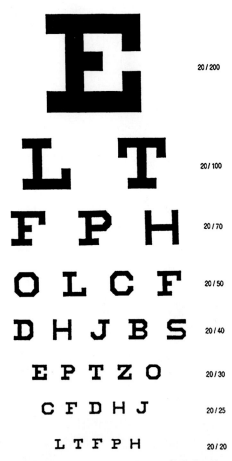

E                    20 / 200

L  T                 20 / 100

F  P  H              20 / 70

O  L  C  F           20 / 50

D  H  J  B  S        20 / 40

E  P  T  Z  O        20 / 30

C  F  D  H  J        20 / 25

L  T  F  P  H        20 / 20

Hold chart in good light 6 feet from eyes (approximately the foot of the
patient's bed). Check eyes separately both with and without glasses.
Chart based on a visual angle of 1'.

*FIGURE A-8* ● Snellen test chart.

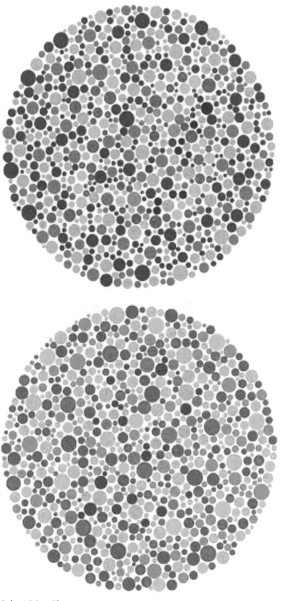

*FIGURE B-1* ● Color Vision Plate

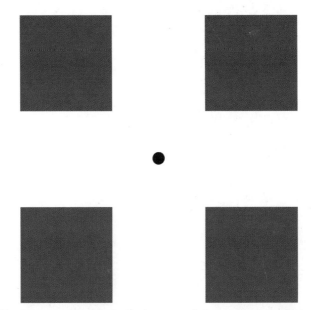

***FIGURE B-2*** ● Red Desaturation Screen: Testing monocularly, have the patient fixate on the central dot and compare the brightness and intensity of the red squares in each visual quadrant.